FOURTH EDITION

PARAMEDIC CARE

VOLUME **7** | **OPERATIONS**

PRINCIPLES & PRACTICE

FOURTH EDITION

PARAMEDIC CARE

CARE VOLUME **7** | **OPERATIONS**

PRINCIPLES & PRACTICE

BRYAN E. BLEDSOE, DO, FACEP, FAAEM, EMT-P

Professor of Emergency Medicine
Director, Prehospital and Disaster Medicine Fellowship
University of Nevada School of Medicine
Attending Emergency Physician
University Medical Center of Southern Nevada
Medical Director, MedicWest Ambulance
Las Vegas, Nevada

ROBERT S. PORTER, MA, EMT-P

Senior Advanced Life Support Educator
Madison County Emergency Medical Services
Canastota, New York

RICHARD A. CHERRY, MS, EMT-P

Director of Training
Northern Onondaga Volunteer Ambulance
Liverpool, New York

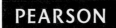

Boston Columbus Indianapolis New York San Francisco Upper Saddle River
Amsterdam Cape Town Dubai London Madrid Milan Munich Paris Montreal Toronto
Delhi Mexico City São Paulo Sydney Hong Kong Seoul Singapore Taipei Tokyo

Library of Congress Cataloging-in-Publication Data

Bledsoe, Bryan E., (Date)
  Paramedic care: principles & practice / Bryan E. Bledsoe,
    Robert S. Porter, Richard A. Cherry. — 4th ed. p. ; cm.
  Includes bibliographical references and index.
  ISBN-13: 978-0-13-211234-5 (v. 7 : alk. paper)
  ISBN-10: 0-13-211234-5 (v. 7 : alk. paper)
  I. Porter, Robert S., (Date) II. Cherry, Richard A. III. Title.
  [DNLM: 1. Emergencies. 2. Emergency Medical Services.
    3. Emergency Medical Technicians. 4. Emergency Treatment. WB 105]
  616.02'5—dc23
                                                    2011034904

Publisher: Julie Levin Alexander
Publisher's Assistant: Regina Bruno
Editor-in-Chief: Marlene McHugh Pratt
Senior Managing Editor for Development: Lois Berlowitz
Editorial Project Manager: Deborah Wenger
Assistant Editor: Jonathan Cheung
Director of Marketing: David Gesell
Marketing Manager: Brian Hoehl
Marketing Specialist: Michael Sirinides
Managing Editor for Production: Patrick Walsh
Production Liaison: Faye Gemmellaro
Production Editor: Mary Tindle, S4Carlisle Publishing Services
Manufacturing Manager: Ilene Sanford

Creative Director: Blair Brown
Cover and Interior Design: Kathryn Foot
Interior Photographers: Nathan Eldridge, Michael Gallitelli, Michal Heron, Ray Kemp/Triple Zilch Productions, Carl Leet, Kevin Link, Richard Logan, Scott Metcalfe
Cover Image: © corepics/Shutterstock
Managing Photography Editor: Michal Heron
Editorial Media Manager: Amy Peltier
Media Project Manager: Lorena Cerisano
Composition: S4Carlisle Publishing Services
Manufactured in the Unites States by RR Donnelley
Cover Printer: RR Donnelley/Kendallville

Notice

The author and the publisher of this book have taken care to make certain that the information given is correct and compatible with the standards generally accepted at the time of publication. Nevertheless, as new information becomes available, changes in treatment and in the use of equipment and procedures become necessary. The reader is advised to carefully consult the instruction and information material included in each piece of equipment or device before administration. Students are warned that the use of any techniques must be authorized by their medical advisor, where appropriate, in accordance with local laws and regulations. The publisher disclaims any liability, loss, injury, or damage incurred as a consequence, directly or indirectly, of the use and application of any of the contents of this book.

Brady
is an imprint of

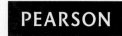

www.bradybooks.com

V011
12 11 10
ISBN 10:   0-13-211234-5
ISBN 13: 978-0-13-211234-5

DEDICATION

This text is respectfully dedicated to all EMS personnel who have made the ultimate sacrifice. Their memory and good deeds will forever be in our thoughts and prayers.

BEB, RSP, RAC

DETAILED CONTENTS

Preface to Volume 7 xi

Acknowledgments xiii

About the Authors xv

CHAPTER 1 ● Ground Ambulance Operations 1

Introduction 2
  Ambulance Standards 2 | Ambulance Design 2 | Medical Equipment Standards 3 |
  Additional Guidelines 4
Checking Ambulances 4
Ambulance Deployment and Staffing 5
  Traffic Congestion 5 | Operational Staffing 6
Safe Ambulance Operations 6
  Educating Providers 6 | Reducing Ambulance Collisions 7 | Standard Operating
  Procedures 8 | The Due Regard Standard 8 | Lights and Siren: A False Sense of
  Security 9 | Escorts and Multiple-Vehicle Responses 9 | Parking and Loading the
  Ambulance 9 | The Deadly Intersection 10

CHAPTER 2 ● Air Medical Operations 14

Introduction 15
History 17
Aircraft 17
  Fixed-Wing Aircraft 18 | Rotor-Wing Aircraft 18
Role in EMS 20
  Uses 20 | Limitations 21 | Staffing 25 | Controversies 26
Scene Operations 26
  Initial Information 27 | Landing Zone 27 | Helicopter Approach 28 | Patient
  Handoff 29 | Aircraft Loading 29 | Aircraft Departure 30

CHAPTER 3 ● Multiple-Casualty Incidents and Incident Management 34

Introduction 36
Origins of Emergency Incident Management 37
  Regulations and Standards 38 | A Uniform, Flexible System 39
Command 39
  Establishing Command 40 | Incident Size-Up 40 | Singular versus Unified
  Command 41 | Identifying a Staging Area 41 | Incident Communications 42 |
  Resource Utilization 42 | Command Procedures 42 | Termination of Command 43
Support of Incident Command 43
  Command Staff 44 | Finance/Administration 45 | Logistics 45 | Operations 45 |
  Planning/Intelligence 45
Division of Operations Functions 45
  Branches 45 | Groups and Divisions 45 | Units 45 | Sectors 46
Functional Groups with an EMS Branch 46
  Triage 46 | Morgue 51 | Treatment 52 | On-Scene Physicians 54 |
  Staging 54 | Transport Unit 54 | Extrication/Rescue Unit 55 | Rehabilitation (Rehab)
  Unit 55 | Communications 55
Disaster Management 56
  Mitigation 56 | Planning 56 | Response 56 | Recovery 56
Meeting the Challenge of Multiple-Casualty Incidents 56
  Common Problems 57 | Preplanning, Drills, and Critiques 57 | Disaster Mental Health
  Services 57

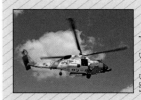

US Coast Guard

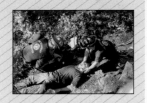

CHAPTER 4 • Rescue Awareness and Operations 61

Introduction 62

Role of the Paramedic 63

Protective Equipment 63

    Rescuer Protection 64 | Patient Protection 65

Safety Procedures 66

    Rescue SOPs 66 | Crew Assignments 66 | Preplanning 66

Rescue Operations 66

    Phase 1: Arrival and Size-Up 67 | Phase 2: Hazard Control 67 | Phase 3: Patient Access 68 | Phase 4: Medical Treatment 68 | Phase 5: Disentanglement 70 | Phase 6: Patient Packaging 70 | Phase 7: Removal/Transport 71

Surface Water Rescues 71

    General Background 71 | Moving Water 72 | Flat Water 74

Hazardous Atmosphere Rescues 76

    Confined-Space Hazards 78 | Confined-Space Protections in the Workplace 79 | Cave-Ins and Structural Collapses 79

Highway Operations and Vehicle Rescues 80

    Hazards in Highway Operations 80 | Auto Anatomy 82 | Rescue Strategies 82 | Rescue Skills Practice 83 | Hybrid Vehicles 84

Hazardous Terrain Rescues 84

    Types of Hazardous Terrain 84 | Patient Access in Hazardous Terrain 85 | Patient Packaging for Rough Terrain 85 | Patient Removal from Hazardous Terrain 86 | Extended Care Assessment and Environmental Issues 87

CHAPTER 5 • Hazardous Materials 91

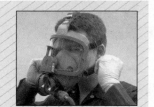

Introduction 93

Role of the Paramedic 93

    Requirements and Standards 94 | Levels of Training 94

Incident Size-Up 94

    IMS and Hazmat Emergencies 94 | Incident Awareness 95 | Recognition of Hazards 96 | Identification of Substances 98 | Hazardous Materials Zones 99

Specialized Terminology 101

    Terms for Medical Hazmat Operations 101 | Toxicologic Terms 103

Contamination and Toxicology Review 103

    Types of Contamination 103 | Routes of Exposure 103 | Cycles and Actions of Poisons 103 | Treatment of Common Exposures 104

Approaches to Decontamination 105

    Methods of Decontamination 106 | Decontamination Decision Making 106 | Field Decontamination 107

Hazmat Protection Equipment 108

Medical Monitoring and Rehabilitation 109

    Entry Readiness 109 | Post-Exit Rehab 109 | Heat Stress Factors 110

Importance of Practice 110

CHAPTER 6 • Crime Scene Awareness 112

Introduction 113

Approach to the Scene 114

    Possible Scenarios 114

Specific Dangerous Scenes 116

    Highway Encounters 116 | Violent Street Incidents 116 | Drug-Related Crimes 117 | Clandestine Drug Laboratories 118 | Domestic Violence 119

Tactical Considerations 119

    Safety Tactics 119 | Tactical Patient Care 121

EMS at Crime Scenes 122

    EMS and Police Operations 122 | Preserving Evidence 122

CHAPTER 7 ● Rural EMS 126

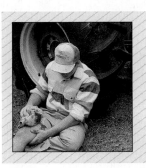

Introduction 128

Practicing Rural EMS 128

    Special Problems 128 | Creative Problem Solving 130

Typical Rural EMS Situations and Decisions 131

    The Distance Factor 131 | Agricultural Emergencies 132 | Recreational Emergencies 136

CHAPTER 8 ● Responding to Terrorist Acts 141

Introduction 143

Explosive Agents 143

Nuclear Detonation 144

    A Nuclear Incident Response 145 | Radioactive Contamination 145

Chemical Agents 145

    Nerve Agents 146 | Vesicants (Blistering Agents) 146 | Pulmonary
    Agents 147 | Biotoxins 147 | Incapacitating Agents 147 | Other Hazardous
    Chemicals 148 | Recognition of a Chemical Agent Release 148 | Management
    of a Chemical Agent Release 148

Biological Agents 148

    Pneumonia-Like Agents 149 | Encephalitis-Like Agents 149 | Other
    Agents 150 | Protection against Biological Agent Transmission 150

General Considerations Regarding Terrorist Attacks 151

    Scene Safety 151 | Recognizing a Terrorist Attack 151 | Responding to a Terrorist
    Attack 152

Precautions on Bloodborne Pathogens and Infectious Diseases 155

Suggested Responses to "You Make the Call" 157

Answers to Review Questions 161

Glossary 162

Index 166

Today's paramedics are professional health care clinicians and practitioners of emergency field medicine. The present paramedic curriculum provides both a broad-based medical education and a specific intensive training program designed to prepare paramedics to perform their traditional role as providers of emergency field medicine. The curriculum also provides a broad foundation in anatomy and physiology, patient assessment, pathophysiology of disease, and pharmacology that allows paramedics to expand their roles in the health care industry. The seven-volume *Paramedic Care: Principles & Practice* and, in particular, *Volume 7, Operations,* reflect these broad and specific purposes.

This volume provides paramedic students with the principles of paramedic operations. The first two chapters discuss ground and air medical transport, respectively. The rest of the book examines special circumstances that the paramedic may face at any time, including multiple-casualty incidents, rescue operations, hazardous materials, crime scenes, rural practice, and terrorist incidents.

OVERVIEW OF THE CHAPTERS

CHAPTER 1 Ground Ambulance Operations discusses the special world of EMS ambulance operations, in which patient care begins long before the call is received. The paramedic is responsible for keeping the ambulance and medical equipment in a constant state of readiness. In addition, the paramedic must understand the various EMS system operations to be able to act appropriately.

CHAPTER 2 Air Medical Operations looks at the use of aircraft for emergency patient transport. Both rotor-wing and fixed-wing aircraft have become vital assets in the emergent transport of seriously ill or injured patients from the scene or between health care facilities, as well as bringing specialty teams to remote locations. Aircraft are also essential for organ transport, search and rescue missions, and disaster assistance. Air medical transport should be considered a medical procedure with benefits and risks that must be weighed against each other. Like any other asset or tool, air medical transport must be used responsibly and EMS providers must be familiar with their capabilities and protocols.

CHAPTER 3 Multiple-Casualty Incidents and Incident Management provides an overview of situations that can result in multiple-casualty incidents. The chapter then presents a detailed discussion of the National Incident Management System (NIMS)—a system developed and mandated by the U.S. Department of Homeland Security for managing resources at the scene of a multiple-casualty incident, particularly at scenes involving many ambulances and multiple agencies. Paramedics must intimately understand the workings of the Incident Management System and apply them in daily operations.

CHAPTER 4 Rescue Awareness and Operations presents a comprehensive discussion of rescue operations. The level of EMS involvement with rescue operations varies significantly. In many EMS systems, paramedics are responsible for rescue operations. In others, paramedics are primarily responsible for patient care, whereas rescue operations are carried out by specially trained and equipped rescue teams. Regardless, the modern paramedic must have a thorough understanding of rescue operations, with an emphasis on scene safety.

CHAPTER 5 Hazardous Materials recognizes that more and more emergency scenes involve hazardous materials (hazmat). Although most hazardous materials scenes are handled by specialized hazmat teams, paramedics are often responsible for recognizing a hazmat incident, for activating the proper response and resources, and, of course, for patient care during the incident. Because the hazardous materials scene can be extremely dangerous, the paramedic must have a fundamental understanding of various hazardous materials and of hazmat operations.

CHAPTER 6 Crime Scene Awareness details the importance of protecting the crime scene. EMS personnel are often the first to arrive at a crime scene. Although their principal responsibilities are personal safety and patient care, they should take great effort to avoid disturbing important aspects of the crime scene. This chapter provides an overview of crime scene operations essential for effective paramedic functioning at the scene.

CHAPTER 7   Rural EMS provides an overview that enhances awareness of the special challenges, such as distance, faced by rural EMS personnel and the creative problem solving necessary to provide high-quality care to those who live or pursue recreation in rural or wilderness areas.

CHAPTER 8   Responding to Terrorist Acts discusses the types of agents likely to be used in terrorist attacks (conventional explosives, nuclear devices, chemical agents, and biological agents) with emphasis on the strategies paramedics need to ensure scene safety and the skills necessary to recognize and respond to a terrorist attack.

WHAT'S NEW IN THE FOURTH EDITION?

The Fourth Edition of *Paramedic Care: Principles & Practice* is the most extensive revision to date and reflects the dynamic and evolving world of paramedicine.

GLOBAL CHANGES/FEATURES

- Text follows the *National EMS Education Standards* and the *Paramedic Instructional Guidelines.*
- Terminology is consistent throughout the new Instructional Guidelines Gs (e.g., primary assessment).
- Reflects current 2010 American Heart Association Emergency Cardiac Care Guidelines.
- Embraces evidence-based emergency care with footnoted peer-review references to the major applicable world literature on the topic.
- Extensive review and editing.
- New design offers a fresh and professional text designed for the modern paramedic student.
- Extensive changes throughout are related to increased concerns about the detrimental effects of hyperoxia and the trend to limited oxygen administration.
- Terminology changed, when applicable, to assure consistency and reflect terms used in the AHA standards as well as the Instructional Guidelines.
- Reformatted into 7 volumes
  o *Volume 1: Introduction to Paramedicine*
  o *Volume 2: Paramedicine Fundamentals*
  o *Volume 3: Patient Assessment*
  o *Volume 4: Medicine*
  o *Volume 5: Trauma*
  o *Volume 6: Special Patients*
  o *Volume 7: Operations*

ACKNOWLEDGMENTS

INSTRUCTOR REVIEWERS

The reviewers of *Paramedic Care: Principles & Practice, Fourth Edition, Volume 7* have provided many excellent suggestions and ideas for improving the text. The quality of the reviews has been outstanding, and the reviews have been a major aid in the preparation and revision of the manuscript. The assistance provided by these EMS experts is deeply appreciated.

R Scott Crawford, NREMT-P, CCEMT-P, EMSI
EMS Instructor/Firefighter/Paramedic
Omaha Fire Department
Omaha, NE

Michael G. Hunter, NREMT-P, CCEMT-P
Primary Instructor and Education Coordinator
Harrison County Hospital
Corydon, IN

Michael Joseph Macedonia, BHA, EMT-P
Director of Paramedic Training Institute
Lackawanna College
Scranton, PA

Janis J. McManus, MS, NREMT-P
Clinical Coordinator
Virtua
Mt. Laurel, NJ

Keith A. Monosky, PhD, MPM, EMT-P
Associate Professor, Department of Nutrition, Exercise, and Health Sciences Director, EMS Paramedicine Program
Central Washington University
Ellensburg, WA

Deborah M. Roebuck, RN, BSN, NREMT-P
Paramedic Program Director
Itawamba Community College
Tupelo, MS

We also wish to express appreciation to the following EMS professionals who reviewed the third edition of Paramedic Care: Principles & Practice. *Their suggestions and perspectives helped to make this program a successful teaching tool.*

Mike Dymes, NREMT-P
EMS Program Director
Durham Technical Community College
Durham, NC

Joyce Foresman-Capuzzi, RN, BSN, CEN, CPN, CTRN, EMT-P
Temple Health System Transport Team
Philadelphia, PA

Darren P. Lacroix
Del Mar College
Emergency Medical Service Professions
Corpus Christi, TX

Greg Mullen, MS, NREMT-P
National EMS Academy
Lafayette, LA

Deborah L. Petty, BS, EMT-P I/C
Training Officer
St. Charles County Ambulance District
St. Peters, MO

B. Jeanine Riner, MHSA, BS, RRT, NREMT-P
GA Office of EMS and Trauma
Atlanta, GA

Mark A. Simpson, AS, BS, MSN, RN, NREMT-P
Program Director
Northwest-Shoals Community College
Muscle Shoals, AL

Allen Walls
Department of Fire & EMS
Colerain Township, OH

Brian J. Wilson, BA, NREMT-P
Education Director
Texas Tech School of Medicine
El Paso, TX

PHOTO ACKNOWLEDGMENTS

All photographs not credited adjacent to the photograph or in the photo credit section below were photographed on assignment for Brady/Prentice Hall/Pearson Education.

Organizations

We wish to thank the following organizations for their valuable assistance in creating the photo program:

Bound Tree University
Dublin, OH. www.boundtreeuniversity.com

Canandaigua Emergency Squad
Canandaigua, NY

Flower Mound Fire Department
Flower Mound, TX

Children's Hospital St. Louis/BJC Health Care
St. Louis, MO

Christian Hospital/BJC Health Care
St. Charles, MO

Chris Postiglione, Chief Clinical Supervisor

Austin/Travis County STAR Flight
Austin, TX

Pat Songer, Director of Emergency Medical Services

Humboldt General Hospital/ Ambulance/Rescue
Winnemucca, NV

Tyco Health Care/Nellcor Puritan Bennet
Pleasanton, CA

Wolfe Tory Medical
Salt Lake City, UT

Winter Park Fire-Rescue
Winter Park, FL
Chief James E. White
Deputy Chief Patrick McCabe

City of Winter Park, FL
Kenneth W. Bradley, Mayor

Technical Advisors

Thanks to the following people for providing technical support during the photo shoots in Winter Park, Florida.

Andrew Isaacs, EMS Captain
Tod Meadors, EMS Captain
Dr. Tod Husty, Medical Director

Richard Rodriguez, EMS Captain
Jeff Spinelli, Engineer-Paramedic

Models

Thanks to the following people from the Flower Mound Fire Department, Flower Mound, Texas, and from Winter Park Fire-Rescue, Winter Park, Florida, who provided locations and/or portrayed patients and EMS providers in our photographs.

FAO/Paramedic Wade Woody
FF/Paramedic Tim Mackling
FF/Paramedic Matthew Daniel
FF/Paramedic Jon Rea
FF/Paramedic Waylon Palmer
FF/EMT Jesse Palmer
Captain/EMT Billy McWhorter
Linda Kirk, Director, Winter Park Towers, Winter Park, FL

Andrew Isaacs
Richard Rodriguez
Tod Meadors
Jeff Spinelli
Mark Vaughn
Victoria Devereaux
Teresa George

BRYAN E. BLEDSOE, DO, FACEP, FAAEM, EMT-P

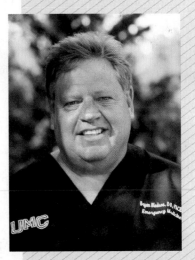

Dr. Bryan Bledsoe is an emergency physician, researcher, and EMS author. Presently he is Professor of Emergency Medicine and Director of the EMS Fellowship program at the University of Nevada School of Medicine and an Attending Emergency Physician at the University Medical Center of Southern Nevada in Las Vegas. He is board-certified in emergency medicine. Prior to attending medical school, Dr. Bledsoe worked as an EMT, a paramedic, and a paramedic instructor. He completed EMT training in 1974 and paramedic training in 1976 and worked for six years as a field paramedic in Fort Worth, Texas. In 1979, he joined the faculty of the University of North Texas Health Sciences Center and served as coordinator of EMT and paramedic education programs at the university.

Dr. Bledsoe is active in emergency medicine and EMS research. He is a popular speaker at state, national, and international seminars and writes regularly for numerous EMS journals. He is active in educational endeavors with the United States Special Operations Command (USSOCOM) and the University of Nevada at Las Vegas. Dr. Bledsoe is the author of numerous EMS textbooks and has in excess of 1 million books in print. Dr. Bledsoe was named a "Hero of Emergency Medicine" in 2008 by the American College of Emergency Physicians as a part of their 40th anniversary celebration and was named a "Hero of Health and Fitness" by *Men's Health* magazine as part of their 20th anniversary edition in November of 2008. He is frequently interviewed in the national media. Dr. Bledsoe is married and divides his time between his residences in Midlothian, TX, and Las Vegas, NV.

ROBERT S. PORTER, MA, EMT-P

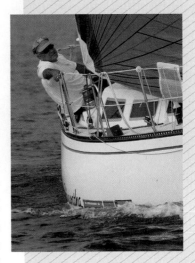

Robert Porter has been teaching in emergency medical services for 38 years and currently serves as the Senior Advanced Life Support Educator for Madison County (New York) Emergency Medical Services. Mr. Porter is a Wisconsin native and received his bachelor's degree in education from the University of Wisconsin. He completed his paramedic training at Northeast Wisconsin Technical Institute in 1978 and earned a master's degree in health education at Central Michigan University in 1990.

Mr. Porter has been an EMT and an EMS educator and administrator since 1973 and obtained his certification and national registration as an EMT-Paramedic in 1978. He has taught both basic and advanced EMS courses in the states of Wisconsin, Michigan, Louisiana, Pennsylvania, and New York. Mr. Porter conducted one of the nation's first rural paramedic programs and developed a university-based, two-year paramedic program. Mr. Porter served for more than ten years as a paramedic program accreditation-site evaluator for the American Medical Association and is a past chair of the National Association of EMTs—Society of EMT Instructor/Coordinators. Mr. Porter also served for 15 years as a flight paramedic with the Onondaga County Sheriff's Department air medical service, AirOne. He has authored Brady's *Paramedic Care: Principles & Practice, Essentials of Paramedic Care, Intermediate Emergency Care: Principles & Practice, Tactical Emergency Care,* and *Weapons of Mass Destruction: Emergency Care,* as well as the workbooks accompanying this text. When not writing or teaching, Mr. Porter enjoys offshore sailboat racing and home restoration.

RICHARD A. CHERRY, MS, EMT-P

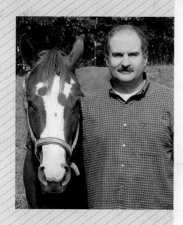

Richard Cherry is the Director of Training for Northern Onondaga Volunteer Ambulance (NOVA) in Liverpool, New York, a suburb of Syracuse. He recently retired from the Department of Emergency Medicine at Upstate Medical University where he held the positions of Director of Paramedic Training, Assistant Emergency Medicine Residency Director, Clinical Assistant Professor of Emergency Medicine, and Technical Director for Medical Simulation. His experience includes years of classroom teaching and emergency fieldwork. A native of Buffalo, Mr. Cherry earned his bachelor's degree at nearby St. Bonaventure University in 1972. He taught high school for the next ten years while he earned his master's degree in education from Oswego State University in 1977. He holds a permanent teaching license in New York State.

Mr. Cherry entered the emergency medical services field in 1974 with the DeWitt Volunteer Fire Department, where he served his community as a firefighter and EMS provider for more than 15 years. He took his first EMT course in 1977 and became an ALS provider two years later. He earned his paramedic certificate in 1985 as a member of the area's first paramedic class.

Mr. Cherry has authored several books for Brady. Most notable are *Paramedic Care: Principles & Practice, Essentials of Paramedic Care, Intermediate Emergency Care: Principles & Practice,* and *EMT Teaching: A Common Sense Approach.* He has made presentations at many state, national, and international EMS conferences on a variety of teaching topics. He and his wife, Sue, run a summer horse-riding camp for children with special needs on their property in West Monroe, New York. He also plays guitar in a Christian band.

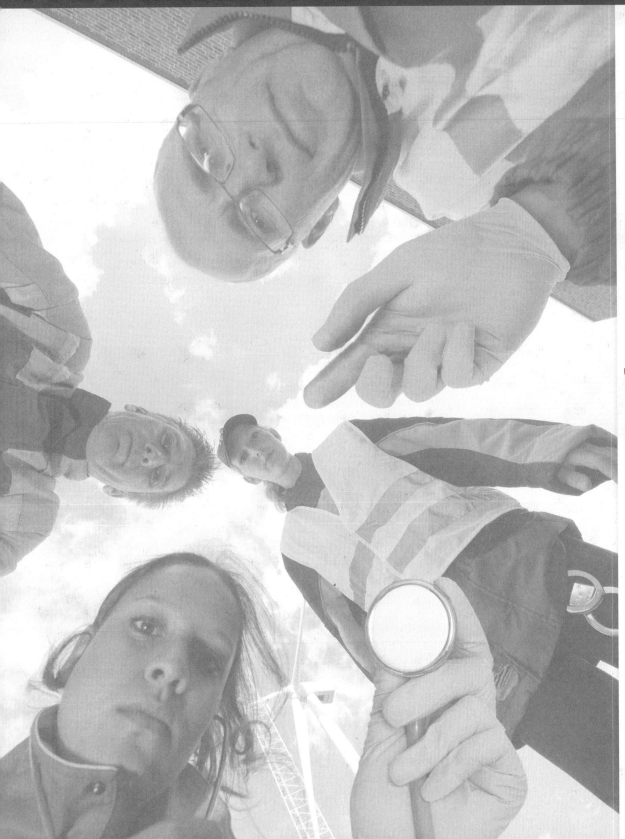

Welcome to

PARAMEDIC CARE PRINCIPLES & PRACTICE

FOURTH EDITION

A Guide to Key Features

Emphasizing Principles

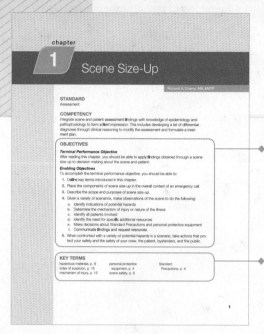

CHAPTER OBJECTIVES

Terminal Performance Objectives and a separate set of Enabling Objectives are provided for each chapter.

KEY TERMS

Page numbers identify where each key term first appears, boldfaced, in the chapter.

TABLES

A wealth of tables offers the opportunity to highlight, summarize, and compare information.

TABLE 4-2	Common Infectious Diseases		
Disease	**Mode of Transmission**	**Incubation Period**
AIDS (acquired immune deficiency syndrome)	AIDS- or HIV-infected blood via intravenous drug use, semen and vaginal fluids, blood transfusions, or (rarely) needlesticks. Mothers also may pass HIV to their unborn children.	Several months or years
Hepatitis B, C	Blood, stool, or other body fluids, or contaminated objects.	Weeks or months
Tuberculosis	Respiratory secretions, airborne or on contaminated objects.	2 to 6 weeks
Meningitis, bacterial	Oral and nasal secretions.	2 to 10 days
Pneumonia, bacterial and viral	Oral and nasal droplets and secretions.	Several days
Influenza	Airborne droplets, or direct contact with body fluids.	1 to 3 days
Staphylococcal skin infections	Contact with open wounds or sores or contaminated objects.	Several days
Chicken pox (varicella)	Airborne droplets, or contact with open sores.	11 to 21 days
German measles (rubella)	Airborne droplets. Mothers may pass it to their unborn children.	10 to 12 days
Whooping cough (pertussis)	Respiratory secretions or airborne droplets.	6 to 20 days
SARS (severe acute respiratory syndrome)	Airborne droplets and personal contact.	4 to 6 days

CONTENT REVIEW

Screened content review boxes set off from the text are interspersed throughout the chapter. They summarize key points and serve as a helpful study guide—in an easy format for quick review.

PHOTOS AND ILLUSTRATIONS

Carefully selected photos and a unique art program reinforce content coverage and add to text explanations.

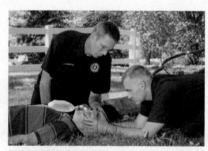

● **Figure 3-3** During the primary assessment of your patient, you will look for and immediately treat any life-threatening conditions.

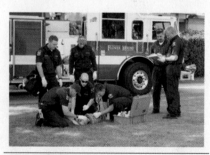

● **Figure 3-7** As leader of the EMS team, the paramedic must interact with patients, bystanders, and other rescue personnel in a professional and efficient manner.

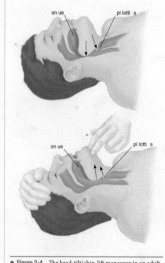

● Figure 2-4 The head-tilt/chin-lift maneuver in an adult.

SUMMARY

This end-of-chapter feature provides a concise review of chapter information.

 SUMMARY

The scene size-up is the initial step in the patient care process. Sizing up the scene and situation begins at your initial dispatch and does not end until you are clear of the call. As the call unfolds, you should be making constant observations and adjustments to your plan of action. Remember that your safety and the safety of your partner are paramount—it is hard to effectively treat both yourself and others.

Scene size-up should be practiced so much that it becomes second nature to you. It is like noticing veins on people in public after you begin starting IVs. (You have all done it—looked across the room at the back of someone's hand and noticed what nice veins they had.) Sizing up a scene is no different. After a while you begin to notice mechanisms of injury and other important details almost subconsciously. But be careful and do not get complacent! Always make it a point to pause for just a few seconds and consciously look around the scene before proceeding into any situation.

Scene size-up is not a step-by-step process, but a series of decisions you make when confronted with a variety of circumstances that are often beyond your control. It is a way to make order out of chaos, keep yourself and your crew safe, and ensure that all necessary resources are focused on patient care and outcomes. With time and experience, you will learn to perform a scene size-up quickly and focus on important issues. Your careful size-up lays the foundation for an organized and timely approach toward patient care and scene management.

REVIEW QUESTIONS

These questions ask students to review and recall key information they have just learned.

REVIEW QUESTIONS

1. Which of the following is *not* a component of the scene size-up?
   a. Standard Precautions
   b. mechanism of injury
   c. primary assessment
   d. location of all patients

2. The HEPA mask is designed to protect you from _____.
   a. tuberculosis
   b. AIDS
   c. hepatitis
   d. meningitis

3. The top priority in any emergency situation is _____.
   a. patient assessment
   b. bystander cooperation
   c. customer service
   d. your personal safety

4. As you approach a scene, something just does not seem right. It is not anything you can put your finger on, just a sense that something is wrong or is about to happen. What should you do about it?
   a. Wait until law enforcement arrives before entering.
   b. Ignore your feelings and enter the scene.
   c. Enter the scene with something with which to protect yourself.
   d. Call out for the patient to come outside.

5. You are responding to a shooting at a well-known bar. How should you approach the scene?
   a. Stage outside the bar until the police arrive.
   b. Wait for another ambulance or rescue crew before entering.
   c. Just enter the scene.
   d. Stage your ambulance a few blocks away until law enforcement arrives.

6. You arrive on the scene and see that a power line lies close to your pediatric patient. You are fairly sure the line is live and decide to move it with a dry piece of equipment. Which of the following should you use?
   a. a wooden-handled ax
   b. a fallen tree branch
   c. a nylon rope
   d. none of the above

7. When you and your partner arrive at a multiple-patient incident, you should _____.
   a. begin assessing and treating the first patient you encounter
   b. establish command and begin triage
   c. provide intensive emergency care to the most critical patient
   d. start at opposite ends and begin assessing patients

REFERENCES

This listing is a compilation of source material providing the basis of updated data and research used in the preparation of each chapter.

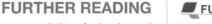 **REFERENCES**

1. U.S. Department of Transportation/National Highway Traffic Safety Administration. *National EMS Scope of Practice Model.* Washington, DC, 2006.
2. National Registry of Emergency Medical Technicians. 2004 National EMS Practice Analysis. Columbus, OH: National Registry of EMTs, 2005.
3. American College of Surgeons. *Verified Trauma Centers.* [Available at: http://www.facs.org/trauma/verified.html]
4. Feldman, M. J., J. L. Lukins, P. R. Verbeek, et al. "Use of Treat-and-Release Directives for Paramedics at a Mass Gathering." *Prehosp Emerg Care* 9 (2005): 213–217.
5. American College of Emergency Physicians. "Interfacility Transportation of the Critical Care Patient and Its Medical Direction." *Ann Emerg Med* 47 (2006): 305.
6. Harkins, S. "Documentation: Why Is It So Important?" *Emerg Med Serv* 31 (2002): 93–94.
7. Lerner, E. B., A. R. Fernandez, and M. N. Shah. "Do Emergency Medical Services Professionals Think They Should Participate in Disease Prevention?" *Prehosp Emerg Care* 13 (2009): 64–70.
8. Poliafico, F. "The Role of EMS in Public Access Defibrillation." *Emerg Med Serv* 32 (2003): 73.
9. Streger M. R. "Professionalism." *Emerg Med Serv* 32 (2003): 35.
10. Klugman, C. M. "Why EMS Needs Its Own Ethics. What's Good for Other Areas of Healthcare May Not Be Good for You." *Emerg Med Serv* 36 (2007): 114–122.
11. Touchstone, M. "Professional Development. Part 1: Becoming an EMS Leader." *Emerg Med Serv* 38 (2009): 59–60.
12. Bledsoe, B. E. "EMS Needs a Few More Cowboys." *JEMS* 28 (2003): 112–113.

FURTHER READING

This list features recommendations for books and journal articles that go beyond chapter coverage.

FURTHER READING

Bailey, E. D. and T. Sweeney. "Considerations in Establishing Emergency Medical Services Response Time Goals." *Prehosp Emerg Care* 7 (2003): 397–399.

Bledsoe, B. E. "Searching for the Evidence behind EMS." *Emerg Med Serv* 31 (2003): 63–67.

Heightman, A. J. "EMS Workforce. A Comprehensive Listing of Certified EMS Providers by State and How the Workforce Has Changed Since 1993." *JEMS* 5 (2000): 108–112.

Jaslow, D. J., J. Ufberg, and R. Marsh. "Primary Injury Prevention in an Urban EMS System." *J Emerg Med* 25 (2003): 167–170.

National Academy of Sciences, National Research Council. *Accidental Death and Disability: The Neglected Disease of Modern Society.* Washington, DC:
U.S. Department of Health, Education, and Welfare, 1966.

Page, J. O. *The Magic of 3 AM.* San Diego, CA: JEMS Publishing, 2002.

Page, J. O. *The Paramedics.* Morristown, NJ: Backdraft Publications, 1979. [No longer available for purchase except as a used book. Entire book can be viewed online at www.JEMS.com/Paramedics.]

Page, J. O. *Simple Advice.* San Diego, CA: JEMS Publishing, 2002.

Persse, D. E., C. B. Key, R. N. Bradley, et al. "Cardiac Arrest Survival as a Function of Ambulance Deployment Strategy in a Large Urban Emergency Medical Services System." *Resusc* 59 (2003): 97–104.

CASE STUDY

This feature at the start of each chapter draws students into the reading and creates a link between text content and real-life situations.

CASE STUDY

On a quiet afternoon, paramedic Dean Barker hears the tones for a person slumped over the steering wheel of his car. He and his partner, Kyle Peeper, a new EMT, respond immediately. En route, Dean emphasizes to his rookie partner the need to put safety first and not to rush in without a quick evaluation of the scene. His partner nods agreeably but is obviously both excited and nervous about his first real emergency call.

When they arrive, Dean notices a very unusual and troubling scene. Dean grabs his partner and stops him from jumping out of the vehicle. He asks him to stop and look around. "Tell me what you see," he says. His partner nervously answers, "Right, OK, I see one car parked alongside a cemetery and it looks like someone might be inside. There seems to be a white cloud inside the car and I smell a strong odor of sulfur or rotten eggs. I also see a sign on the driver's side window with what looks like a hazard emblem on it."

"So, is there anything we should do before jumping out and entering this scene? What is our first priority? asks Dean. "Patient care." answers his partner. "No, safety first. We'll park our vehicle upwind from the car and I'll make a quick report to dispatch and call for more help. We already know this is more than we can handle by ourselves."

Dean assumes the role of incident commander; he calls for the fire department's hazmat team, cordons off the area, and alerts all responding personnel that the potential for fire and explosion exists. There also may be a need to evacuate the area. Waiting for the fire department to arrive seems like hours to his energetic partner. Dean asks him what they can do until they arrive. Kyle responds that they can shut down the road and secure the scene from bystanders.

When the hazmat team arrives, they read the signs that someone left on three of the four windows. They appear to be suicide notes and a warning to rescuers of the toxic atmosphere inside the car. The hazmat team begins the arduous process of identifying the toxic substance, containing the exposure, and decontaminating the victim and all rescuers. Dean and his partner are released and head back to the station.

Kyle asks Dean what the substance was inside that car and asks why they didn't try to extricate and resuscitate the driver. Dean calmly explains that the white cloud and rotten-egg odor strongly suggested a deadly asphyxiant, hydrogen sulfide, and if they had opened the door to extricate him, they would have been just as dead as their victim. This day a rookie learned a crucial lesson—on an EMS call, nothing is more important than his safety. Nothing.

YOU MAKE THE CALL

A scenario at the end of each chapter promotes critical thinking by requiring students to apply principles to actual practice.

YOU MAKE THE CALL

On a rainy and windy evening, you hear the tones for a car crash on the interstate highway just five minutes from the station. You are the only ambulance dispatched along with fire department rescue and fire apparatus. On arrival you see three cars smashed up, one on its side, smoke rising from the crash, and what looks like fluid leaking from one vehicle. By the time you arrive, traffic is backed up for three blocks. You realize that the decisions you make in the first few minutes will have a major effect on safety, patient care, and overall operations.

Describe how you would size up this scene. Make sure you cover the following areas:

- Vehicle placement
- Initial radio report
- Assuming incident command
- Safety
- Hazard control
- Standard Precautions
- Location and triaging of patients
- Resource determination
- Mechanisms of injury

See Suggested Responses at the back of this book.

PROCEDURE SCANS

Visual skill summaries provide step-by-step support in skill instruction.

Procedure 5–22 ● Reassessment

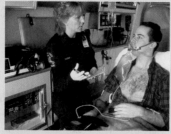

5-22a ● Reevaluate the ABCs.

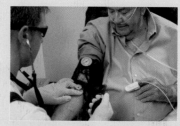

5-22b ● Take all vital signs again.

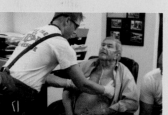

5-22c ● Perform your focused assessment again.

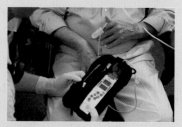

5-22d ● Evaluate your interventions' effects.

Special Features

PATHO PEARLS

Offer a snapshot of pathological considerations students will encounter in the field.

PATHO PEARLS

Patient assessment actually starts as soon as you approach the scene. Clues about the patient's underlying pathophysiology might be evident from such things as positioning of the vehicle, downed power lines, or the appearance and actions of bystanders. However, your safety, and that of your fellow rescuers, is always paramount. Never approach a scene that appears unsafe. With time, you will develop a "sixth sense" about emergency scenes and bystanders.

As you begin the patient encounter, process all that you see into your patient assessment and care. For example, consider this scenario: A car with two 16-year-old girls fails to negotiate a turn on a country road and overturns into a flowing creek adjacent to the road. Although the ambient temperature is in the 60s, you know that the temperature of the water in this area often is in the 40s. Thus, you should immediately suspect the possibility of hypothermia.

As the girls are removed from entrapment, no obvious injuries are noted. Vital signs are normal other than slight tachycardia. However, peripheral pulses are weak and the skin is pale and cool. Is it shock? Is it hypothermia? Is it both? Your index of suspicion is high for both hypothermia and blunt force trauma. You follow local protocols with regard to immobilization, fluid therapy, and monitoring. Once in the ambulance and wrapped in blankets, both girls start to show signs that blood flow to the skin is improving. By the time you reach the hospital, their skin has a normal color and their pulse rates are normal.

Following a comprehensive assessment in the emergency department, the girls are discharged to their parents with no apparent injuries. Thus, your instincts were right. The potential for shock was a greater risk to the girls than the potential for hypothermia, and you had to treat based on this risk. But hypothermia turned out to be the principal problem. Integrating information from the scene size-up, patient history, and patient examination gave you a clear picture of the patients' underlying pathophysiologic process.

CULTURAL CONSIDERATIONS

Provide an awareness of beliefs that might affect patient care.

CULTURAL CONSIDERATIONS

Eye contact is a major form of nonverbal communication. Short eye contact is often seen as friendly, whereas prolonged eye contact may be interpreted as threatening. Thus, timing is an important factor in how a person interprets eye contact.

One's culture also influences how eye contact is interpreted. Eye contact can mean respect in one culture and disrespect in another. Often, Asians will avoid eye contact even when they have nothing to hide. Eye contact between people of different sexes is problematic in Muslim cultures, in which a prolonged look in the face of a member of the opposite sex might be misinterpreted. Because of this, people in Middle Eastern countries might look a person of the same sex in the eye and not look into the eyes of a person of the opposite sex.

If you work in a culturally diverse community, you should learn the customs of eye contact and other forms of nonverbal communication of those you might encounter during the course of your work.

LEGAL NOTES

Present instances in which legal or ethical considerations should be evaluated.

LEGAL CONSIDERATIONS

Gatekeeper to the Health Care System. *The EMS system is often the initial point of contact for a person entering the health care system. Thus, to a certain extent, a paramedic frequently functions as a sort of gatekeeper to the health care system as a whole.*

Part of a paramedic's responsibility is to ensure that a patient is taken to a facility that can appropriately care for the patient's condition. Today, hospitals have become more specialized. That is, some hospitals have chosen to provide certain services and not provide others. For example, one hospital may elect to specialize in cardiac care, another in stroke care, another in burn care, and so on. This is especially true in communities with multiple hospitals. Because of this, it is essential that paramedics understand the capabilities of the hospitals in the system where they work. Also, with overcrowding in modern emergency departments, diversion of ambulances by hospitals whose emergency departments are full has become commonplace.

For all these reasons, local EMS system protocols must be available to guide prehospital personnel in ensuring that each patient is delivered to a facility that can adequately care for the patient's condition.

ASSESSMENT PEARLS

Offer tips, guidance, and information to aid in patient assessment.

ASSESSMENT PEARLS

Chest pain is a common reason that people summon EMS. However, the causes of chest pain are numerous. In emergency medicine or EMS, we often look to exclude the most serious causes before determining whether chest pain is of a benign origin. Internal organs do not have as many pain fibers as do such structures as the skin and other areas. Pain arising from an internal organ tends to be dull and vague. This is because nerves from various spinal levels innervate the organ in question. The heart, for example, is innervated by several thoracic spinal nerve segments. Thus, cardiac pain tends to be dull and is sometimes described as pressure. It also tends to cause referred pain (i.e., pain in an area somewhat distant to the organ), such as pain in the left arm and jaw. Dull pain that is hard to localize (or to reproduce with palpation) may be due to cardiac disease. One sign often seen with patients suffering cardiac disease is Levine's sign. With Levine's sign, the patient will subconsciously cle... *pain. Levine's sign is a...* *(e.g., angina or acute c...*

ASSESSMENT PEARLS

Assessing skin abnormalities in dark-skinned people can be a challenge. Try the following techniques:

Jaundice *Look for a yellow color in the sclera and hard palate.*

Erythema *Look for an ashen color in the sclera, conjunctiva, mouth, tongue, lips, nail beds, palms, and soles.*

Pallor *Feel for warmth in the affected area.*

Petechiae *Look for tiny purplish dots on the abdomen.*

Cyanosis *Look for a dull, dark coloring in the mouth, tongue, lips, nail beds, palms, and soles.*

Rashes *Feel for abnormal skin texture.*

Edema *Look for decreased color and feel for tightness.*

Student Workbook

A student workbook with review and practice activities accompanies each volume of the Paramedic Care series. The workbooks include multiple-choice questions, other exercises, case studies, and special projects, along with an answer key with text page references.

REVIEW OF CHAPTER OBJECTIVES

Tied to chapter objectives, content summaries review important information and concepts.

CASE STUDY REVIEW

An in-depth analysis at the start of each chapter highlights essential information and applied principles.

CONTENT SELF-EVALUATION

Multiple-choice, matching, and short-answer questions test reading comprehension.

SPECIAL PROJECTS

Experiences have been designed to help students remember information and principles.

PATIENT SCENARIO FLASHCARDS

Flashcards present scenarios with signs and symptoms and information to make field diagnoses.

DRUG FLASHCARDS

A special set of flashcards represents drugs commonly used in paramedic care.

MyBRADYLab™

www.mybradylab.com

WHAT IS MyBRADYLab?

MyBRADYLab is a comprehensive online program that gives you the opportunity to test yourself on basic information, concepts, and skills to see how well you know paramedic course material. From the test results, the program builds a self-paced, personalized study plan unique to your needs. Remediation in the form of e-text pages, illustrations, animations, exercises, and video clips is provided for those areas in which you may need additional instruction or reinforcement. You can then work through the program until material is learned and mastered. **MyBRADYLab** is available as a standalone program or with an embedded e-text.

   MyBRADYLab maps objectives created from the National EMS Education Standards for the Paramedic level to each learning module. With **MyBRADYLab**, you can track your own progress through the entire course. The personalized study plan material supports you as you work to achieve success in the classroom and on certification exams.

HOW DO STUDENTS BENEFIT?

MyBRADYLab helps you:

- Keep up with the new, complex information presented in the text and lectures.
- Save time by focusing study and review on just the content you need.
- Increase understanding of difficult concepts with study material for different learning styles.
- Remediate in areas in which you need additional review.

KEY FEATURES OF MyBRADYLab

Pre-Tests and Post-Tests Using questions aligned to Paramedic Standards, quizzes measure your understanding of topics and expected learning outcomes.

Personalized Study Material Based on the topic pre-test results, you will receive a personalized study plan highlighting areas where you may need improvement. Study tools include:

- Skills and animation videos
- Links to specific pages in the e-text
- Images for review
- Interactive exercises
- Audio glossary
- Access to full chapters of the e-text

HOW DO INSTRUCTORS BENEFIT?

- Save time by providing students with a comprehensive, media-rich study program
- Track student understanding of course content in the program Gradebook
- Monitor student activity with viewable student assignments

What Resources Are Available to Instructors?

Visit **www.bradybooks.com** to log onto Brady's Resource Central website for the Paramedic Care series. Your Brady sales representative will assist with access codes. At Resource Central instructors will find a wealth of curriculum management material to support class presentations, student assessment, and administrative functions.

Where Do I Get More Information?

Contact your local Brady representative for more information.

1

Ground Ambulance Operations

Bryan Bledsoe, DO, FACEP, FAAEM, EMT-P

STANDARD
EMS Operations (Principles of Safely Operating a Ground Ambulance)

COMPETENCY
Applies knowledge of operational roles and responsibilities to ensure patient, public, and personnel safety.

OBJECTIVES

Terminal Performance Objective
After reading this chapter, you should be able to place patient care tasks in the context of ground ambulance operations to safely respond to calls and transport patients.

Enabling Objectives
To accomplish the terminal performance objective, you should be able to:

1. Define key terms introduced in this chapter.
2. Describe the roles of standards, trends, and administrative rules and regulations on the design of ambulances and the equipment they carry.
3. Identify the types of ambulance design according to the General Services Administration federal specifications for ambulances.
4. Describe the roles of the Commission on Accreditation for Ambulance Services and the American College of Surgeons Committee on Trauma with respect to ambulance equipment and supplies.
5. Describe the role and responsibilities of the paramedic in checking the ambulance at the beginning of each shift.
6. Identify components of typical ambulance checklists.
7. Describe considerations in ambulance deployment and staffing configurations.
8. Discuss the significance of ambulance collisions.
9. Identify strategies for reducing the risk of ambulance collisions and associated deaths and injuries.
10. Implement safety measures related to driving, parking, and loading the ambulance.

KEY TERMS
demographic, p. 5
deployment, p. 2
DOT KKK 1822F specs, p. 2

due regard, p. 8
essential equipment, p. 2
gold standard, p. 2

minimum standards, p. 2
peak load, p. 5

primary areas of responsibility   spotter, p. 6   tiered response
  (PARs), p. 5   system status management   system, p. 6
reportable collisions, p. 6   (SSM), p. 6
reserve capacity, p. 6

CASE STUDY

It's 6:00 A.M., the start of another shift. You and your partner have just arrived to relieve the overnight crew. As you check and sign out the narcotics with the outgoing paramedic, the tones go off for a priority one call on the other side of town. You quickly finish the paperwork and rush out the door. As you load your personal protective equipment, you shout to the outgoing crew: "How's the rig?" The paramedic responds, "Fine. We just restocked."

You feel confident that the ambulance has everything you will need. Your service is dedicated to ensuring that each shift fills in ambulance checklists and that replacement supplies are easily obtained. In this case, you arrive at the scene to find that the patient is having difficulty breathing, most likely from an acute exacerbation of asthma. The call runs smoothly, and the patient actually improves en route to the hospital.

You quickly wrap up the paperwork and return to the station. On the way, you and your partner recall the haphazard ambulance operations of a few years ago. The former management team looked the other way when some medics failed to restock the supplies and equipment that they used. Imagine not having enough oxygen or a bronchodilator for an asthma patient. You and your partner both agree—things have gotten a lot better since the new management has insisted that crews take the tour checklists seriously.

INTRODUCTION

Good ambulance operations involve some of the knowledge and skills that you have already established in your EMT training and through field experience. However, because the safety of so many people—the EMS team, the patient, and bystanders—depends on effective ambulance maintenance and operation, it is important for you to review this information regularly so that it becomes second nature. In addition to the communication and dispatch skills learned in Volume 1, Chapter 9, you should keep in mind these topics: ambulance standards, maintenance of ambulance equipment and supplies, ambulance stationing, and safe ambulance operations.

Ambulance Standards

Various standards, as well as administrative rules and regulations, influence the design of ambulances and the medical equipment carried on each unit. Similar guidelines determine staffing levels and **deployment** of EMS agencies (see information later in this chapter).

Because the oversight for EMS usually falls to state governments, many of the requirements for ambulance service are written in state statutes or regulations. However, national standards and trends do have an influence on the development of these laws. Typically, state laws are broad, whereas corresponding regulations provide more specific guidelines or rules. For example, a public health law may authorize the state department of health to issue regulations through its EMS Bureau. These regulations, known as the "state EMS code," might then handle such matters as the **essential equipment** to be carried on every ambulance.

In most cases, state standards tend to be generic enough that they are "palatable," affordable, and politically feasible to all EMS agencies throughout the state. State standards usually set **minimum standards**, rather than a **gold standard**, for operation. In other words, they establish the lowest level at which units will be allowed to operate. When local and/or regional EMS systems get involved in regulation, their lists tend to be much more detailed and often approach a gold standard, which is the goal when ample resources are provided.

Ambulance Design

The U.S. General Services Administration's Automotive Commodity Center issues the federal regulations that specify ambulance design and manufacturing requirements. These specifications, known as the **DOT KKK 1822F specs**, attempt to influence safety standards as well as standardize the look of ambulances.[1]

Over the years, the "KKK specifications" have had a significant influence on ambulance manufacturing. The specs describe the following three basic ambulance designs:

- *Type I*—conventional truck cab-chassis with a modular ambulance body
- *Type II*—standard van, forward control integral cab-body ambulance
- *Type III*—specialty van, forward control integral cab-body ambulance

In addition to these three designs, there is also a medium-duty ambulance rescue vehicle (Figure 1-1 ●) that is designed to handle heavier loads and has a gross weight of approximately 24,000 pounds.

The federal specifications not only provide standards for the purchase of ambulances used by the federal government, but they also provide guidelines for the states to follow. Massachusetts, for example, refers to the federal specifications in its own state regulations. In such cases, the federal specifications become the state standard for ambulance services to follow when purchasing vehicles.

Some states, including Connecticut, Vermont, and New Jersey, have chosen to develop their own standards. Often these states use the federal specifications as the basis or starting point for their own regulations. A few states, such as New York, use neither federal nor state specifications. Instead, the decisions for ambulance purchases are determined on a local or regional basis.

There has been a recent push over the last decade to improve the safety of ground ambulances. The National Highway Traffic Safety Administration (NHTSA) and the National Institute for Occupational Safety and Health (NIOSH) are collaborating on a four-year research-based project to improve existing standards to make patients and EMS workers safer in the rear compartment of ambulances. Several ambulance manufacturers and EMS operators have developed concept vehicles to explore and test new ambulance safety systems and designs (Figure 1-2 ●).

In addition to the U.S. Department of Transportation (DOT), other federal agencies and national organizations influence standards. Air ambulance standards, for example, are usually designed with input from representatives of the Air and Surface Transport Nurses Association (ASTNA), the International Association of Flight and Critical Care Paramedics (IAFCCP), and the Association of Air Medical Services (AAMS). The Federal Communications Commission (FCC), which is discussed in Volume 1, Chapter 9, specifies the radio bands and types of equipment that may be used in ambulances.

Medical Equipment Standards

With increases in the presence of hazardous materials and awareness of infectious diseases, the Occupational Safety and Health Administration (OSHA) has become more and more involved in ambulance standards. As the agency charged with protecting worker safety, OSHA has helped ensure the use of

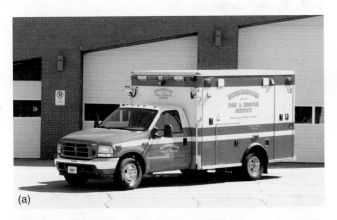

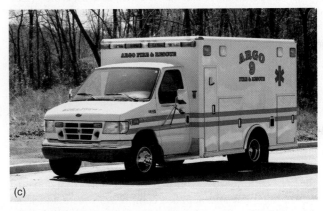

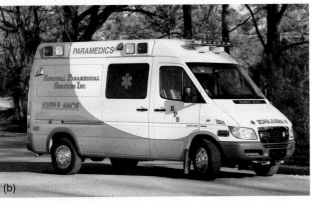

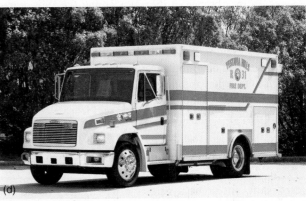

● **Figure 1-1** Four types of ambulances. (a) Type I, (b) Type II, (c) Type III, and (d) medium-duty rescue vehicle.

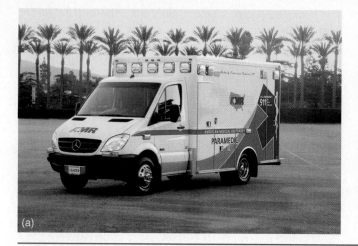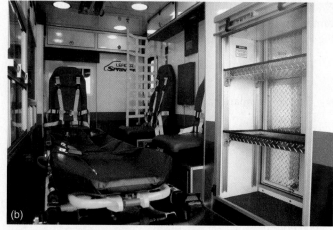

● **Figure 1-2** Many safety concept ambulances are under evaluation as safety becomes a paramount concern for EMS. (a) Exterior view. (b) Interior view with safety harness. *(Photos courtesy of American Medical Response and American Emergency Vehicles)*

equipment lists calling for disinfecting agents, sharps containers, red bags, HEPA masks, and personal protective equipment. The National Institute for Occupational Safety and Health (NIOSH) has established similar standards.

Other voluntary standards have been set by peer organizations, such as the National Fire Protection Association (NFPA). In many cases, these standards are referenced in local ordinances and thus have become the standard for a given municipality.

In addition to city, county, and/or district ambulance ordinances, local medical direction boards sometimes list the medications that paramedics can carry. These boards, which issue indirect medical direction, may also list the specific advanced life support (ALS) equipment and supplies that should be on every ambulance. For example, in areas where the paramedics are trained to obtain a 12-lead ECG, the medical direction board may have specified the actual brand of equipment in an effort to standardize care on a system-wide or regional basis.

Additional Guidelines

At the national level, the Commission on Accreditation of Ambulance Services (CAAS) provides a voluntary "gold standard" for the EMS community to follow. CAAS requires that onboard medical equipment and supplies comply with state and local guidelines. In the absence of these guidelines, CAAS requires services to develop guidelines that meet or exceed those established by the American College of Surgeons (ACS). The ACS Committee of Trauma issued its first list of "essential equipment" to be carried on ambulances in 1970 and revised the list in 1994. Of note is that as long ago as 1970 the list included the ALS equipment, emergency drugs, and fluids commonly used on ALS calls today.

CHECKING AMBULANCES

On each shift, an essential part of a paramedic's duties includes completion of the ambulance equipment and supply checklist. Aside from reminding the personnel exactly where

all equipment and supplies are stored on the ambulance, the shift checklist helps ensure that all equipment and supplies will be available and in working order when needed for patient care. The checklist also makes the work environment safer by ensuring mechanical maintenance and the availability of personal protective equipment.

The components of a typical vehicle/equipment checklist include the following:

- Patient infection control, comfort, and protection supplies
- Initial and focused assessment equipment
- Equipment for the transfer of the patient
- Equipment for airway maintenance, ventilation, and resuscitation
- Oxygen therapy and suction equipment
- Equipment for assisting with cardiac resuscitation
- Supplies and equipment for immobilization of suspected bone injuries
- Supplies for wound care and treatment of shock
- Supplies for childbirth
- Supplies, equipment, and medications for the treatment of acute poisoning, snakebite, chemical burns, and diabetic emergencies
- ALS equipment, medications, and supplies
- Safety and miscellaneous equipment
- Information on the operation and inspection of the ambulance itself

Routine detailed shift checks of the ambulance can minimize the issues associated with risk management. Many services, for example, hold a "stretcher day" once a week. By performing and documenting preventive maintenance on stretchers, it is less likely that a faulty stretcher will cause a patient to be dropped or EMS personnel to injure their backs. Medications carried on the paramedic unit expire. Therefore, expiration dates should be checked each shift, and the older, unexpired drugs marked appropriately so that they will be used first. In services that use

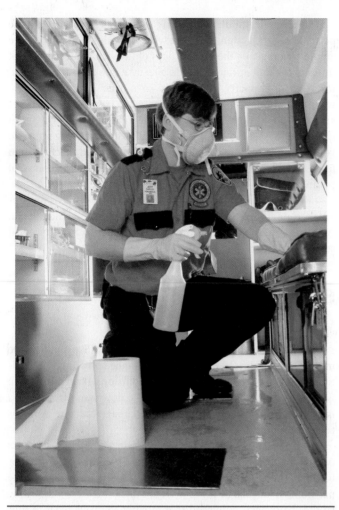

● **Figure 1-3**   Disinfecting the ambulance.

- Cardiac monitor
- Capnograph
- Oxygen systems
- Automated transport ventilator (ATV)
- Pulse oximeter
- Suction units
- Laryngoscope blades
- Lighted stylets
- Penlights
- Any other battery-operated equipment

CONTENT REVIEW

▶ Deployment Factors
- Location of facilities to house ambulances
- Location of hospitals
- Anticipated volume of calls
- Local geographic and traffic considerations

scheduled medications such as narcotics, the paramedics should sign for these medications at the beginning and at the end of each shift.

As mentioned, the vehicle itself should be regularly checked so that it is always in safe working order. If the ambulance or any equipment needs repair, it is your responsibility to report the failure to your supervisor in a manner prescribed by the standard operating procedures (SOPs) for your service.

To meet OSHA requirements, you must also make sure that the ambulance has been properly disinfected after the transport of any patients with potentially communicable diseases (Figure 1-3 ●). Most services routinely clean the ambulance after every call, and some agencies document the procedure. All services are required, either by OSHA or the state equivalent of OSHA, to have an exposure control plan that specifies cleaning requirements and the methods of cleaning up blood spills in the ambulance. If there is no specific SOP in your agency, you should document cleaning and disinfecting on the shift checklist.

Finally, you should do all scheduled tests, maintenance, and calibrations on specific medical equipment. Items that should be regularly checked include:

- Automated external defibrillator (AED)
- Glucometer

AMBULANCE DEPLOYMENT AND STAFFING

The strategy used by an EMS agency to maneuver its ambulances and crews in order to reduce response times is known as *deployment*. Deployment is based on a number of factors: location of the facilities to house ambulances, location of hospitals, anticipated volume of calls, and the specific geographic and traffic considerations of your area.

Most services must develop deployment strategies based on current station locations. Few agencies are in a position to move their stations to better locations. Such moves require years of budgeting, land acquisition, community education, building design, and financing of a capital construction project.

The ideal deployment decisions must take into account two sets of data: past community responses and projected **demographic** changes. The highest volume of calls, or **peak load**, should be described both in terms of the day of the week and the time of day.

In communities that do not have multiple strategically located stations, services often deploy ambulances to wait for calls at specific high-volume locations. Such stationing locations are known as **primary areas of responsibility (PARs)**. These ambulances may be relocated throughout the day as the population moves—to work or to school—and as other ambulances in the community respond to calls. The size of a PAR can vary from a few city blocks to a larger location, such as "northeast sector of town." The PAR size depends on the number of ambulances available and the expected call volume.

Some technologically sophisticated systems use computers to assist the dispatch center in relocating the ambulances. Vehicle tracking systems tell the computer exactly where each ambulance is located at a given time.

Traffic Congestion

In determining deployment strategies, traffic congestion must be taken into account, as well as special situations such as a ground-level railroad. Some communities, for example, must station an ambulance on the other side of the tracks before a freight train splits the town in half for perhaps 15 minutes or more. Other special deployment considerations include the ongoing daily activities within the community, especially commuter traffic and school bus schedules. Additional vehicles and crews may be required for these time periods. Other traffic (and potential patient) considerations include sporting events, VIP appearances, mass gatherings, and community days.

One deployment strategy that has become popular in recent years is known as system status management (SSM). SSM is a computerized personnel and ambulance deployment system designed to meet service demands with fewer resources and to ensure appropriate response times and vehicle locations.

The EMS response time can make the difference between life and death for the citizens of a community—especially in the setting of cardiac arrest. However, recent research has shown that only response times of less than 4 minutes are associated with improved outcomes.[2] Several studies have shown that an 8-minute response time, a de facto industry standard, is not uniformly associated with better patient outcomes overall.[3-5] In most areas, a routine response time of 4 minutes is either impossible or cost-prohibitive. Thus, appropriate response times must be determined by each community and its available resources.[6] A system's standards for reliability must take into account the time frames for such high-priority calls. The medical director should have direct input into setting these standards. An example of such a reliability standard might be response within 4 minutes to 90 percent of the priority-one calls (cardiac arrests, respiratory complaints, and motor vehicle collisions).

To meet reliability standards, many communities use a tiered response system in which public safety agencies trained as first responders carry an AED to a patient's side. The first tier of response, which helps ensure arrival within the 4-minute window, is then backed up by a second tier that brings an ALS unit to the patient within 8 minutes. Some communities add a third tier of response by separating their paramedics from their ambulances. No one system works best for all communities. The system that is ideal for your specific area will depend on such considerations as available personnel, available training, and many other factors.

Operational Staffing

For as long as paramedics have been trained, controversy has existed over the number of paramedics that should be assigned to a unit. This is a complex decision. Clearly, an ambulance with two paramedics onboard is limited in the amount of care these two highly trained personnel can provide if they are the only available responders to cardiac arrests (meaning no backup for simultaneous additional emergencies). As a result, some communities prefer to combine an Advanced EMT with a paramedic to make an ALS unit. Other communities, such as New York City, specify that an ALS unit must have two paramedics so that they can back up each other in making on-scene decisions. Because communities and available resources vary so widely, the controversy will in all likelihood be settled locally based on particular needs and available resources.

In general, ambulance staffing should take into account the peak load of the system. Some services vary shift times to ensure ample coverage for the busiest days of the week and the busiest times of the day. Services should also take into account the need for reserve capacity—the ability to muster additional crews when all ambulances are on call or when a system's resources are taxed by a multiple-casualty incident. Some services fulfill this need by asking off-duty personnel to carry pagers or to volunteer for backup. Whatever plan is adopted, each system must consider how they will deal with establishing a reserve of paramedics.

Finally, each service needs to determine standards for ambulance operators (drivers) and for driving the vehicle itself. As a rule, these standards are usually spelled out at the local service level.

SAFE AMBULANCE OPERATIONS

Patients, family members, motorists, and EMS providers are injured—sometimes fatally—in ambulance collisions. In addition to personal injuries, ambulance collisions exact a high toll: vehicle repair or replacement, lawsuits, downtime from work, increased insurance premiums, and damage to your agency's reputation in the community.

No national database has been set up to provide statistics on ambulance collisions in all 50 states. As a result, it is difficult to establish any form of "acceptable" ambulance collision rate per number of calls or miles driven. Furthermore, few scientific studies have been published that attempt to prove what, if any, strategies effectively reduce ambulance collisions. However, you can be certain of one thing: If your agency does experience a serious ambulance collision, questions will undoubtedly arise about the agency's training of drivers and its collision prevention program.[7, 8]

Educating Providers

The first part of any proactive collision prevention program is the recognition and definition of the problem. In the absence of a national database, this is easier said than done. However, some states do keep data, and their examples can provide a starting point. The following statistics come from an analysis of 22 years of reportable collisions—collisions involving more than $1,000 in vehicle damage or a personal injury—in New York State. The data are not intended to be scientific evidence that can be generalized to the other 49 states. The data also do not include many of the crashes that have resulted from backing up the ambulances, resulting in crashes that could be avoided by use of a spotter. Rather, the data, which come from a large number of cases, are used for purposes of illustration.

There has been a marked increase in the frequency of ground ambulance accidents over the past decade. The exact cause is unclear although several theories have been proposed. First, modern automobiles are better sealed and more soundproof than even cars of a decade ago. This can make it difficult for persons to hear an approaching ambulance. In addition, ambulances have increased in size and weight. The performance characteristic of modern ambulances is quite different from older models. Modern ambulances tend to be on a truck chassis and have characteristics more consistent with a large truck than a car. They accelerate poorly, are less responsive, and have a much greater braking distance. Also, the center of gravity is quite different from that of automobiles. Although the first rule in medical practice is "Do no harm," these collisions by emergency vehicles have harmed a considerable number of people.[9]

An analysis of the data collected by New York provides a profile of the typical ambulance collision. Inclement weather accounted for a relatively small number of the accidents. About 18 percent occurred on rainy days, 16 percent on cloudy days, and 6 percent on days with snow, sleet, hail, or freezing rain. The majority of collisions (55 percent) took place on clear days. Of all the collisions, some 67 percent took place during daylight hours.

Although head-on collisions can be very serious, they accounted for only 1 percent of the accidents. The largest number of collisions (41 percent) occurred when the ambulance struck another vehicle laterally or at a right angle or was struck itself. Approximately 21 percent of the collisions resulted from sideswiping or overtaking another vehicle. Another 12 percent occurred while making a right or left turn.

Probably the most important observation from the data is that nearly three-quarters (72 percent) of all collisions took place at intersections. Most safety-minded ambulance operators agree that the days of "blowing through" an intersection at high speeds with lights blaring and siren blasting have come and gone. Yet nearly half of all accidents took place at locations with a traffic control device. Another third took place at locations with no traffic device or sign at all.

Based on the statistics from New York, the profile of a typical ambulance collision might read as follows: *A lateral collision that takes place on a dry road during daylight hours on a clear day in an intersection with a traffic light.* Typically, when ambulance operators respond in poor weather conditions, they try to drive with a bubble of safety around the vehicle. Maybe the bubble should be there all the time, instead of reserving it for poor road conditions when ambulance collisions rarely occur!

Reducing Ambulance Collisions

What is your EMS agency doing to reduce ambulance collisions? Do you have an aggressive, proactive driver training program? Or does the agency follow a "we'll deal with it when it becomes a problem" kind of approach? All too often, the latter approach can result in news bulletins such as this one from the Associated Press: "Ambulance collides with car, killing three small children and seriously injuring their mother and sister; ambulance driver arrested on three counts of manslaughter."

As mentioned, such situations can be prevented by determining when and where they are most likely to occur. That is why the New York profile—or better yet, a profile from your own state—can be helpful in directing your own personal attitudes and training. Instead of confining your practice to skidding around wet or snowy parking lots, consciously practice safe driving under normal conditions.[10]

If you have the opportunity to develop programs to reduce ambulance collisions in your community, consider implementing the following actions or standards:

- Routine use of driver qualification checklists and driver's license checks, either through the local police or the Department of Motor Vehicles

- Demonstrated driver understanding of preventive mechanical maintenance, including a vehicle operator checklist and a procedure for reporting any problems found during the check or while driving the vehicle

- Provision of adequate hands-on driver training, using experienced and qualified field officers. (A 10,000- to 24,000-pound ambulance has a much longer stopping distance than the 2,500-pound pickup truck that an operator drove to work. One goal, for instance, would be to prevent an inexperienced driver from being stopped by a light pole—or another car—after sliding through an intersection [Figure 1-4 ●].)

- Implementation of a slow-speed course to ensure that operators know how to use mirrors, back up, park, and handle ambulance-sized vehicles, including accurate estimation of braking distance and turn radius

- Training that ensures operators know how to react to emergency situations such as the loss of brakes, loss of power steering, a stuck accelerator, a blown-out tire, or a vehicle breakdown

- Demonstrated driver knowledge of both the primary and backup routes to all hospitals in your service response area

- Demonstrated driver understanding of the rules, regulations, and laws that your Department of Motor Vehicles has established for drivers in general and for ambulance operators in particular

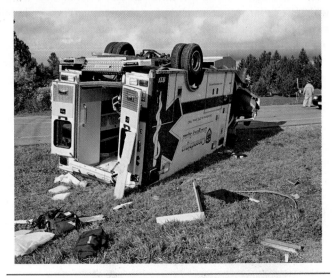

● **Figure 1-4** Ambulance collision. (© *Canandaigua Emergency Squad*)

Standard Operating Procedures

Each EMS agency should have standard operating procedures pertaining to the operation of its vehicles. At a minimum, SOPs should spell out the following:

- Procedure for qualifying as an ambulance operator
- Procedure for handling and reporting an ambulance collision
- Process for investigating and reviewing each collision
- Process for implementing quality assurance in the aftermath of a collision
- Method for using a spotter when backing up a vehicle (Figure 1-5 ●)
- Use of seat belts in the ambulance, and the procedure for transporting a child passenger under 40 pounds
- Guidelines on what constitutes an emergency response and the exemptions that may be taken under state laws
- Guidelines on prudent speed; proper travel in, and the circumstances for using, oncoming lanes; and safe negotiation of intersections
- Circumstances and procedures for use of escorts
- A zero-tolerance policy for driving the vehicle under the influence of alcohol or any drugs

The Due Regard Standard

The motor vehicle laws enacted by most states are based on a model law. As might be expected, state laws pertaining to ambulance operation tend to be similar. One similarity centers on the legal concept of **due regard**. Essentially, due regard exempts ambulance drivers from certain laws but at the same time holds them to a higher standard.

State laws typically exempt ambulance drivers who are operating in an emergency from posted speed limits, posted directions of travel, parking regulations, and requirements to wait at red lights. There are, however, certain situations from which ambulances are rarely or never exempt. They include passing over a railroad crossing with the gates down and passing a school bus with flashing red lights. In the latter case, you

should wait until the bus driver secures the safety of the children and turns off the red lights. Only then should you proceed past the bus.

Although the laws are often liberal in their exemptions, they place the responsibility for deciding when and where these exemptions should be applied squarely on the shoulders of drivers. The laws often say, for example, "the foregoing provisions and exemptions do not relieve the operator of an emergency vehicle from acting with due regard for the safety of all persons." Such language sets a higher standard for ambulance operators than for almost any other driver on the road. Nowhere in the motor vehicle laws are other drivers held accountable for the safety of all other motorists!

To see how this higher standard might affect you, consider a situation that could occur in any community. It's 7:00 P.M. in a suburban neighborhood. After a dry, clear, warm day, the sun has started to set. A five-year-old child takes one last ride on a Big Wheel, a low-profile, plastic tricycle. The child pedals down a slightly inclined driveway past a pine tree obstructing the view of oncoming motorists and rolls into the street. A midsized car with four adults on their way to dinner and a movie is headed toward the driveway. The driver is sober, traveling at the speed limit, and having a normal conversation. Suddenly the child darts into view from behind the pine tree. The driver immediately steps on the brakes, but it is too late. The car strikes the child, who later dies from multiple trauma in the emergency department.

When the police arrive, they take statements from all involved, ensure the driver is sober, make sure the vehicle's inspection sticker is up to date, and measure skid marks. In all likelihood, they issue no tickets. The family of the child may decide to sue the driver for the loss of their child, but the police usually take no action unless a specific motor vehicle law has been violated.

Now imagine the same situation, except it is your ambulance headed toward the child. An emergency call has brought you into the neighborhood. You have lights on, siren off, and are not exceeding the posted speed limit. As you and your partner search for house numbers, a child suddenly darts into view. You strike the brakes immediately, but unfortunately the child instantly dies from multiple trauma.

When the police arrive, they take statements from all involved, ensure you are sober, check the vehicle's inspection documentation, and measure the skid marks. They then turn the case over to the county grand jury for further investigation. You will appear before the jury, which will scrutinize your personal and professional driving record, service SOPs, rules of the road, and perhaps even your personal habits. In the meantime, the local newspaper has run a front-page story, complete with your name and that of your service. The headline implies that you killed the child as you raced through town in your ambulance.

By now, some of your neighbors have begun to throw dirty looks at you while you empty your mailbox. The reputation of your service has been indelibly tarnished in the public's mind. Members of other crews say their patients have questioned the safety of riding in your service's ambulances. But you can't really respond. Your service has suspended you from driving pending the results of the hearing.

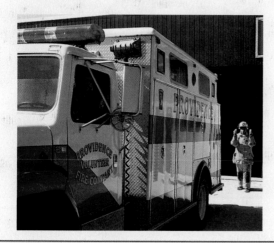

● **Figure 1-5** Use of a spotter.

After more than a week of deliberations, the grand jury clears you of all responsibility. It has found that you were sober, attentive, and doing your job. There was nothing you could have done, says the jury, to have prevented the child's death. If the newspaper even carries the final chapter of the story, it appears inside the paper in a small follow-up piece.

The moral is this: As an ambulance driver, you will always be held to a higher standard than other drivers. You must be attentive and prepared to shoulder the responsibilities that come with the profession that you have chosen.

Lights and Siren: A False Sense of Security

As a general rule, do not rely solely on lights and siren to alert other motorists of your approach. Studies have shown that most motorists do not see or hear your ambulance until it is within 50 to 100 feet of their vehicles. Even so, the siren is the most commonly used—and abused—audible warning device. Before you decide to turn on the siren, consider the following points:

- Motorists are less inclined to yield to an ambulance when the siren is sounded continuously.
- Many motorists feel that the right-of-way privileges given to ambulances are abused when sirens are sounded.
- Inexperienced motorists tend to increase their driving speeds by 10 to 15 miles per hour when a siren is sounded.
- The continuous sound of a siren can possibly worsen the condition of sick or injured patients by increasing their anxiety.
- Ambulance operators may also develop anxiety, not to mention the possibility of hearing problems, from sirens used on long runs.

Some states and services have specific laws and/or SOPs that address the use of sirens. Consider these useful guidelines:

- Use the siren sparingly and only when you must.
- Never assume that all motorists will hear your siren.
- Assume that some motorists will hear your siren but choose to ignore it.
- Be prepared for panic and erratic maneuvers when drivers do hear your siren.
- Never use the siren to scare someone.

Whenever the ambulance is on the road, day or night, turn on the headlights to increase its visibility. Alternating headlamps should be used at night only if they are installed in a secondary lamp. Probably the most useful light is the one in the center of the cowling on the front hood. This light can usually be easily seen in the rearview mirror of the car in front of you.

Each corner of the ambulance should have large flashers that blink in tandem or unison to help oncoming vehicles identify the location and size of the ambulance. Although the controversy over the use of strobes continues, consider the latest research on the subject when designing or choosing the lighting on your ambulance. At present, recommendations lean toward the use of single-beam bulbs and strobes instead of relying on one type of lighting system. The most important point is visibility. The vehicle must be clearly visible from 360 degrees to all other motorists and pedestrians.

Interestingly, several studies have shown that the use of lights and sirens reduced response times only a modest amount—an amount that may not be clinically significant. Because of the risk associated with lights and siren usage, EMS must ensure that the potential benefits afforded the patient by a lights and siren response are not offset by the risks imposed on the crew and the public.[11-13]

Escorts and Multiple-Vehicle Responses

Most EMS agencies no longer suggest the use of a police escort for ambulances, except in circumstances in which the ambulance is providing service to an unfamiliar district and needs to be taken to the patient and/or the hospital. There are several reasons for this. First, ambulances and police cars have different braking distances. If an ambulance follows a police car too closely, it can easily rear-end the car if they both stop quickly. Second, the two vehicles have different acceleration speeds. As a result, an ambulance operator may have trouble keeping up with a police car. A gap often develops, allowing other vehicles to pull in between. Finally, other motorists are not likely to realize that the two emergency vehicles are traveling together. After the police car speeds by, a vehicle may pull in front of an ambulance, assuming the coast is clear.

In multiple-vehicle responses, the dangers are the same as for an escort. In addition, another danger occurs when two emergency vehicles approach an intersection at the same time. Besides totally confusing motorists and pedestrians, the potential for an intersection collision increases dramatically. Motorists often fail to yield the right of way to the first emergency vehicle, the second emergency vehicle, or, in some instances, both vehicles.

It is a good idea to pay attention to other calls taken in your district. However, do not assume that you know all the responses that are taking place. To avoid warning the perpetrators of crimes, for example, the police often respond to incidents without announcing their approach. As a general rule, always negotiate an intersection assuming that you may meet another emergency vehicle.

Parking and Loading the Ambulance

Whenever you arrive first at the site of a motor vehicle collision, take steps to size up the scene for potential hazards to you, your crew, and the patients. Consider establishing a danger zone, parking at least 100 feet from the wreckage upwind and uphill (if possible) to avoid fire or any escaping hazardous liquids or fumes. If there are no fire or escaping liquids or fumes, park at least 50 feet from the wreckage. If possible, assign a member of the crew to handle traffic until the police arrive to take control of the task.

If your ambulance is the first emergency vehicle on the scene, make sure you park in front of the wreckage so your warning lights can alert approaching motorists. Then set up flares, or nonincendiary warning devices, as quickly as possible.

If the scene has already been secured, park beyond the wreckage to prevent your ambulance from being exposed to traffic (Figure 1-6 ●). If command has already been established by an on-scene EMS unit, you may receive prearrival instructions. In the case of multiple-casualty incidents, for example, the commander may tell you where to park and who you should report to.

Always be aware of potential traffic hazards at the scene of a call. Many EMS providers have been seriously injured—and some even killed—after being struck by passing motorists. As much as possible, try not to expose either your crew or your patient to traffic. Keep in mind that the rear ambulance doors often obstruct the warning lights when they are opened to load the patient. Also remember that studies have shown that red revolving lights attract drunk or tired drivers. Consider pulling off the road, turning off your headlights, and using just the amber rear sealed blinkers that flash in tandem or in unison. These lights, as noted, will help oncoming motorists to identify both the size and the location of your vehicle.

The Deadly Intersection

Recall that New York statistics reveal that 72 percent of all ambulance collisions occur in intersections. Clearly the intersection is a very unsafe, if not deadly, place to be. Exercise extreme caution whenever you approach one of these hazards. Keep in mind the braking distance of your ambulance, the effectiveness of lights and siren, the rules of the road, the SOPs of your service, the acceleration needed to get through the intersection safely, and more. Helpful tips for negotiating an intersection include the following:

● Stop at all red lights and stop signs and then proceed with caution.

● Always proceed through an intersection slowly.

● Make eye contact with other motorists to ensure they understand your intentions.

● If you are using any of the exemptions offered to you as an emergency vehicle, such as passing through a red light or a stop sign, make sure you warn motorists by appropriately flashing your lights and sounding the siren.

● Remember that lights and siren only "ask" the public to yield the right of way. If the public does not yield, it may be because they misunderstand your intentions, cannot hear the siren because of noise in their own vehicles, or cannot see your lights. Never assume that other motorists have a clue to what you plan on doing at the intersection.

● Always go around cars stopped at the intersection on their left (driver's) side. In some instances, this may involve passing into the oncoming lane, which should be done slowly and very cautiously. You invite trouble when you use a clear right lane to sneak past a group of cars at an intersection. If motorists are doing what they should do under motor vehicle laws, they may pull into the right lane just as you attempt to pass.

● Know how long it takes for your ambulance to cross an intersection. This will help you judge whether you have enough time to pass through safely.

● Watch pedestrians at an intersection carefully. If they all seem to be staring in another direction, rather than at your ambulance, they may well be looking at the fire truck headed your way.

● Remember that there is no such thing as a rolling stop in an ambulance weighing more than 10,000 pounds or a medium-duty vehicle weighing some 24,000 pounds. Even at speeds as slow as 30 miles per hour, these vehicles will not stop on a dime. When negotiating an intersection, consider "covering the brake" to shorten the stopping distance.

PATHO PEARLS

Rooting EMS Practice in Sound Science

During the development of emergency medical services, most of its practices were based on common sense, current medical practices, or rational conjecture. In the late 1990s, the National Highway Traffic Safety Administration (NHTSA), in conjunction with the Health Resources and Services Administration, developed The EMS Agenda for the Future, *published by the NHTSA in 1996.* The EMS Agenda for the Future *provided an opportunity to examine what had been learned during the past three decades and created a vision for the future. This opportunity has come at an important time—when the agencies, organizations, and individuals that affect EMS are evaluating their role in the context of a rapidly evolving health care system. See Volume 1, Chapter 2 for a more extensive discussion of* The EMS Agenda for the Future.

Furthermore, the government and third-party payers (Medicare, Medicaid, private insurance companies) are going to pay only for prehospital care interventions that can be proven to improve patient care and patient outcome. Because of this, all current EMS practices must come under scrutiny. For example, medical helicopters may not provide the patient benefit once thought. The quality of prehospital care has improved to a degree that there is often little difference between the quality of care a helicopter crew can provide when compared to a ground EMS crew. Likewise, we are learning that speed makes a difference for very few patients. Because of this and other issues, it is important that we specifically define the role and utilization criteria for expensive resources such as medical helicopters and similar interventions. This is all a part of the natural evolution of modern EMS.

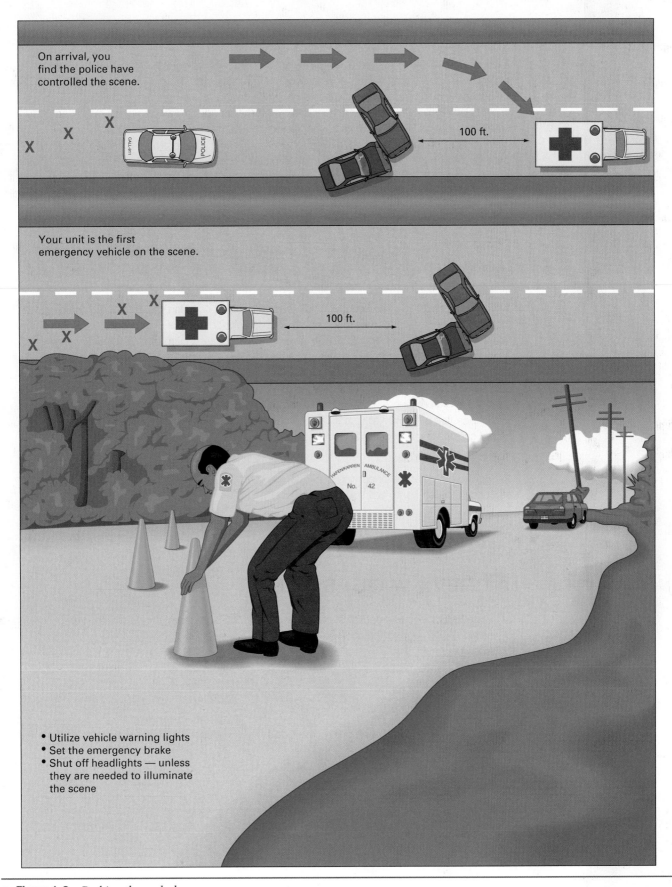

On arrival, you find the police have controlled the scene.

100 ft.

Your unit is the first emergency vehicle on the scene.

100 ft.

HAFENKARREN AMBULANCE No. 42

- Utilize vehicle warning lights
- Set the emergency brake
- Shut off headlights — unless they are needed to illuminate the scene

● **Figure 1-6** Parking the ambulance.

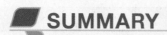

SUMMARY

Even though you have learned about ambulance operations in your EMT training and in your everyday experience, good safety habits grow stronger with review and practice. As a paramedic, you should be familiar with standards that influence ambulance design, equipment requirements, and staffing. You should also regularly complete all checklists, whether they apply to the vehicle, onboard equipment, or essential supplies. Be aware of items that require routine maintenance or calibration, as well as the expiration dates on all drugs. Keep in mind OSHA requirements that promote the safety of personnel and patients and know how to report equipment problems or failures to your supervisor.

As you know, ambulance operators have a special responsibility whenever they take the wheel. It is your professional duty to recognize the profile of a typical ambulance collision and to develop strategies for preventing it from occurring. You should also be aware of the issues surrounding the staging and staffing of ambulances and determine your agency's policies on these matters.

YOU MAKE THE CALL

You and your partner are working on Medic Ambulance 622 covering the west portion of town. It's your turn to drive when a call comes in for an automobile collision. Responding priority one, lights and siren, you travel eastbound on Central Avenue, approaching the intersection of Wolf Road. You know that this is probably one of the busiest intersections in town. It has two through lanes and two turn lanes in each direction. As a result, there are almost always two moving lanes of traffic.

About 250 feet from the intersection, you notice that the light has turned red. Cars have stopped in both of the left turn lanes. There are a few cars in the center lane, and no cars at all in the right lane. As usual, there are a number of cars traveling northbound through the intersection. There are also southbound cars waiting to turn left and proceed eastbound.

1. Should you drive down the open eastbound right lane with your lights and siren on? Explain.

2. Should you enter the oncoming traffic by going around the left side of the vehicle that is currently stopped in the left-hand, eastbound lane? Explain.

3. How can you best deal with this very dangerous intersection?

See Suggested Responses at the back of this book.

REVIEW QUESTIONS

1. State EMS agencies establish state standards called _____ standards for ambulance operation.
   a. gold
   b. optimal
   c. minimum
   d. maximum

2. Which of the following describes a Type II ambulance design?
   a. medium-duty ambulance rescue vehicle
   b. standard van, forward control integral cab-body ambulance
   c. specialty van, forward control integral cab-body ambulance
   d. conventional truck cab-chassis with a modular ambulance body

3. The agency charged with protecting worker safety is _____.
   a. ASTNA
   b. FCC
   c. OSHA
   d. CAAS

4. At the national level, _____ provides a voluntary "gold standard" for the EMS community to follow.
   a. ACS
   b. NHTSA
   c. OSHA
   d. CAAS

5. The strategy used by an EMS agency to maneuver its ambulances and crews in order to reduce response times is known as _____.

a. assignment
b. calibration
c. deployment
d. maintenance

6. _____ is a computerized personnel and ambulance deployment system designed to meet service demands with fewer resources and to ensure appropriate response time and vehicle location.

a. SSM   c. SAR
b. PAR   d. AED

See Answers to Review Questions at the back of this book.

REFERENCES

1. United States General Services Administration. *Federal Specification for the Star-of-Life Ambulance (KKK-A-1822F)*. Washington, DC. Government Printing Office, 2007.

2. De Maio, V. J., I. G. Stiell, G. A. Wells, D. W. Spaite, Ontario Prehospital Advanced Life Support Study Group. "Optimal Defibrillation Response Intervals for Maximum Out-of-Hospital Cardiac Arrest Survival Rates." *Ann Emerg Med* 42 (2003): 242–250.

3. Pons, P. T., J. S. Haukoos, W. Bludworth, T. Cribley, K. A. Pons, and V. J. Markovchick. Paramedic Response Time: Does It Affect Patient Survival? *Acad Emerg Med* 12 (2005): 594–600.

4. Blackwell, T. H., J. Kline, J. Willis, et al. Lack of Association between Prehospital Response Times and Patient Outcomes. *Prehosp Emerg Care* 11(1) (2007): 115.

5. Vukmir, R. and L. Katz, Sodium Bicarbonate Study Group. The Influence of Urban, Suburban, or Rural Locale on Survival from Refractory Cardiac Arrest. *Am J Emerg Med* 22 (2004): 90–93.

6. Valenzuela, T. D., D. J. Roe, G. Nichol, L. L. Clark, D. W. Spaite, and R. G. Hardman. Outcomes of Rapid Defibrillation by Security Officers after Cardiac Arrest in Casinos. *N Engl J Med* 343 (2000): 1206–1209.

7. Berger, E. Nothing Gold Can Stay? EMS Crashes, Lack of Evidence Bring the Golden Hour Concept under New Scrutiny. *Ann Emerg Med* 56 (2010): A17–A19.

8. Studnek, J. R. and A. R. Fernandez. Characteristics of Emergency Medical Technicians Involved in Ambulance Crashes. *Prehosp Disaster Med* 23 (2008): 432–437.

9. Custalow, C. B. and C. S. Gravitz. Emergency Medical Vehicle Collisions and Potential for Preventive Intervention. *Prehosp Emerg Care* 8 (2004): 175–184.

10. De Grave, K., K. F. Deroo, P. A. Calle, et al. How to Modify the Risk-Taking Behaviour of Emergency Medical Services Drivers. *Eur J Emerg Med* 10 (2003): 111–116.

11. Marques-Baptista, A., P. Ohman-Strickland, K. T. Baldino, M. Prasto, and M. A. Merlin. Utilization of Warning Lights and Siren Based on Hospital Time-Critical Interventions. *Prehosp Disaster Med* 25 (2010): 335–339.

12. Brown, L. H., C. L. Whitney, R. C. Hunt, M. Addario, and T. Hogue. Do Warning Lights and Sirens Reduce Ambulance Response Times? *Prehosp Emerg Care* 4 (2000): 70–74.

13. Hunt, R. C., L. H. Brown, E. S. Cabinum, et al. Is Ambulance Transport Time with Lights and Siren Faster Than That Without? *Ann Emerg Med* 25 (1995): 507–511.

FURTHER READING

Limmer, D., and M. F. O'Keefe. *Emergency Care*. 12th ed. Upper Saddle River, NJ: Pearson/Prentice Hall, 2011.

Lindsey, J. T., and R. W. Patrick. *Emergency Vehicle Operations*. Upper Saddle River, NJ: Pearson/Prentice Hall, 2007.

Mistovich, J. J., and K. J. Karren. *Prehospital Emergency Care*. 9th ed. Upper Saddle River, NJ: Pearson/Prentice Hall, 2010.

2

Air Medical Operations

Bryan Bledsoe, DO, FACEP, FAAEM, EMT-P
Mike Abernethy, MD, FAAEM
Ryan J. Wubben, MD, FAAEM

STANDARD
EMS Operations (Air Medical)

COMPETENCY
Applies knowledge of operational roles and responsibilities to ensure patient, public, and personnel safety.

OBJECTIVES

Terminal Performance Objective
After reading this chapter, you should be able to place patient care tasks in the context of air ambulance operations to safely interact with or operate within air medical services to respond to calls and transport patients.

Enabling Objectives
To accomplish the terminal performance objective, you should be able to:

1. Define key terms introduced in this chapter.

2. Describe the roles and uses that helicopters and fixed-wing aircraft can play in the care and transport of ill or injured patients.

3. Describe the evolution of air medical transport over time, including key events that led to the development of air medical transport as it exists today.

4. Describe the characteristics and capabilities of fixed-wing and rotor-wing aircraft.

5. Discuss limitations, concerns, and controversies about the use of air medical transport.

6. Discuss the staffing and crew configurations of air medical transport craft.

7. Given a scenario involving air medical response, take the actions needed to ensure effective and safe ground operations.

8. Given a scenario involving air medical response, obtain and communicate information needed for safe and effective interaction between the air medical crew and ground personnel.

KEY TERMS
ADAMS, p. 26

fixed-wing aircraft, p. 17

instrument flight rules (IFR), p. 20

night-vision goggles (NVG), p. 16

rotor-wing aircraft, p. 17

visual flight rules (VFR), p. 19

On a rural Nevada highway, approximately 75 miles north of Las Vegas, a small sports car pulls around a slow-moving recreational vehicle (RV) to pass. However, as the driver is alongside the RV, he sees a motorcycle approaching quickly in the oncoming lane. He hits the brakes and tries to return to his prior position behind the RV. However, he is unable to get back before striking the motorcycle. The motorcyclist, seeing the impending accident, tries to avoid a head-on collision by laying the bike on its side. Thus, at approximately 60 miles per hour, the bike and the motorcyclist are tumbling down the highway. The bike hits the sports car and the motorcyclist tumbles into the desert.

The driver of the sports car screeches to a halt. The elderly couple in the RV see the accident in their rearview mirrors and return to the scene. The motorcyclist is about 30 meters off the road. He is unresponsive with gurgling respirations. Despite the fact he is wearing a helmet and leathers, he has sustained multiple significant injuries. The couple from the RV and the driver involved in the accident run to the victim. Unsure of what to do, they retrieve a small first aid kit from the RV. The driver of the sports car tries to use his cell phone but cannot get a signal. The couple in the RV try as well—to no avail. About this time, another motorcyclist arrives. He is a friend of the victim. He cannot get a cell phone signal either. He decides to drive down the road to a roadside emergency phone and summon the police and EMS.

After about 20 minutes, a volunteer fire department staffed with first responders arrives. After a quick look, they summon a medical helicopter. The closest hospital is about an hour away by ground. They provide initial stabilizing care and, along with the highway patrol, establish a safe landing zone for the incoming helicopter.

The helicopter lands and the medical crew assesses the patient. The crew members perform a rapid secondary assessment and rapidly prepare the patient for transport. The patient is moved to the helicopter and transported to a trauma center in Las Vegas. On arrival at the trauma center, the patient is treated promptly. He is found to have a subdural hematoma, multiple facial fractures, a fractured spleen, and multiple lower-extremity fractures. He is taken immediately to surgery for an exploratory laparotomy and splenectomy. He requires 8 units of blood. He remains intubated and on mechanical ventilation in the trauma ICU for four days. He is eventually extubated and transferred to a standard floor bed. He undergoes numerous operations to repair his facial fractures and orthopedic injuries. Finally, after six weeks in the hospital, he is discharged to return to his home in Montana. His prognosis is very good.

INTRODUCTION

The use of aircraft for emergency patient transport has become a critical component of modern EMS practice. Both helicopters and airplanes (fixed wing) have proved to be vital assets in the emergent transport of the ill or injured patient. These include:

- *Scene responses.* The first major use of aircraft, specifically helicopters, was for flying directly to an incident scene and then transporting the patient to a definitive care facility (Figure 2-1 ●). Scene responses may be primary (air medical crew is first on the scene) or secondary (summoned by ground personnel).[1, 2]

- *Interfacility transport.* One of the most rapidly expanding areas of air medical transport is the emergent transfer of patients between health care facilities (Figure 2-2 ●). In the rural setting, patients often require a level of specialty care that is unavailable locally. When dealing with critically ill patients, significant prehospital time can be minimized through air transport. The type of aircraft used is based on the distance to be traveled and the patient's condition. Generally speaking, helicopters are limited to distances less than 150 to 200 miles.[3–5]

- *Specialty care.* Air medical transport can bring specialty teams to community hospitals for care of selected patients (Figure 2-3 ●). The most common example is that of neonatal transport. Neonates, especially preterm infants, can require sophisticated specialized care. In some systems, a neonatal team is transported to the community hospital where initial stabilization is completed. Following that,

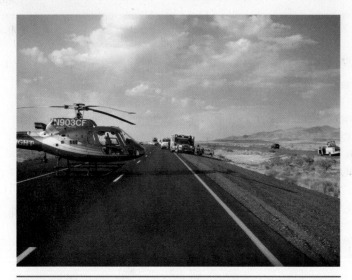

● **Figure 2-1** A helicopter can fly directly to an incident scene and transport a patient to a definitive care facility. (© *Pat Songer*)

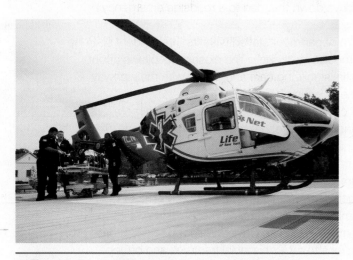

● **Figure 2-2** A rapidly expanding area of air medical transport is the emergent transfer of patients between facilities. (© *Mark Foster*)

transport may or may not be by aircraft. In some systems, the neonatal team is transported to the community hospital by helicopter but return to the tertiary care facility is often by ground ambulance.[6,7]

● *Organ procurement.* The transplantation of human organs has evolved significantly over the past two decades. The procurement of human organs is a time-sensitive endeavor. Because of this, organ procurement teams often use aircraft to respond to the site of the donor and subsequently transport the organs back to the transplant center.

● *Search and rescue.* The use of aircraft for search and rescue has been a part of aviation virtually since its inception. Medical aircraft, including both fixed-wing aircraft and helicopters, are sometimes used in search-and-rescue operations. Although this can be system dependent, it is not an uncommon practice. Medical helicopter pilots and crews are often intimately familiar with local geography and can provide much-needed assistance in search-and-rescue operations. The addition of technology such as high-intensity spotlights, forward-looking infrared (FLIR), and **night vision goggles (NVG)** makes helicopters a valuable asset in these situations (Figure 2-4 ●).

● *Disaster assistance.* Disaster situations often impact or destroy the infrastructure of the community and region affected. In many instances, ingress and egress are restricted because of the destruction of roads. This is commonly seen following both earthquakes and hurricanes. However, it is also seen in tornadoes and similar events. Aircraft, particularly helicopters, can provide access to disaster regions not accessible by ground ambulances. The role of helicopters proved crucial and lifesaving, for example, following Hurricane Katrina, which struck New Orleans and southern Louisiana as well as adjoining states in the 2005 Atlantic hurricane season.[8]

Air medical transport is an important asset to any EMS system. It should be considered a medical procedure with benefits and risks. These risks and benefits must be weighed. However, like any other asset or tool, air medical transport must be used responsibly. EMS providers should be familiar with local medical capabilities and those protocols for usage.

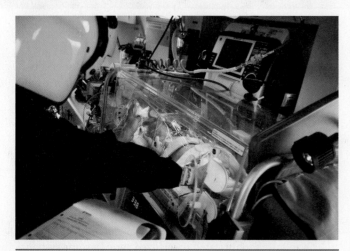

● **Figure 2-3** Helicopters can bring neonatal specialty teams to community hospitals. (© *Austin/Travis County STAR Flight*)

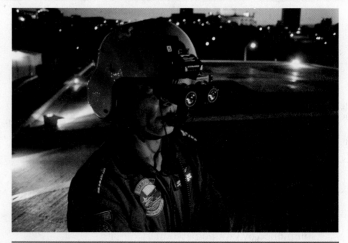

● **Figure 2-4** Night vision goggles are useful in helicopter search-and-rescue operations. (© *Austin/Travis County STAR Flight*)

HISTORY

Like most aspects of emergency medicine, air medical transport's origins and development are deeply rooted within the military. The first recorded use of an airplane to evacuate wounded casualties was during World War I by a French aircraft in Serbia. Later in that same war, the British used aircraft to evacuate casualties in the Turkish theater. Subsequently, a fully organized air ambulance operation was used by both the French and British during the African and Middle Eastern colonial wars of the 1920s. During Germany's involvement in the Spanish Civil War, casualties from its "Condor Legion" expeditionary force were evacuated by Junkers Ju-52 trimotors back to Germany for care.

The first successful operational helicopter was the Sikorsky YR-4, built in the United States in 1942. These were then deployed in an experiment to Burma by the U.S. Army in 1944–1945. Initially they were intended to be used in a search-and-rescue function for downed aircrew, but on January 26, 1945, the first documented medical evacuation by helicopter took place in the jungles of Burma that otherwise would have taken 10 days on foot to accomplish.

By the time the United States entered the Korean War in 1950, helicopter usage had become more common both as an aerial observation platform and for the medical evacuation of infantry casualties. In Korea, patients were evacuated from the battlefield to Mobile Army Surgical Hospital (MASH) units and battalion aid stations for emergency medical and surgical care. As the patients were transported on the skids of the aircraft, medical care during transport was nonexistent. Critically ill or injured casualties were later transported to well-equipped hospital ships for definitive care and repatriation.

By 1960, the mass production of more powerful gas turbine engines allowed the design of larger, more powerful helicopters. For the first time, battlefield casualties could ride inside the helicopter and receive in-flight care from medical personnel.

The helicopter in the military serves several nonmedical roles. Medical evacuation of battlefield casualties by helicopter, often referred to as "dust off," was heavily used during the Vietnam War and was responsible for a significant improvement in the outcome of wounded soldiers (Figure 2-5 ●). In modern warfare, medical evacuation by both helicopter and fixed-wing aircraft plays an important role in the safety of military personnel.[9]

The civilian use of aircraft for medical evacuation and care was initiated in rural areas, such as those in Australia and Canada. Most notably, Australia developed the Royal Flying Doctor Service (RFDS) that provided medical care to the inhabitants of rural Australia. The RFDS continues to operate today. The first dedicated air ambulance service in the United States was begun by Schaeffer Ambulance Service in Los Angeles. The service opened in 1947 and was the first to use Federal Aviation Administration (FAA)-certified aircraft in an ambulance role. By the late 1960s, the helicopter had proven itself as an effective means of transport for critically injured military casualties. However, this lifesaving technology saw little, if any, use in the civilian sector.

In 1970, Congress passed legislation creating the Military Assistance to Safety and Traffic (MAST) program. This authorized the U.S. military to use the battle-proven system of

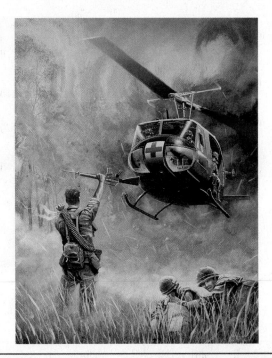

● **Figure 2-5**   The medevac (also called the "dust off") helicopter played a major role in decreasing mortality in Vietnam by rapidly moving injured soldiers from the battlefield to definitive care. *(Dustoff © 2000, Joe Kline Aviation Art)*

simultaneous helicopter evacuation and medical care to augment existing U.S. civilian EMS. MAST programs were established at 12 active army bases, as well as several National Guard and Army Reserve installations.

In 1970, the Maryland State Police established the first nonmilitary helicopter medical evacuation program. Two years later, St. Anthony's Hospital in Denver founded the first civilian helicopter EMS (HEMS) program, called Flight for Life (Figure 2-6 ●).

Over the next 30 years, there was a gradual, expected growth in the HEMS industry. The majority of the new programs were hospital based, mainly because of the cost of such an endeavor. In 2001, Medicare increased the reimbursement for HEMS transport, allowing a huge growth in the community (nonhospital)-based sector of the industry. As of 2010, there were approximately 730 HEMS bases with 900 aircraft in the United States.

AIRCRAFT

The types of aircraft used in air medical transport have changed considerably over the past several decades. Much of this was in response to developments and improvements in aviation technology. The two types of aircraft used in air medical transport are **fixed-wing aircraft** (airplanes) and **rotor-wing aircraft** (helicopters). Fixed-wing aircraft provide comfort, speed, and significant range, especially when compared with ground ambulances. Rotor-wing aircraft can access hard-to-reach situations and provide transport that is often quicker than that available in ground ambulances. The choice of aircraft type is usually based on the distance of transport, medical needs, patient condition, and availability.

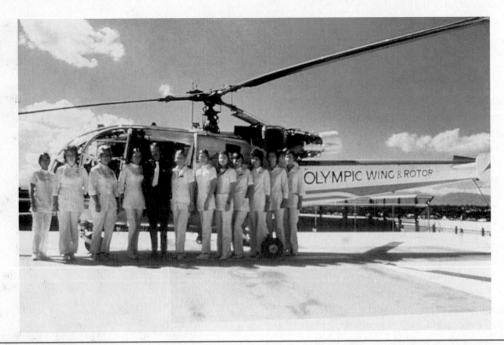

● **Figure 2-6** The first U.S. civilian helicopter devoted exclusively to patient care was St. Anthony's Flight for Life in Denver. *(© Flight For Life Colorado)*

Fixed-Wing Aircraft

Fixed-wing aircraft, commonly referred to as airplanes, are vehicles capable of flight that use fixed wings to generate lift (Figure 2-7 ●). Generally speaking, the speed of an airplane is greater than that of most helicopters. Either a turbine engine or a piston engine typically powers fixed-wing aircraft. Some turbine-powered airplanes have a propeller (turboprop) to provide propulsion, whereas others are jet powered. In the turboprop system, most of the energy derived from the turbine goes to power the propeller. In the jet propulsion system, the turbine powers a rotary air compressor that compresses incoming air and exhaust gases and ejects these via a duct. The ejected gases generated by the turbine are the propulsion used to move the aircraft.

Most air ambulances are turbine powered and usually have at least two engines. Many fixed-wing aircraft contain pressurized cabins that allow safe and comfortable travel at altitudes that are inaccessible by aircraft without a pressurized cabin. Generally speaking, fixed-wing aircraft are somewhat larger than helicopters, with many being capable of transporting several patients at the same time. Jet airplanes have a much greater range and speed than helicopters.

The limitation of airplanes as air ambulances is that they must land and take off from established airports. Such airports are not always in close proximity to the patient or hospital. Thus, the patient must also be transported by ground ambulance to the airport to meet the aircraft, which incurs delays to definitive care.

Rotor-Wing Aircraft

Helicopters, which by definition are rotary-wing aircraft, are commonly used in modern EMS (Figure 2-8 ●). Helicopters use rotating blades, referred to as a *rotor*, to provide lift and

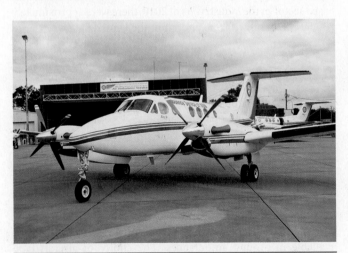

● **Figure 2-7** Fixed-wing fleet operated as part of the New South Wales, Australia, ambulance service. *(© Dr. Bryan E. Bledsoe)*

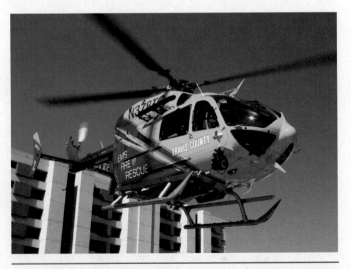

● **Figure 2-8** Helicopters (rotary-wing aircraft) are commonly used in modern EMS. *(© Austin/Travis County STAR Flight)*

propulsion. The main rotor system is supplemented by a tail rotor to counteract the natural torque produced by the rotor; without the tail rotor, the cabin and fuselage would spin in the opposite direction from the main rotors. Essentially, all helicopters used in an EMS role in the United States are powered by a turbine (jet) engine. As of 2009, 46 percent of the EMS helicopter fleet had single engines, whereas 54 percent used twin-engine aircraft.[10] Most EMS helicopters are considered small to medium in size (Figures 2-9 ● through 2-13 ●). Others use a larger airframe (Figure 2-14 ●). In the United States, most EMS helicopters have a single pilot. Some medical helicopters in the United States are capable of instrument flight rule usage.

One of the most significant limitations that all helicopters face is the weather. There are very specific rules that all pilots must follow in regard to the weather when making decisions to fly or to continue flying once they are in the air. The basic dichotomy is between flying under **visual flight rules (VFR)** or

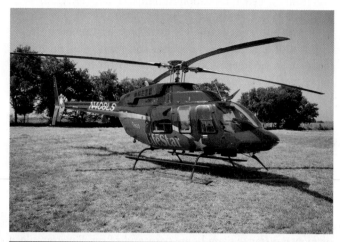

● **Figure 2-12** Bell 407 helicopter.

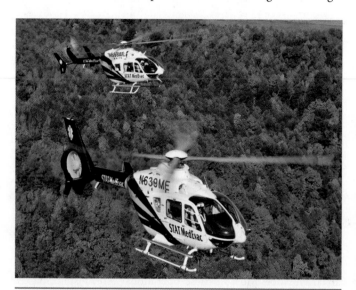

● **Figure 2-9** Eurocopter EC135 helicopter. (© *STAT MedEvac/ Mike Reyno*)

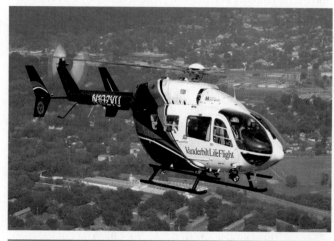

● **Figure 2-13** Eurocopter EC145 helicopter. (© *Vanderbilt LifeFlight*)

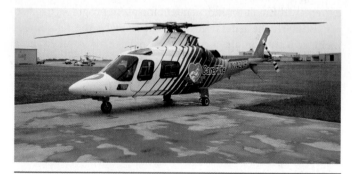

● **Figure 2-10** Agusta 109 Power helicopter.

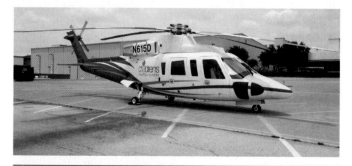

● **Figure 2-11** Sikorsky S76 helicopter. (*Courtesy of Children's Medical Center, Dallas*)

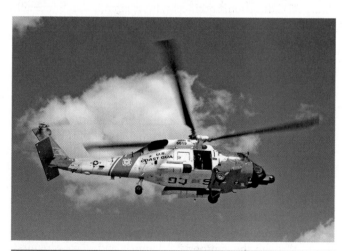

● **Figure 2-14** The U.S. Coast Guard uses larger-frame helicopters. (*US Coast Guard*)

under **instrument flight rules (IFR)**. The difference between the two is whether the pilot can fly visually (without instruments) and be able to see a visible horizon for orientation. This is contrasted with conditions such as flying in the clouds or in marginal weather and relying on aircraft instruments and direction from the Federal Aviation Administration's (FAA) Air Traffic Control (ATC) system.

Most programs in the United States are limited to flying under VFR conditions at all times and train to fly on instruments in an emergency only when poor weather conditions are inadvertently encountered. A few helicopter EMS programs in the United States have made the investment to train their pilots and equip their aircraft to fly in IFR conditions intentionally with patients on board. The vast majority of EMS helicopters in the United States only have one pilot, which then requires sophisticated autopilot and ground positioning system (GPS) navigation systems to fly safely in the clouds.

The weather conditions that an EMS helicopter requires before it can fly safely vary from program to program and vary with the expected terrain that will be encountered, lighting (day or night), distance from home base, and so on. For example, a VFR helicopter program may need to have at least 3 miles of horizontal visibility and there must be at least 1,000 feet of clearance between the ground and lowest level of clouds before they can accept a flight. All the variables mentioned here can change the minimum conditions required before a pilot can accept a flight. All aircraft must give thunderstorms a wide berth; in certain parts of the country at certain times of the year, these storms can be a common problem, limiting the ability to fly.

Even helicopter programs that have the capability and training to fly under IFR conditions have significant limitations. For example, most civilian helicopters are not certified by the FAA to fly knowingly in conditions in which ice may form on the airframe of the helicopter (which adds weight and drag, seriously degrading aircraft performance and handling), making this a significant safety issue that has caused many accidents. In northern climates, this may mean that flights may be prohibited whenever there are clouds in winter, or when the temperatures at altitude are below freezing and precipitation may be encountered. Programs that fly IFR are also limited in where they can fly under ATC direction. Specifically, these aircraft usually are able to fly only from airport to airport, or from hospital to hospital if the hospital is near an airport or has an approved instrument approach directly to the hospital.

Helicopters are also not generally able to fly on instruments to random points on the ground, such as accident scenes on the highway, because of the limitations of current technology and the ATC system. In this situation, it may be best as the paramedic on the ground to transport your patient to the nearest hospital. Despite these limitations, the ability to fly IFR provides far more options should weather conditions change, and affords an added layer of safety in a constantly changing environment.

For the paramedic in the field, it is difficult under the best of circumstances to know all the variables that go into a helicopter service's decision to accept or deny a flight. Thus, it is best to call through the appropriate channels and make a request, rather than try to guess whether a helicopter can fly or not. This will allow the pilot to evaluate the situation using the resources at his disposal and make an informed decision. Even if there is fog, driving snow, thunderstorms, or tornadoes, it is still best to make the call because weather is a constantly changing phenomenon and conditions may improve in a time frame when a helicopter may still be able to provide assistance.

The obvious advantage of a helicopter as an air ambulance is that it is not limited to an airport as its only point of takeoff or landing. Thus, helicopters have become an important part of the modern trauma system. Weather permitting, they can land almost anywhere, retrieve a patient, and transport directly to a trauma center or hospital. In many instances, this can shorten the patient's out-of-hospital time.

ROLE IN EMS

In many EMS systems, air medical transport has been an important part of system operation for decades. Most Australian ambulance services, for instance, have air medical divisions. These operations are often a mix of airplanes and helicopters. Because Australia is such a rural nation, these aircraft are used on a daily basis to move patients between rural areas and the major cities. In the coastal states of Australia, helicopters are used primarily for rescue. In London, the helicopter service is intimately linked with the ground EMS system.

The use of helicopters and airplanes in the U.S. EMS system has evolved in the past 40 years. In the 1970s, several hospitals and other entities established air medical operations. By the mid-1980s, virtually every major community had access to an air ambulance. Most of these operations were hospital based, whereas some, such as the Maryland State Police, were government operations. Because of poor reimbursement, without the backing of a large medical institution or government, it was extremely difficult for independent for-profit programs to exist.

In 2001, the federal government changed the reimbursement scheme for air medical transport. This resulted in a significant increase in the number of air ambulances in the United States. Following this, there has been a transition from a hospital-based model to a community-based model. With that, there has been a transition from hospital-operated models to for-profit models as well.

Uses

There is no doubt that air medical transport plays an important role in the modern EMS system. However, the exact role that helicopter EMS plays in the United States is somewhat loosely defined and unregulated. Because of the rapid growth of air medical operations in the United States and the shift from hospital-based to for-profit models, there has been a proportionate increase in usage. There has been a recent push to better determine and define the role of air ambulances.

The initial use of medical helicopters in EMS was for trauma care. Much of this was based on the work and writings of Dr. R. Adams Cowley, the founder of the Shock Trauma Center in Baltimore. As Dr. Cowley developed the Maryland system, he introduced two concepts that have helped to drive modern trauma care. One was the concept of the "Golden Hour."[11, 12]

The second was the establishment of a network of helicopters, operated by the Maryland State Police, who would transport trauma patients from the scene directly to the Shock Trauma Center in Baltimore. These two principles became a fundamental tenet of modern trauma care. However, subsequent research has shown that these two factors are less important than originally thought. Despite this, recent research has demonstrated that a specific subset of patients—those with significant injuries—appears to benefit from helicopter transport.[13–19]

Today, there is no doubt that medical helicopters still play a critical role in the prehospital management of trauma. However, they are now also used for nontrauma situations. Although scene responses have remained a major and important use of medical helicopters, there has been a significant expansion of medical helicopter usage for interfacility transport. Much of this has resulted from the specialization of hospitals. The concept of a general hospital is now uncommon. Thus, it has become common practice to move patients, even those who are seriously ill or injured, between facilities. Many institutions have found air medical transport an effective, efficient, and timely method of moving these patients to minimize the inherently risky out-of-hospital time. This is particularly true in the care of patients with a recent stroke and for patients suffering a more severe, identifiable type of acute myocardial infarction (STEMI).[20]

Several studies have shown limited benefit from many helicopter transports. Strategies are being investigated to help prehospital and hospital personnel identify which patients stand to benefit from air medical transport. The American College of Emergency Physicians (ACEP) has endorsed a strategy to guide decision making in regard to selecting a medical helicopter for patient transport (Table 2–1). This statement supplements a prior position paper that defines criteria, developed by the National Association of EMS Physicians (NAEMSP) and ACEP, under which air medical dispatch might be considered (Table 2–2). Table 2–2 does not, however, reflect utilization criteria. One must not confuse the criteria for transfer to a trauma and/or burn center with the need for air transport to those facilities. Simply because a patient needs the care of a specialized center does not necessarily mean the patient must be transported by helicopter or airplane. In addition, patients with traumatic cardiac arrest have such a poor prognosis that helicopter transport is generally not warranted.

The benefits of air medical transport include speed, decreased out-of-hospital time, and, in some instances, the quality of care provided. Patients who do not need rapid transport or a reduced out-of-hospital time, or who can receive adequate quality of care by ground transport personnel, should be transported by ground units, if available. If patients need a decreased out-of-hospital time, quality of care that is unavailable by ground transport, or rapid access to specialty care, air medical transport should be considered seriously.

Limitations

Despite the potential benefits, air medical transport has its limitations. First and foremost, especially with regard to helicopter operations, flights may be impossible during periods of inclement weather, as described earlier. In these cases, ground transport may be the only option.

Air medical transport is an expensive endeavor. Costs routinely exceed $10,000 to $20,000 per transport. Insurance may cover some of these costs, but it is not uncommon for patients and

---

TABLE 2–1 | Appropriate Utilization of Air Medical Transport in the Out-of-Hospital Setting*

As an adjunct to this policy statement, the ACEP's Air Medical Transport Section developed a Policy Resource and Education Paper (PREP) titled Guidelines for Air Medical Dispatch.

The American College of Emergency Physicians (ACEP) recognizes that helicopter air medical care is a crucial component in a tiered response (including all levels of EMS providers, BLS and ALS ground services, rescue, etc.) for the expeditious initial care and delivery of the patient to an appropriate health care facility. An air medical helicopter should be an appropriately equipped and licensed ambulance that is staffed with adequate personnel to provide rapid and stabilizing care under various conditions. The air ambulance personnel should provide this care with the supervision of a qualified emergency physician cognizant of the unique features of air evacuation and use approved protocols for direct on-line as well as off-line medical control. Dispatch of the air ambulance should be under the direction of the appropriate emergency medical response entities.

Appropriate reasons to use an air medical helicopter in the out-of-hospital setting include:

1. Patient has a significant potential to require the high level life support available from an air medical helicopter, which is not available by ground transport.
2. Patient has a significant potential to require a time-critical intervention and an air medical helicopter will deliver the patient to an appropriate facility faster than ground transport.
3. Patient is located in a geographically isolated area which would make ground transport impossible or greatly delayed.
4. Local EMS resources are exceeded.

The air ambulance should be recognized as a regional resource that is available to every person needing care, at any time (weather permitting), regardless of the ability to pay. The patient should have initial stabilization and preparation for flight, then be expeditiously transported to the closest appropriate facility.

*American College of Emergency Physicians, Policy Statement Approved 1999; Revised 2008.

TABLE 2–2 | Guidelines for Air Medical Dispatch

Guidelines for Air Medical Dispatch*

1. General
   a. Patients requiring critical interventions should be provided those interventions in the most expeditious manner possible.
   b. Patients who are stable should be transported in a manner that best addresses the needs of the patient and the system.
   c. Patients with critical injuries or illnesses resulting in unstable vital signs require transport by the fastest available modality, and with a transport team that has the appropriate level of care capabilities, to a center capable of providing definitive care.
   d. Patients with critical injuries or illnesses should be transported by a team that can provide intratransport critical care services.
   e. Patients who require high-level care during transport, but do not have time-critical illness or injury, may be candidates for ground critical care transport (i.e., by a specialized ground critical care transport vehicle with level of care exceeding that of local EMS) if such service is available and logistically feasible.

2. Comparative considerations for air transport modes
   a. Rotor-wing
      i. Advantages
         1. In general, decreased response time to the patient (up to approximately 100 miles distance depending on logistics such as duration of ground transfer leg)
         2. Decreased out-of-hospital transport time
         3. Availability of highly trained medical crews and specialized equipment
      ii. Disadvantages
         1. Weather considerations (e.g., icing conditions, weather minimums)
         2. Limited availability as compared with ground EMS
   b. Fixed-wing
      i. Advantages
         1. In comparison with rotor-wing, decreased response time to patients when transport distances exceed approximately 100 miles
         2. In comparison with ground transport, decreased out-of-hospital transport time
         3. Availability of highly trained medical crews and specialized equipment
         4. In comparison with rotor-wing, less susceptibility to weather constraints
      ii. Disadvantages
         1. Requires landing at airport, with two extra transport legs between airports and the patient origin and destination
         2. In comparison with ground transport, more subject to weather-related unavailability (e.g., icing, snow)
         3. Overall, less desirable as a transport mode for severely ill or injured patients (though extenuating circumstances may modify this relative contraindication to fixed-wing use)

3. Logistical issues that may prompt the need for air medical transport
   a. Access and time/distance factors
      i. Patients who are in topographically hard-to-reach areas may be best served by air transport.
         1. In some cases patients may be in terrain (e.g., mountainside) not easily accessible to surface transport.
         2. Other cases may involve the need for transfer of patients from island environs, for whom surface water transport is not appropriate.
      ii. Patients in some areas (e.g., in the western United States) may be accessible to ground vehicles, but transport distances are sufficiently long that air transport (by rotor-wing or fixed-wing) is preferable.
   b. Systems considerations
      i. In some EMS regions, the air medical crew is the only rapidly available asset that can bring a high level of training to critically ill/injured patients. In these systems, there may be a lower threshold for air medical dispatch.
      ii. Systems in which there is widespread advanced life support (ALS) coverage, but such coverage is sparse, may see an area left "uncovered" for extended periods if its sole ALS unit is occupied providing an extended transport. Air medical dispatch may be the best means to provide patient care and simultaneously avoid deprivation of a geographic region of timely ALS emergency response.
      iii. Disaster and mass casualty incidents offer important opportunities for air medical participation. These roles, too complex for detailed discussion here, are outlined elsewhere.

(Continued)

TABLE 2–2 | Guidelines for Air Medical Dispatch *Continued*

4. Clinical situations for scene triage to air transport (also known as "primary" air transport) are outlined below. In some cases (e.g., flail chest), the diagnosis can be clearly established in the prehospital setting; in other cases (e.g., cardiac injury suggested by mechanism of injury and/or cardiac monitoring findings), prehospital care providers must use judgment and act on suspicion. Absent unusual logistical considerations as an overriding factor, scene air response involves rotor-wing vehicles rather than airplanes. As a general rule, air transport scene response should be considered more likely to be indicated when use of this modality, as compared with ground transport, results in more rapid arrival of the patient to an appropriate receiving center or when helicopter crews provide rapid access to advanced level of care (e.g., when a ground basic life support team encounters a multiple trauma patient requiring airway intervention).

  a. Trauma: Scene response to injured patients probably represents the mode of helicopter utilization with the best supporting evidence.

    i. General and mechanism considerations
1. Trauma Score <12
2. Unstable vital signs (e.g., hypotension or tachypnea)
3. Significant trauma in patients <12 years old, >55 years old, or pregnant patients
4. Multisystem injuries (e.g., long-bone fractures in different extremities; injury to more than two body regions)
5. Ejection from vehicle
6. Pedestrian or cyclist struck by motor vehicle
7. Death in same passenger compartment as patient
8. Ground provider perception of significant damage to patient's passenger compartment
9. Penetrating trauma to the abdomen, pelvis, chest, neck, or head
10. Crush injury to the abdomen, chest, or head
11. Fall from significant height

    ii. Neurologic considerations
1. Glasgow Coma Scale score <10
2. Deteriorating mental status
3. Skull fracture
4. Neurologic presentation suggestive of spinal cord injury

    iii. Thoracic consideration
1. Major chest wall injury (e.g., flail chest)
2. Pneumothorax/hemothorax
3. Suspected cardiac injury

    iv. Abdominal/pelvic considerations
1. Significant abdominal pain after blunt trauma
2. Presence of a "seatbelt" sign or other abdominal wall contusion
3. Obvious rib fracture below the nipple line
4. Major pelvic fracture (e.g., unstable pelvic ring disruption, open pelvic fracture, or pelvic fracture with hypotension)

    v. Orthopedic/extremity considerations
1. Partial or total amputation of a limb (exclusive of digits)
2. Finger/thumb amputation when emergent surgical evaluation (i.e., for replantation consideration) is indicated and rapid surface transport is not available
3. Fracture or dislocation with vascular compromise
4. Extremity ischemia
5. Open long-bone fractures
6. Two or more long-bone fractures

    vi. Major burns
1. >20% body surface area
2. Involvement of face, head, hands, feet, or genitalia
3. Inhalational injury
4. Electrical or chemical burns
5. Burns with associated injuries

    vii. Patients with near drowning injuries

  b. Nontrauma: At this time the literature support for primary air transport of noninjured patients is limited to logistical considerations. It is conceivable that clinical indications for scene air response may be identified in the future. However, at this time prehospital providers should incorporate logistical considerations, clinical judgment, and medical oversight in determining whether primary air transport is appropriate for patients with nontrauma diagnoses.

(Continued)

TABLE 2–2 | Guidelines for Air Medical Dispatch *Continued*

5. Clinical situations for air transport in interfacility transfers are best summarized as being present when (1) patients have diagnostic and/or therapeutic needs which cannot be met at the referring hospital, and (2) factors such as time, distance, and/or intratransport level of care requirements render ground transport nonfeasible.

   a. Trauma: Injured patients constitute the diagnostic group for which there is best evidence to support outcome improvements from air transport.

      i. Depending on local hospital capabilities and regional practices, any diagnostic consideration (suspected, or confirmed as with referring hospital radiography) listed above under "scene" guidelines may be sufficient indication for air transport from a community hospital to a regional trauma center.

      ii. Additionally, air transport (short- or long-distance) may be appropriate when initial evaluation at the community hospital reveals injuries (e.g., intra-abdominal hemorrhage on abdominal computed tomography) or potential injuries (e.g., aortic trauma suggested by widened mediastinum on chest x-ray; spinal column injury with potential for spinal cord involvement) requiring further evaluation and management beyond the capabilities of the referring hospital.

   b. Cardiac: Due to regionalization of cardiac care and the time-criticality of the disease process, patients with cardiac diagnoses often undergo interfacility air transport. Patients with the following cardiac conditions may be candidates for air transport:

      i. Acute coronary syndromes with time-critical need for urgent interventional therapy (e.g., cardiac catheterization, intra-aortic balloon pump placement, emergent cardiac surgery) unavailable at the referring center

      ii. Cardiogenic shock (especially in presence of, or need for, ventricular assist devices or intra-aortic balloon pumps)

      iii. Cardiac tamponade with impending hemodynamic compromise

      iv. Mechanical cardiac disease (e.g., acute cardiac rupture, decompensating valvular heart disease)

   c. Critically ill medical or surgical patients: These patients generally require a high level of care during transport, may benefit from minimization of out-of-hospital transport time, and may also have time-critical need for diagnostic or therapeutic intervention at the receiving facility. Ground critical care transport is frequently a viable transfer option for these patients, but air transport may be considered in circumstances such as the following examples:

      i. Pretransport cardiac/respiratory arrest

      ii. Requirement for continuous intravenous vasoactive medications or mechanical ventricular assist to maintain stable cardiac output

      iii. Risk for airway deterioration (e.g., angioedema, epiglottitis)

      iv. Acute pulmonary failure and/or requirement for sophisticated pulmonary intensive care (e.g., inverse-ratio ventilation) during transport

      v. Severe poisoning or overdose requiring specialized toxicology services

      vi. Urgent need for hyperbaric oxygen therapy (e.g., vascular gas embolism, necrotizing infectious process, carbon monoxide toxicity)

      vii. Requirement for emergent dialysis

      viii. Gastrointestinal hemorrhages with hemodynamic compromise

      ix. Surgical emergencies such as fasciitis, aortic dissection or aneurysm, or extremity ischemia

      x. Pediatric patients for whom referring facilities cannot provide required evaluation and/or therapy

   d. Obstetric: In gravid patients, air transport's advantage of minimized out-of-hospital time must be balanced against the risks inherent to intratransport delivery. If transport is necessary in a patient in whom delivery is thought to be imminent, then a ground vehicle is usually appropriate, although in some cases the combination of clinical status and logistics (e.g., long driving times) may favor use of an air ambulance. Air transport may be considered if ground transport is logistically not feasible and/or there are circumstances, such as the following:

      i. Reasonable expectation that delivery of infant(s) may require obstetric or neonatal care beyond the capabilities of the referring hospital

      ii. Active premature labor when estimated gestational age is <34 weeks or estimated fetal weight <2,000 grams

      iii. Severe preeclampsia or eclampsia

      iv. Third-trimester hemorrhage

      v. Fetal hydrops

      vi. Maternal medical conditions (e.g., heart disease, drug overdose, metabolic disturbances) exist that may cause premature birth

      vii. Severe predicted fetal heart disease

      viii. Acute abdominal emergencies (i.e., likely to require surgery) when estimated gestational age is <34 weeks or estimated fetal weight <2,000 grams

   e. Neurologic: In addition to those with need for specialized neurosurgical services, this category is being expanded to include patients requiring transfer to specialized stroke centers. Examples of neurologic conditions where air transport may be appropriate include:

      i. Central nervous system hemorrhage

      ii. Spinal cord compression by mass lesion

(Continued)

TABLE 2–2 | Guidelines for Air Medical Dispatch *Continued*

  iii. Evolving ischemic stroke (i.e., potential candidate for lytic therapy)
  iv. Status epilepticus
  f. Neonatal: Regionalization of neonatal intensive care has prompted the development of specialized (air and/or ground) services focusing on transport for this population. Given the fact that, in neonates, rapid transport is often less of a priority than (time-consuming) stabilization at referring institutions, some systems have found that the best means for incorporating air vehicles into neonatal transport is to use them to rapidly get a stabilization/transport team to the patient; the actual patient transport is then performed by a ground vehicle. In some systems, patients are transported (usually with a specialized neonatal team) by air when the ground transport out-of-hospital time exceeds 30 minutes. Examples of instances where air medical dispatch may be appropriate for neonates include:
  i. Gestational age <30 weeks, body weight <2,000 grams, or complicated neonatal course (e.g., perinatal cardiac/respiratory arrest, hemodynamic instability, sepsis, meningitis, metabolic derangement, temperature instability)
  ii. Requirement for supplemental oxygen exceeding 60%, continuous positive airway pressure (CPAP), or mechanical ventilation
  iii. Extrapulmonary air leak, interstitial emphysema, or pneumothorax
  iv. Medical emergencies such as seizure activity, congestive heart failure, or disseminated intravascular coagulation
  v. Surgical emergencies such as diaphragmatic hernia, necrotizing enterocolitis, abdominal wall defects, intussusception, suspected volvulus, or congenital heart defects
  g. Other: Air medical dispatch may also be appropriate in miscellaneous situations such as the following:
  i. Transplant
  1. Patient has met criteria for brain death and air transport is necessary for organ salvage.
  2. Organ and/or organ recipient requires air transport to the transplant center in order to maintain viability of time-critical transplant.
  ii. Search-and-rescue operations are generally outside the purview of air medical transport services, but in some instances helicopter EMS may participate in such operations. Since most search-and-rescue services have limited medical care capabilities, and since most air medical programs have similarly limited search-and-rescue training, cooperative effort is necessary for optimizing patient location, extrication, stabilization, and transport.
  iii. Patients known to be in cardiac arrest are rarely candidates for air medical transport.
  1. A previous NAEMSP position paper has addressed situations in which resuscitation efforts should be ceased in the field for adult nontraumatic cardiac arrest victims. In such cases air transport should not be considered an alternative to discontinuing (futile) efforts at resuscitation.
  2. In situations where patients are in cardiac arrest and do not meet local criteria for cessation of resuscitative efforts, or in jurisdictions in which prehospital providers cannot cease such efforts, air transport is an option only in very rare cases (e.g., pediatric cold-water drowning where helicopter transport to a cardiac-bypass center is considered).

*Excerpt, Policy Resource and Education Paper, of the National Association of EMS Physicians (NAEMSP); American College of Emergency Physicians (ACEP), 2006.

their families to bear the full burden if they are uninsured or underinsured. The expense is derived from the high costs of aircraft maintenance, initial and recurrent training for medical and aviation crew, 24/7 staffing and availability, fuel, and insurance. Thus, it is incumbent on providers to ensure that air medical transport is used only for patients who stand to benefit from such care.

There are significant space limitations within most small to medium-sized helicopters, which are markedly smaller than even the smallest ground ambulance. In some instances, and on some airframes, the ability to carry morbidly obese patients is quite limited, not so much from the weight itself (as in the case of one of the most popular light twin EMS helicopters in use, the Eurocopter EC-135) but from the girth that prevents safe loading through clamshell doors at the rear of the fuselage. Unfortunately, our population is slowly becoming more obese. Patients who are morbidly obese unfortunately may not be candidates for medical transport. Likewise, depending on the aircraft type, patients who are quite tall or who have a traction splint applied may not fit into the helicopter. Providers should be familiar with local weight restrictions and limitations of the services that provide air medical transport in their service areas. In some aircraft, access to parts of the patient is limited. In these situations, ground transport may afford better access and room.

Staffing

The staffing and crew configuration of air ambulances varies significantly—both in the United States and around the world. In most instances, modern medical helicopters are staffed by a three-person crew consisting of the pilot and two medical providers. In some operations, two pilots are used, increasing the crew size to four. In the United States, approximately 95 percent of HEMS programs use a crew configuration consisting of a paramedic and a nurse. However, there are multiple variations of crew staffing, ranging from nurse–nurse to nurse–respiratory therapist, nurse–doctor, or two paramedics. Occasionally, in specialty care situations, specifically trained personnel, such as a pediatric respiratory therapist or a neonatal nurse, will replace one of the regular flight crew members. In some rare instances in the United States, certain flight programs have a nurse–physician crew configuration. Most commonly, these are emergency physicians or emergency medicine residents functioning under the direction of an attending-level emergency physician.[20-24] A crew composed of a pilot and a single medical provider (nurse, paramedic, or physician) is generally inadequate except for the transport of extremely stable patients.

The physician–nurse staffing model is much more common outside the United States, including in Europe, Australia, Japan, and South Africa—where the physicians are often anesthesiologists, intensivists, emergency physicians, or general practitioners. In some helicopter EMS operations in the United Kingdom and New Zealand, ground providers will staff medical helicopters as the need arises. Typically, staffing is based on local tradition and availability. It is very much country and system specific.

Controversies

Even though air medical transport, especially helicopter EMS, has become a fixture in modern EMS systems, it has not been without controversy. Significant concern has been raised by many, including the National Transportation Safety Board, regarding a perceived increase in the rate and incidence of crashes involving medical helicopters.

As of 2009, there were almost 900 helicopters in service in the United States, according to the most up-to-date information from the **ADAMS** (Atlas and Database of Air Medical Services) database. This brisk expansion has come under increasing scrutiny in recent years, as many helicopters are based in close proximity to one another, raising significant questions of medical necessity. There has also been increasing concern about this near-exponential expansion outside the medical community. Specifically, even federal transportation agencies, such as the National Transportation Safety Board (NTSB), have begun to look into the number of helicopters with growing concern that competition may lead to poor aeronautical decision making or subliminal pressures that influence the decision to accept a flight.[25, 26] Although many of these aircraft are flying in very rural areas with long distances between the scene of an accident and the hospital, or between rural hospitals and tertiary higher-level care, many helicopter programs are being developed in areas of the country that already have adequate air medical coverage.

Another area of significant concern arose following a series of crashes in 2008 that marred the safety record of helicopter EMS. That year there were 13 accidents that resulted in 29 fatalities (Figure 2-15 ●). This was a significant increase in the accident and fatality rate when compared with the previous year.[27] There was also an initiative from within the air medical community to develop and embrace strategies to improve the safety of helicopter EMS. As a result, the Patient First Air Ambulance Alliance (PFAA), a grassroots organization of medical and aviation providers, was formed. The organization is committed to ensuring that critically ill and injured patients have access to the safest and highest quality air medical system possible.[28]

In many respects, the HEMS industry has been the beneficiary of tools developed in the military to aid their mission. Specifically, more and more programs are using night vision goggle (NVG)

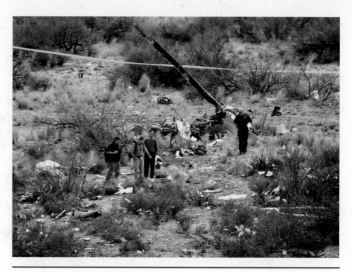

● **Figure 2-15** Medical helicopter operations have come under greater scrutiny because of an increased incidence of accidents. (© AP Images/Odessa American, Paul Zoeller)

technology, especially for night scene responses. In the past several years, in response to accidents in which helicopters have collided with terrain, the adoption of GPS-based helicopter-specific terrain avoidance warning systems (HTAWS) and enhanced ground proximity warning systems (EGPWS), as well as radar altimeters that precisely measure the aircraft's altitude from the ground, are all tools that improve safety. Even in 2011, however, none of these tools was mandated by the FAA to be on all EMS helicopters.

Unlike the fairly heavily regulated ground EMS industry, local and state governments have little, if any, authority to regulate air ambulances. The authority to regulate operation of air ambulances (helicopter and fixed-wing) is exclusively that of the FAA. Air ambulances fall under the authority and purview of the Airline Deregulation Act, which was signed into law in 1978. As a direct result of this act, states have been prohibited from overseeing the "quality, accessibility, availability, and acceptability" of air ambulance services. This has prevented local and state governments from developing rules and regulations for air ambulance usage. Currently, there is no one, uniformly recognized, certifying organization for the air medical industry. Air ambulance services (as well as critical care ground services) can be accredited by the Commission on Accreditation of Medical Transport Services (CAMTS), a private nongovernmental entity.

SCENE OPERATIONS

The decision to summon a medical helicopter should be made early in scene operations. If it is later determined that the patient or patients do not require helicopter transport, then the inbound aircraft can be canceled, frequently at no charge to anyone. It is vital to notify local air medical services as soon as possible, as it takes several minutes to check the weather, prepare to fly, and cover the distance to the scene of the accident. Unlike ground EMS and fire operations, which are often dispatched with an urgency that results in only seconds or minutes before they are out the door, flight crews must be careful to properly assess all the variables, such as weather, hazards, and terrain, before accepting a flight.

Initial Information

Most EMS agencies will be familiar with the requirements and needs of their local HEMS providers. However, the following general concepts apply to most EMS systems:

- Location of scene:
  - ○ GPS coordinates (longitude and latitude), including degrees, minutes, and decimals of minutes (e.g., 37° 14.50 N and 115° 48.50 W). There are several conventions with regard to how GPS coordinates are displayed, so check with local programs to determine the local convention, whether degrees/minutes/decimals of minutes (the convention in the aviation world) *or* degrees/minutes/seconds and decimals of seconds.
  - ○ Closest cross street or roads. Many helicopter communication centers have commercially available computer mapping programs (Deloreme) that will automatically show GPS coordinates when the cursor is hovered over an intersection or spot on the computer screen.
  - ○ Closest city/town.
  - ○ Actual address of location.
  - ○ Well-known landmarks (e.g., water tower, high school, local airports).
- Launch information:
  - ○ Requesting agency identity, contact radio frequencies, and a call-back cell phone number on location, if possible.
  - ○ Local weather conditions.
  - ○ Presence of hazardous materials.
  - ○ Number of patients and basic medical description (e.g., rollover with ejection, 30-foot fall with LOC, GSW to chest).

Landing Zone

The early establishment of a landing zone (LZ) is important. As a part of NIMS and the ICS, an LZ officer should be designated. The LZ officer should coordinate the incoming aircraft operations with the incident commander (IC). The responsibilities of the LZ officer include:

- Selection of site
- Site preparation
- Site protection and control
- Air-to-ground communications with incoming aircraft
- Updating IC on estimated time of arrival (ETA) of aircraft

When establishing an LZ, look for an area that is (ideally) 100 feet by 100 feet square (Figure 2-16 ●). An LZ of this size will accommodate most EMS helicopters. There should be little, if any, slope to the LZ, and it should be clear of any readily visible debris or obstructions. If the area is dusty, consider wetting the area with a light water fog pattern to prevent blowing dust (brownout) from obscuring the pilot's view during landing. It is never necessary to routinely have a charged fire hose pointing at the aircraft, as is the custom with some fire services at LZs (and makes many flight

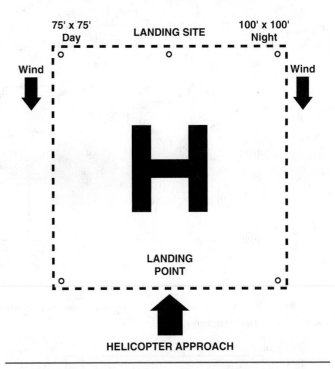

● **Figure 2-16** The helicopter landing zone should be at least 100 × 100 feet (at night) and clear of obstacles.

crews nervous). In most circumstances, the approach and landing will be made as near into the wind as practical, keeping in mind obstructions and terrain. A marker on the upwind side of the LZ (such as a cone or strobe) is conventional practice (Figure 2-17 ●).

Mark the LZ with cones (day) and strobes (night). As an alternative to strobes, consider laying the cones down, pointing toward the center of the LZ, with a flashlight placed inside each cone. Avoid shining lights up toward the approaching aircraft. Lights should be directed across the LZ away from the approaching aircraft (Figure 2-18 ●). Different services may use different-colored strobes for night scene operations, but it should be kept in mind that certain colored strobes (green and blue) are difficult to see with NVGs. Red and white strobes are much easier to see at night with NVGs. Aircraft equipped with NVGs may actually ask that bright scene lights be turned off, as they may interfere with their ability to see the periphery of the lit area where wires, trees, and poles may hide. Avoid using flares.

LZ security is of critical importance from the time of initial approach until the aircraft departs. Nonessential personnel and all vehicles and equipment must be kept clear of the LZ during this period. Have personnel walk the LZ looking for debris, obstructions, or other dangers. The mnemonic HOTSAW is sometimes used to remind crews of potential hazards:

- **H**azards
- **O**bstructions
- **T**errain
- **S**urface
- **A**nimals
- **W**ind/Weather

It is also important not only to look around an LZ, but also to look up! Many forget that aircraft work in a three-dimensional

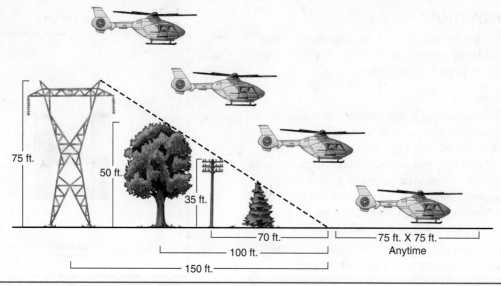

● **Figure 2-17** When selecting a landing zone, always consider wind direction and nearby obstacles such as trees, buildings, towers, and other structures.

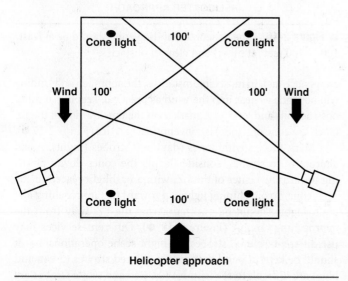

● **Figure 2-18** Lighting of helicopter landing zones must not interfere with the pilot's vision. Never point lights up toward the approaching aircraft.

environment and are of course approaching from above, so be sure to look up and assess the LZ for any obstructions above, such as wires, poles, and trees.

Helicopter Approach

The LZ officer should remain in contact with the incoming aircraft and respond to any requests made by the pilot. Ideally, during night landings, as the helicopter approaches, ensure the following:

● Turn off flashing white lights (the pilot may request that other lights be turned off).

● Use spotlights to mark any possible obstacles (e.g., overhead wires, trees, poles).

● Do not shine lights (or lasers) at the helicopter.

Many medical helicopters use night vision imaging systems (i.e., NVGs) during night operations. These devices significantly increase visible light. If these are being used, the crew may request that many scene lights be turned off to ensure a safe landing.

Generally speaking, the crew of the inbound aircraft will notify you when they are close to the scene (generally 5 minutes out). In turn, notify them when you hear the aircraft and when you are able to see it. Although you can see the aircraft, its crew may not be able to see you.

If necessary to provide guidance to the approaching aircraft, use clock-based directional terms. Always consider the point of reference for the pilot (the nose of the aircraft) to be the 12 o'clock position. When the aircraft is on final approach, limit communications to safety concerns. If at any time the LZ becomes unsafe (e.g., a person wanders onto the LZ), say, "Abort landing!" The LZ officer should move to a safe distance and continue to watch for hazards.

Never allow anyone to approach the aircraft until the crew has indicated it is safe to do so. Modern turbine aircraft require anywhere from 30 seconds to 2 minutes to cool off the engines before they can be shut down. Always remain well outside the rotor perimeter and LZ until it is safe to approach (as indicated by the flight crew), as rotors can "droop" when the engines are spooling down; they are much more subject to flexing in the wind and hence may actually be much lower than they are at rest. The pilot may or may not leave the helicopter running. Under no circumstances should anyone approach the tail of a helicopter, even if it has a shrouded or ducted tail rotor, as it can easily be forgotten and unseen and is very dangerous.

Personnel should approach the aircraft only from the front and while in direct view of the flight crew (Figure 2-19 ●). If the aircraft is on unlevel ground, always approach from the downhill side. Walk away from the aircraft in the same direction from which you approached it (Figure 2-20 ●). Allow the crew to open the doors and remove any needed equipment.

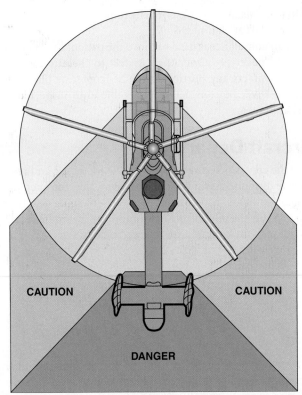

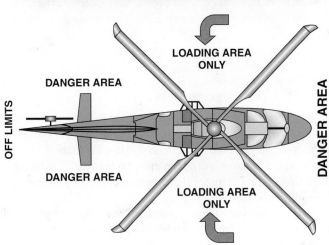

● **Figure 2-19** Personnel should approach the aircraft when requested to do so by the flight crew. They should approach only from the front and while in direct view of the flight crew.

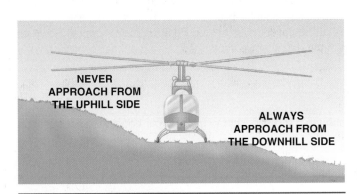

● **Figure 2-20** Always approach a helicopter from the downhill side if the landing zone has an incline.

Patient Handoff

Do not bring the patient directly to the helicopter. The flight crew will typically come to the patient to ensure adequate assessment and packaging for transport. After exiting the aircraft, the helicopter flight crew should be directed to the patient. The primary caregiver (paramedic) should give a brief, concise report of the patient's condition, describe any care provided, and detail the response to such care. It is important to report which medications were administered (e.g., fentanyl, sedatives, paralytics), the dose provided, and when the medications were given. If possible, provide a copy of the patient's identification, vital signs, and any other physiologic data (e.g., ECG, capnography). Other important details to relay to the flight crew include the best GCS and neuro exam if the patient has been intubated, what paralytics were given and when, any episodes of hypotension for a trauma patient, and the mechanism of injury. If a patient was intubated, relate the size of the tube used and the location (how many centimeters at the lip).

Aircraft Loading

If asked to do so, assist the flight crew in loading the patient. Again, follow all safety rules for approaching and leaving the aircraft. Do not hold any equipment above shoulder height. Always follow any directions of the flight crew. Some helicopters load from the side, whereas others load from the rear (Figures 2-21 ● and 2-22 ●). Keep an eye on the crew, as verbal communications are often difficult because of the noise. Allow the crew to close and secure the doors and any outside

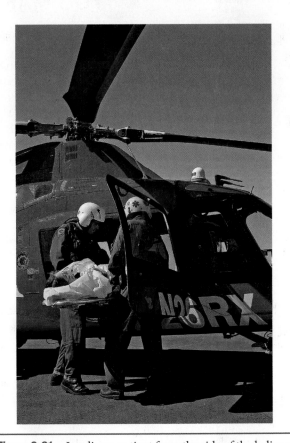

● **Figure 2-21** Loading a patient from the side of the helicopter.

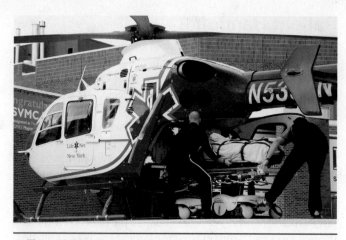

● **Figure 2-22** Loading a patient from the rear of the helicopter.
(© Mark Foster)

compartments. Again, it is critically important to avoid the tail of the aircraft at all times.

If an ambulance is used to move the patient to the aircraft, it should never get closer than 25 feet to the aircraft. If any vehicle contacts any portion of the helicopter or blades, that helicopter will be considered inoperable until inspected by a mechanic.

Aircraft Departure

Once the crew has secured the patient, leave the LZ and remain at a safe distance. Assist the crew by being alert for open doors or compartments. Look for any straps left hanging out. Immediately notify the pilot of any new or unseen hazards. Remain in contact with the aircraft until it is well clear of the area.

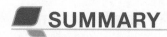 **SUMMARY**

Air ambulances are an important part of the modern EMS system. Like any medical procedure, transporting a patient by helicopter requires considerations of the potential benefits and risks. Because of the inherent danger and cost of using medical aircraft, the potential benefit must clearly outweigh the risks. Patients will be unfamiliar with the role of helicopters in modern EMS. They depend on you, the paramedic, to act in their best interest.

YOU MAKE THE CALL

You and your partner are responding to an injured-person call in a remote part of the county. Little additional information is known. You know that the local first responders, the Red Canyon Volunteer Fire Department, are already en route to the scene. You turn onto a rural road and see the flashing lights of the fire department in the distance. You pull up to the scene and park behind the fire truck. The house is a small rural frame house that is well kept. One of the first responders meets you and your partner and leads you to the patient.

The patient is a 72-year-old woman who tripped over a throw rug and fell. She is complaining of left hip pain. The patient's husband is at her side and is holding her hand. You complete your primary and secondary assessments and feel that the patient is suffering an isolated left hip fracture. You send one of the first responders to the front yard to retrieve your ambulance stretcher. The first responder gives you somewhat of an inquisitive look and states, "We have the helicopter coming." You look at him and ask, "You have a helicopter coming for her?" He replies that the crew felt the patient would be more comfortable in a helicopter as opposed to the 20-minute transport in your ground ambulance. Besides, the husband told the first responders that he had a subscription to one of the local helicopter services.

You and your partner both know that this patient does not require a medical helicopter. However, you want to maintain good relations with the volunteer fire department. Based on the scenario, answer the following questions:

1. Would you go ahead and allow the patient to be transported by helicopter when her condition clearly does not warrant helicopter transport?

2. What would you tell her husband and the first responders to explain your decision to not transport by helicopter?

3. What options are available to you to assist in dealing with the situation?

See Suggested Responses at the back of this book.

REVIEW QUESTIONS

1. The first recorded use of aircraft to evacuate casualties was during _____.
   a. World War I
   b. World War II
   c. the Korean War
   d. the Vietnam War

2. One of the most significant limitations faced by all helicopters is _____.
   a. distance
   b. light conditions
   c. patient condition
   d. weather

3. An aircraft can fly intentionally in weather with poor visibility only if the pilot and aircraft have been equipped to fly under _____ rules.
   a. IFR   c. V4R
   b. VFR   d. GPS

4. The initial use for medical helicopters in EMS was for _____.
   a. cardiac patients
   b. stroke patients
   c. obstetric patients
   d. trauma patients

5. Benefits of air medical transport include _____.
   a. proper medical care
   b. decreased distance of flights
   c. decreased out-of-hospital time
   d. lower quality of care

6. Patient candidates for air medical transport include those with _____.
   a. diving emergencies
   b. cardiac arrest
   c. hazmat exposure
   d. acute strokes

7. Limitations to air medical transport include _____.
   a. cost
   b. lack of fuel
   c. short distances
   d. spinal injuries

8. You are on scene of a head-on collision with pin-in. Your patient is pinned in the vehicle and has a massive head injury and altered level of consciousness. Which of the following factors may prevent the patient from being accepted by air medical services?
   a. head injury
   b. patient size
   c. spinal injury
   d. altered level of consciousness

9. A GPS-based helicopter-specific terrain warning system designed to help pilots avoid flying into terrain is _____.
   a. HTAWS   c. FAA-NVG
   b. GPSWS   d. NVG

10. Air ambulances fall under the authority and purview of _____.
    a. local medical direction
    b. state medical direction
    c. state office of EMS
    d. the Federal Aviation Administration

11. The initial information you provide when requesting an air ambulance includes _____.
    a. distance to the scene
    b. number of patients
    c. your supervisor's name
    d. closest body of water

12. The landing zone officer is responsible for site preparation and selection, updating the incident commander on ETA of aircraft, and _____.
    a. site visibility
    b. ground-to-air communications
    c. rescue scene safety
    d. patient preparation

13. Ideally, a landing zone (LZ) should be free from debris; have a minimum slope, if any; and be _____ in size.
    a. 50 feet by 50 feet
    b. 75 feet by 75 feet
    c. 100 feet by 100 feet
    d. 150 feet by 150 feet

14. The center of the LZ should be marked with _____.
    a. flares   c. flashlights
    b. cones   d. sheets

15. During a night landing the LZ should be marked with _____.
    a. flashing white lights
    b. spotlights on overhead obstacles
    c. flares in a cross-like pattern
    d. lasers fixed on the aircraft

16. You are talking in an approaching aircraft. Which of the following statements would be correct for giving the pilot directions?
    a. "The LZ is to the left of Belmont Road."
    b. "The LZ is marked with Captain Jones' pickup truck on the right edge."
    c. "I have you in sight; the LZ is 50 yards north of my location."
    d. "The LZ is marked with cones on each corner and is at your 3 o'clock position."

17. The most dangerous direction to approach an aircraft while the engines are on is _____.

    a. from the downhill side

    b. from the front

    c. from the pilot's side

    d. from the rear

18. If the flight crew were to ask for assistance with loading, you should _____.

    a. allow the crew to direct you to the aircraft

    b. remove all patient clothing

    c. approach from the uphill side

    d. wait for the copilot to throttle down the engines

19. In the event any debris or foreign object comes in contact with the aircraft, the aircraft _____.

    a. must be rendered inoperable until checked out by a mechanic

    b. will be delayed 20 minutes while the pilots check out the aircraft

    c. will automatically shut down for a 45-minute cool-down

    d. must cool down for 20 minutes before additional patient care

See Answers to Review Questions at the back of this book.

REFERENCES

1. Karanicolas, P. J., P. Bhatia, J. Williamson, et al. "The Fastest Route between Two Points Is Not Always a Straight Line: An Analysis of Air and Land Transfer of Nonpenetrating Trauma Patients." *J Trauma* 61 (2006): 396–403.

2. Talving, P., P. G. Teixeira, G. Barmparas, et al. "Helicopter Evacuation of Trauma Victims in Los Angeles: Does It Improve Survival?" *World J Surg* 33 (2009): 2469–2476.

3. Svenson, J. E., J. E. O'Connor, and M. B. Lindsay. "Is Air Transport Faster? A Comparison of Air versus Ground Transport Times for Interfacility Transfers in a Regional Referral System." *Air Med J* 25 (2006): 170–172.

4. Diaz, M. A., G. W. Hendey, and H. G. Bivins. "When Is the Helicopter Faster? A Comparison of Helicopter and Ground Ambulance Transport Times." *J Trauma* 58 (2005): 148.

5. Fan, E., R. D. MacDonald, N. K. Adhikari, et al. "Outcomes of Interfacility Critical Care Adult Patient Transport: A Systematic Review." *Crit Care* 10 (2006): R6.

6. Werman, H. A. and B. N. Neely. "One-Way Neonatal Transports: A New Approach to Increase Effective Utilization of Air Medical Resources." *Air Med J* 15 (1996): 13–17.

7. Berge, S. D., C. Berg-Utby, and E. Skogvoll. "Helicopter Transport of Sick Neonates: A 14-Year Population-Based Study." *Acta Anaesthesiol Scand* 49 (2005): 999–1003.

8. Thomas, S. H., T. Harrison, S. K. Wedel, and D. P. Thomas. "Helicopter Emergency Medical Services Roles in Disaster Operations." *Prehosp Emerg Care* 4 (2000): 338–344.

9. Martin, T. *Aeromedical Transport: A Clinical Guide.* 2nd ed. Williston, VT: Ashgate Publishing, 2006.

10. Atlas and Database of Air Medical Services (ADAMS). [Available at http://www.aams.org/AAMS/Media_Room/ADAMS_Database/aams/MediaRoom/ADAMSDatabase/ADAMS_Database.aspx?hkey=4cccf748-2bc7-4bb9-b41a-c710366c51dc]

11. Lerner, E. B. and R. M. Moscati. "The Golden Hour: Scientific Fact or Medical "Urban Legend"?" *Acad Emerg Med* 8 (2001): 758–760.

12. Newgard, C. D., R. H. Schmicker, J. R. Hedges, et al. "Emergency Medical Services Intervals and Survival in Trauma: Assessment of the "Golden Hour" in a North American Prospective Cohort." *Ann Emerg Med* 55 (2010): 235–246.

13. Brown, J. B., N. A. Stassen, P. E. Bankey, A. T. Sangosanya, J. D. Cheng, and M. L. Gestring. "Helicopters and the Civilian Trauma System: National Utilization Patterns Demonstrate Improved Outcomes after Traumatic Injury." *J Trauma* 69 (2010): 1030–1034; discussion 1034–1036.

14. Schiller, J., J. E. McCormack, V. Tarsia, et al. "The Effect of Adding a Second Helicopter on Trauma-Related Mortality in a County-Based Trauma System." *Prehosp Emerg Care* 13 (2009): 437–443.

15. Butler, D. P., I. Anwar, and K. Willett. "Is It the H or the EMS in HEMS That Has an Impact on Trauma Patient Mortality? A Systematic Review of the Evidence." *Emerg Med J* 27 (2010): 692–701.

16. Bledsoe, B. E., A. K. Wesley, M. Eckstein, T. M. Dunn, and M. F. O'Keefe. "Helicopter Scene Transport of Trauma Patients with Nonlife-Threatening Injuries: A Meta-Analysis." *J Trauma* 60 (2006): 1257–1265; discussion 1265–1266.

17. Black, J. J., M. E. Ward, and D. J. Lockey. "Appropriate Use of Helicopters to Transport Trauma Patients from Incident Scene to Hospital in the United Kingdom: An Algorithm." *Emerg Med J* 21(3) (2004): 355–361.

18. Thomas, S. H., F. Cheema, S. K. Wedel, and D. Thomson. "Trauma Helicopter Emergency Medical Services Transport: Annotated Review of Selected Outcomes-Related Literature." *Prehosp Emerg Care* 6 (2002): 359–371.

19. Thomas, S. H. "Helicopter EMS Transport Outcomes Literature: Annotated Review of Articles Published 2004–2006." *Prehosp Emerg Care* 11 (2007): 477–488.

20. Bayley, R., M. Weinger, S. Meador, and C. Slovis. "Impact of Ambulance Crew Configuration on Simulated Cardiac Arrest Resuscitation." *Prehosp Emerg Care* 12 (2008): 62–68.

21. Burney, R. E., L. Passini, D. Hubert, and R. Maio. "Comparison of Aeromedical Crew Performance by Patient Severity and Outcome." *Ann Emerg Med* 21 (1992): 375–378.

22. Burney, R. E., D. Hubert, L. Passini, and R. Maio. "Variation in Air Medical Outcomes by Crew Composition: A Two-Year Follow-Up." *Ann Emerg Med* 25 (1995): 187–192.

23. Ray, A. M. and D. P. Sole. "Emergency Medicine Resident Involvement in EMS." *J Emerg Med* 33 (2007): 385–394.

24. Garner, A., S. Rashford, A. Lee, and R. Bartolacci. "Addition of Physicians to Paramedic Helicopter Services Decreases Blunt Trauma Mortality." *Aust N Z J Surg* 69 (1999): 697–701.

25. National Transportation Safety Board. Public Hearing: Helicopter Emergency Medical Services, February 3–6, 2009.

26. Federal Aviation Administration. *Fact Sheet—Helicopter Emergency Medical Services Safety.*

27. National Transportation Safety Board. *EMS Helicopter Safety: Is It an Oxymoron?* [Available at http://www.ntsb.gov/doclib/speeches/sumwalt/aamt.pdf]

28. Patient First Air Ambulance Alliance. [Available at http://www.patientfirstalliance.org/]

FURTHER READING

Air and Surface Transport Nurses Association. *ASTNA Patient Transport: Principles and Practices.* St. Louis: Mosby, 2009.

Bledsoe, B. E., and R. W. Benner. *Critical Care Paramedic.* Upper Saddle River, NJ: Pearson/Prentice Hall, 2006.

Deschamp C. *Introduction to Air Medicine.* Upper Saddle River, NJ: Pearson/Prentice Hall, 2006.

3

Multiple-Casualty Incidents and Incident Management

Bryan Bledsoe, DO, FACEP, FAAEM, EMT-P
Louis Molino, NREMT-I

STANDARD
EMS Operations (Multiple-Casualty Incidents)

COMPETENCY
Applies knowledge of operational roles and responsibilities to ensure patient, public, and personnel safety.

OBJECTIVES

Terminal Performance Objective
After reading this chapter, you should be able to effectively perform the expected functions of EMS personnel in a multiple-casualty incident.

Enabling Objectives
To accomplish the terminal performance objective, you should be able to:

1. Define key terms introduced in this chapter.

2. Anticipate situations that can result in low-impact, high-impact, and disaster-related multiple-casualty incidents (MCIs).

3. Describe the origins and purposes of incident command or incident management systems.

4. Describe the components of the National Incident Management System (NIMS).

5. Describe NIMS as a uniform, yet flexible system.

6. Describe the purpose of a mutual aid coordination center (MACC).

7. Describe the purpose and function of each of the five major functional areas of NIMS or incident command system (ICS).

8. Describe the roles of various personnel within each of the five major functional areas of NIMS/ICS.

9. Apply a system of triage to MCIs.

10. Perform the various functions expected of EMS personnel in the triage, treatment, and transport branch or group in a multiple-casualty incident.

11. Describe special considerations in the response and operating procedures in disasters.

12. Anticipate common problems that occur in MCIs and disasters.

13. Describe the importance of preplanning, drills, and critiques with regard to MCI and disaster response.

14. Describe the role of disaster mental health services.

KEY TERMS

branches, p. 45
C-FLOP, p. 39
closed incident, p. 41
command, p. 39
command staff, p. 43
consensus standards, p. 38
demobilized, p. 43
Department of Homeland
　Security (DHS), p. 38
disaster management, p. 56
domestic incidents, p. 39
emergency operations center
　(EOC), p. 39
EMS communications
　officer, p. 56
extrication, p. 55
facilities unit, p. 45
finance/administration
　section, p. 45
incident command post
　(ICP), p. 41
Incident Command System
　(ICS), p. 38
incident commander (IC), p. 39

Incident Management System
　(IMS), p. 38
information officer (IO), p. 44
liaison officer (LO), p. 44
logistics section, p. 45
medical supply unit, p. 45
morgue, p. 51
morgue officer, p. 52
multiple-casualty incident
　(MCI), p. 36
mutual aid agreement, p. 45
mutual aid coordination center
　(MACC), p. 39
National Incident
　Management System
　(NIMS), p. 38
open incident, p. 41
operations section, p. 45
planning/intelligence section,
　p. 45
primary triage, p. 46
rapid intervention
　team, p. 55
safety officer (SO), p. 44

SALT (sort–assess–lifesaving
　interventions–treatment/
　transport) triage, p. 48
scene-authority law, p. 38
secondary triage, p. 47
section chief, p. 43
sector, p. 46
singular command, p. 41
situational awareness, p. 40
span of control, p. 40
staff functions, p. 44
staging area, p. 54
staging officer, p. 54
START, p. 47
transportation unit
　supervisor, p. 54
treatment group
　supervisor, p. 52
treatment unit leaders, p. 54
triage, p. 46
triage group supervisor, p. 46
triage officer, p. 40
unified command, p. 41
windshield survey, p. 40

CASE STUDY

A charter bus carrying 29 elementary school children is headed northbound on County Road 219 when the driver loses control of the vehicle on a patch of "black ice." The bus swerves off the roadway and strikes a thickly wooded stand of pine trees at approximately 45 miles per hour on the left shoulder of the county road. The bus driver is able to use his cell phone to call the county 911 public safety answering point (PSAP). The PSAP notifies the local police, fire, and EMS agencies, and notifies the school district's administrative headquarters via landline.

The first ambulance arrives shortly after the first police unit. The paramedic in the passenger seat does a windshield survey. She then relays her size-up to dispatch: "Central, Ambulance 21 on scene, assuming County Road 219 Command, we have a school bus that veered off the road into a heavily wooded area on the shoulder of the road, severe damage to the vehicle with a probable extrication problem. Ambulance 21 will be County Road 219 Command." The dispatcher acknowledges the message, "OK, Ambulance 21, you're on scene at 0723 hours, establishing County Road 219 Command."

The lead paramedic, now acting as the incident commander (IC), assigns her partner to be the triage officer. The IC then performs a 360-degree perimeter walk of the scene to assess the entire area, surveying for hazards to responders, rescue problems, and locations for the future staging of incoming resources. Meanwhile, the triage officer, after donning his personal protective equipment (PPE), enters the bus through the rear emergency entrance, as the main entry door is damaged and obscured by debris from the woods. He does a rapid patient count and finds 30 patients—all of whom are children, except for the bus driver. He relays this to the IC via radio. Using the START/JumpSTART system, the triage officer moves quickly from patient to patient, making a rapid assessment of each and tagging each patient while keeping a running count of the patient totals.

The triage officer completes his primary triage and reports to the IC that they have 30 patients in total: 7 red tags, 12 yellow tags, 11 green tags, and 0 black tags. Three patients, including the bus driver, are heavily entrapped.

Outside the bus, the IC calls the dispatcher and reports: "Central, County Road 219 Command, we have a full-size school bus that has run into a heavily wooded area on the left side of County Road 219 about one mile north of State Highway 34. We have a total of 30 patients. All are children except for the bus driver. We have a significant MCI at this location. I am requesting at least ten additional transport units, as well as more fire, heavy rescue, and police units. Have the next due unit establish a staging area on the opposite side of County Road 219 near the open field and have everyone keep the center lane clear for transport units to exit the scene."

The senior dispatcher at the PSAP activates the county's Mutual Aid Coordination Center (MACC) and activates the regional MCI and disaster plan. Additional EMS, fire, police, and other response agencies are mobilized for scene response as well as back-fill coverage for empty stations to ensure adequate coverage for normal call volume. Several mutual aid agencies initiate callbacks of off-duty personnel to staff additional units and provide fill-in coverage. All local hospitals are notified of the incident through use of phones and radio and pager systems and are asked to update the MACC with up-to-date counts of their available beds and specialty beds of all types.

More ambulances arrive and begin to treat the critical patients, focusing their care on life-threatening conditions only, until more resources can reach the scene. Fire and rescue units arrive a short time later, initiating hazard control and rescue operations for the severely entrapped patients. The on-duty EMS field supervisor arrives and meets with the IC, who provides a situation report and then transfers command to the EMS Field Supervisor. She alerts dispatch, "Central, County Road 219 Command. Transferring command from Ambulance 21 to EMS -1." The paramedic from Ambulance 21 is then assigned to the operations section chief position.

As additional EMS units arrive, the operations section chief assigns various functions, such as safety officer, treatment unit manager, and transport unit manager; other personnel provide patient care, gather supplies, or transfer patients to waiting ambulances. Operations run smoothly, with all the various incident management system elements communicating with each other and personnel performing their assigned tasks.

Ambulances transport the first critical patients off the scene at 7:49, just 26 minutes after the first arriving unit established command. The Transportation Officer distributes patients evenly among the three local hospitals, with the patient loads determined by the types of injury and with appropriate care centers such as the designated trauma center receiving the most critical trauma patients. The last patients depart the scene 53 minutes after Ambulance 21 established command. Although the emergency response phase of the incident is now terminated, several units remain on the scene to assist in the investigation of this incident.

During this incident, other EMS units in the county responded to eight emergencies, including one multiple-vehicle collision, which created another smaller-scale MCI event. Although some minor delays were reported on the routine call load, neither of the two multiple-casualty incidents in any way significantly compromised either response times or patient care within the county EMS system.

INTRODUCTION

Traditional paramedic education focuses on the relationship between one or two patient care providers and a single patient. In this setting, a paramedic has the ability to concentrate on the assessment and treatment of the patient. Occasionally, however, paramedics are called on to treat more than one patient at a time. The multiple-patient incident may result from a motor vehicle collision (MVC), an apartment fire, a gang fight, or any number of other scenarios. During your career as a paramedic, you can also expect to respond to a much larger **multiple-casualty incident (MCI)**, also known as a *mass-casualty incident*.

The MCI can involve "everyday" incidents, such as the school bus collision described in the opening case study, or disasters such as tornadoes, train wrecks, airline crashes, or even a terrorist event (Figures 3-1 ●, 3-2 ●, and 3-3 ●). Definitions of an MCI vary from agency to agency and may even vary on a district level within a single jurisdiction or agency. Some agencies define an MCI as any incident involving three or more patients. Other agencies set the level for an MCI at five, seven, or more patients. In situations involving a disaster, the number of patients can reach into the hundreds or thousands. In general practice, the accepted definition of an MCI is any incident that depletes the available on-scene resources at any given time. Using this criterion, a single ambulance with two paramedics that arrives at an MVC with four patients who are all in need of advanced life support (ALS) care would be an MCI by definition.

Each EMS system has a relatively finite capacity to manage an MCI. Some large urban departments can easily manage an MCI that would overwhelm a smaller department. However, generally speaking, an MCI can be classified as follows:

- **Low-impact incident.** A low-impact incident is one that can typically be managed by local emergency personnel. It may tax the local EMS system, but typically will not overwhelm it. Examples include a motor vehicle collision with multiple victims, a shooting with multiple victims, or similar scenarios.

- **High-impact incident.** A high-impact incident is one that stresses local emergency resources including fire, police, and EMS as well as local hospitals. Examples include tornadoes, structural collapse, floods, and similar scenarios.

- **Disaster.** A disaster is an event that overwhelms regional emergency response resources. Examples include hurricanes, earthquakes, and major floods. Terrorist acts can also result in disaster situations.

In this chapter, you will learn about the EMS response to MCIs as well as response to disasters in general, which may or may not generate casualties. The same techniques and tools used to respond to a multiple-patient MVC will be used to manage a more extensive MCI. Command-and-control concepts that have evolved during the past 25 years to help facilitate the organization and eventual control of such responses will be discussed. The special considerations involved in disaster management will appear near the end of the chapter.

ORIGINS OF EMERGENCY INCIDENT MANAGEMENT

Based on the confusion surrounding several major fires and other large-scale incidents in the 1970s, the fire service, particularly in the Southern California area, took the lead in organizing responses to large-scale emergencies. This later evolved into a

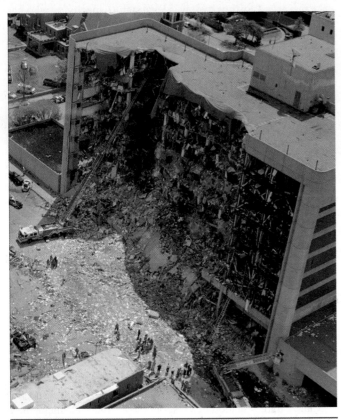

● **Figure 3-1** The scene of the April 19, 1995, bombing of the Alfred P. Murrah Federal Building in Oklahoma City. (© AP Images)

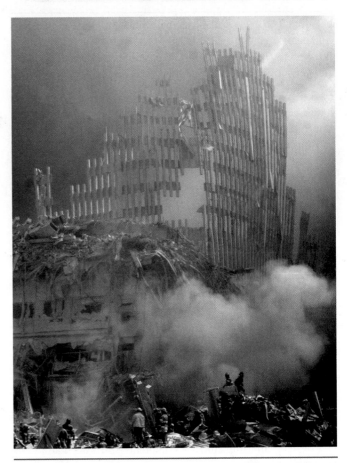

● **Figure 3-2** The attacks on the World Trade Center and the Pentagon on September 11, 2001, will forever change the way mass-casualty incidents are handled. (© AP Images/Shawn Baldwin)

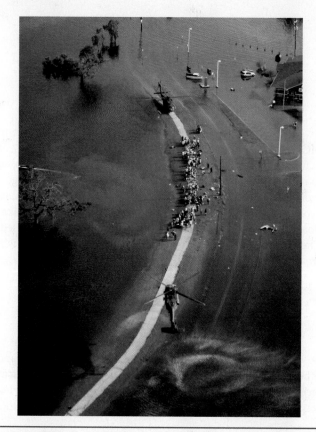

● **Figure 3-3** Hurricane Katrina, which struck the central Gulf coast on August 29, 2005, was one of the worst natural disasters in U.S. history. It also exposed flaws in the national disaster support system. *(© AP Images/David J. Phillip)*

All EMS agencies need to be aware of the requirements for NIMS compliance because, in the future, federal funding for disaster response and other federal funding may be withheld from any jurisdiction that fails to adopt such a system for response to emergencies. The Internet and the speed at which information can now flow is a great tool to learn the needs of your agency's efforts to remain in compliance with the NIMS and to get your agency to the point at which you are able to integrate with any level of response needed, whether it be to a large-scale local-level MCI, such as the school bus accident described in the case study, or an "incident of national significance" such as Hurricanes Katrina and Rita or another territory's attack on America.

Regulations and Standards

The uniform practices followed in incident management stem from a variety of sources. Prior to the Homeland Security Presidential Directive #5 (HSPD5), which prescribed the National Incident Management System, the only federal requirement for use of IMS fell under the Occupational Safety and Health Administration (OSHA) regulations requiring "the use of a site-specific ICS" during an emergency response to the release of hazardous substances, more often known as a hazmat response.[1] The OSHA regulations were mirrored by Environmental Protection Agency regulations that forced the adoption of this type of management system by all states, regardless of their OSHA status.

In addition, various states have passed laws requiring the use of the IMS. As a paramedic, you should research whether such laws exist in your state. Pay particular attention to the presence of a **scene-authority law**, a legal statute specifying who has ultimate authority at an incident.

National **consensus standards**, or widely agreed-on guidelines, have been developed by the National Fire Protection Association (NFPA) and other such entities. Although these standards are not laws, nor are they regulations, some of these may recommend practices for use at MCIs. Many of these standards, with which you should be familiar, include the ones that relate to hazardous materials incidents (as will be discussed in Chapter 5), health and safety, and disaster management. Such standards are being continually reviewed in the post-September 11 world because the rules of the game have changed seemingly overnight with regard to the response to such incidents. To be more prepared for a large-scale event, a robust day-to-day response system needs to be developed and must be practiced in order to be effective when needed.

Although there is no true national standard curriculum for implementing an IMS, several model curricula are available, such as those taught by the National Fire Academy in Emmitsburg, Maryland, and further by the National Wildland Coordinating Group (NWCG), a consortium of wildland firefighting service members from throughout the United States. The reason that many of the concepts of IMS have evolved from the wildland world is simply that the incidents they tend to respond to get very large very fast and then, once controlled, require a rapid fold-up of operations. The use of a solid and standardized IMS allows for the easy and rapid escalation of a response to a large-scale incident.

Since the publication of HSPD5, many pieces of guidance and direction have been issued by the USDHS related specifically to the training requirements for the implementation of NIMS. Many pre-September 11 courses have been updated and/or

statewide system that became known as FIRE SCOPE. This system then began to be exported into other major areas around and throughout the United States. Each area had its own way of doing things and more or less adopted the basic tenets of the system that had become known as the **Incident Command System (ICS)**. In essence, ICS is a management system or philosophy that takes the basic tenets of good, sound management and adapts them to the needs of the emergency scene. ICS was designed for controlling, directing, and coordinating emergency response resources in, as much as possible, an effective manner. Although the ICS was originally developed for use at major fires, a standardized ICS, or **Incident Management System (IMS)**, has been adopted by law enforcement, EMS, hospitals, and industry.

In recent years, particularly in the months since the terrorist attacks against the United States on September 11, 2001, the various versions of the ICS or IMS in use in the United States have been merged into the comprehensive, standardized **National Incident Management System (NIMS)**. NIMS was prescribed by way of a Homeland Security Presidential Directive (HSPD), which will, in time, require that all emergency services agencies develop and implement a comprehensive IMS that adopts the standards as prescribed by the **Department of Homeland Security (DHS)**. Since the NIMS was formally introduced to the United States response community, much guidance and direction have been provided to all manner of response agencies for compliance with the requirements of NIMS.

The National Incident Management System

Following the attacks on the United States on September 11, 2001, and with the establishment of a federal Department of Homeland Security, it became clear that we needed an Incident Management System that was effective for, and understood by, all agencies who might respond to a disaster or MCI. The National Incident Management System (NIMS) was developed to provide a common system that emergency service agencies can use at local, state, and federal levels. It is a model for an IMS that is driven by Homeland Security Presidential Directive #5 (HSPD5), as discussed in the text. This directive was issued on February 28, 2003, and was intended to enhance the ability of the United States to manage **domestic incidents** *by establishing a single, comprehensive National Incident Management System.*

NIMS consists of five major subsystems that collectively provide for a total system approach to all hazards and risk management:

- *The Incident Management System (IMS)—includes operating requirements, eight interactive components, and procedures for organizing and operating an on-scene management structure*
- *Training—standardized teaching that supports the effective operations of NIMS*
- *Qualifications and certification system—provides for personnel across the nation to meet standard training, experience, and physical requirements to fill specific positions in the ICS*
- *Publications management—includes development, publication, and distribution of NIMS materials*
- *Supporting technologies—includes satellite remote imaging, sophisticated communications systems, and geographic information systems that support NIMS operations*

The U.S. Department of Homeland Security has recognized the value that incident management provides in the response both to natural disasters and to potential large-scale terrorist acts. They have used the experiences of the fire and other emergency services to produce and refine a standardized and national approach to major incident response. The concept of a national standard for incident response ensures that when services respond to disasters distant from their normal service area, all parties will be using the same terminology and the same response structure.

NIMS ensures that interservice and incident-wide communications are standardized so agency managers can get an accurate and complete picture of the incident's nature and scope. Additionally, NIMS ensures that communication with the public is timely, accurate, and appropriate. Because much of NIMS is derived from the concepts of the more established IMS and incorporates much of the ICS currently used by the nation's fire and emergency services, this should mean little change for most EMS providers participating in incident responses.

NIMS has the ability to place all members of the response continuum—including those not usually involved in emergency services activities in a field mode, such as public health—on the same page with a common system of command, control, communications, and coordination of emergency incidents.

otherwise revised so that they are now seen as NIMS compliant. Much of that guidance may be found online at the NIMS Integration Center (NIC website). This site (http://www.fema.gov/emergency/nims/index.shtm) should be reviewed periodically by every emergency responder to determine what changes have been made to NIMS and the related compliance documents that are found on the NIC website.

A Uniform, Flexible System

With its uniform terminology and approach, the National Incident Management System has a number of advantages over the multitudes of currently existing IMSs that developed during past decades. First, NIMS recognizes that an incident can and will cross jurisdictional and geographic boundaries, and the use of a standardized and compatible management system will permit a well-organized response to routine and large-scale emergencies. The single best example of this was the devastating hurricane season of 2005 with Hurricanes Katrina and Rita. Many states were affected by these two storms and, in fact, by the end of the response to both of these events all 50 states and all 6 U.S. territories would be integrated into the massive responses. Recovery from those events is still not complete. Second, the NIMS has the flexibility to respond to emergencies in both the public and private sectors and incorporates concepts of business continuity and crisis management employed by the private sector to ensure the necessary continuity and continuance of critical operations.

Also, remember that a key element in the management of any incident that spans jurisdictions is the **mutual aid coordination center (MACC)**, formerly referred to as the **emergency operations center (EOC)**. The MACC is a site from which civil government officials (e.g., municipal, county, state, and/or federal) exercise direction and control in an emergency or disaster. From this site, management and support personnel carry out coordinated emergency response activities. The MACC may be a dedicated facility or an office, conference room, or other predesignated location having appropriate communications and informational materials to carry out the assigned emergency response mission. When possible, the MACC should be located in a secure and protected location.

To familiarize yourself with the concepts, structure, and practices of both NIMS and the ICS, which is the fundamental tenet of NIMS, the following sections of this chapter will focus on the major functional areas of NIMS and ICS. Use the mnemonic **C-FLOP** to keep these areas in mind as you read. The letters stand for:

C—Command

F—Finance/administration

L—Logistics

O—Operations

P—Planning

COMMAND

The most important functional area in the Incident Management System is **command**. The **incident commander (IC)** is the individual who essentially runs the entire incident. The IC has the full legal authority and, in most cases, all of the associated liabilities of dealing with this incident.

The most critical concept to grasp about command is this: *The ultimate authority for decision making rests with the incident commander. The IC is responsible for coordinating the many activities that occur on the emergency scene. Because it would be too confusing or impossible for all on-scene personnel to report directly to the IC, the person charged with command delegates certain functions and responsibilities to others.* In this way, the IC maintains a reasonable **span of control**, or number of people or tasks that a single individual can monitor. Depending on the complexity of a given operation, the overall scope of the incident, and the resources that are available to the IC, the span of control may range from three to seven people, with the optimal span of control for most emergency operations being five.

The important thing to bear in mind regarding span of control is that the more risky any given task or operation is, the more tightly must be the span of control. Those operations that put operational personnel in the greatest physical danger *must* be supervised by both qualified and competent persons and they *must* have the right numbers of the right qualified and competent personnel operating under them to ensure that all operations are conducted in an environment that is as safe as possible.

Establishing Command

As already mentioned, the determination of when to establish command and when to declare an MCI will vary from agency to agency. The formal declaration of an MCI may occur as soon as an incident reaches a certain patient count or when some other predetermined condition has been met that makes scene management challenging or significantly taxes the available resources of a system. Generally, when any two or more units respond to an emergency, when casualties include two or more patients, or if multiple agencies are involved in response to the incident, you should implement IMS.

As a rule, the first-arriving public safety unit should establish command (Figure 3-4 ●). This may or may not be the first-arriving EMS unit, and it may or may not be from the agency that has the legal authority to establish command for the type of incident in question. On arrival, the IC will do a **windshield survey** of the scene. As you already know, EMS providers should never exit the vehicle until they have identified any and all potential hazards of the incident to the extent possible from inside their vehicle. At an MVC, for example, do not miss the vehicle partially hidden in the woods or the pool of gasoline near your vehicle. Once you have determined the visible scope of an incident and any obvious hazards, relay this information to dispatch and all other responding units and agencies.

Incident Size-Up

Size-up is a concept that is widely taught to fire personnel. However, it is often not taught to EMS personnel in this context. Regardless, it has application in any emergency response

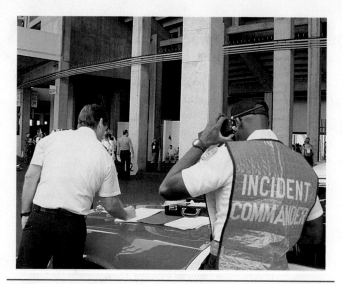

● **Figure 3-4** The first on-scene unit must assume command and direct all rescue efforts at a multiple-casualty incident.

situation. A size-up is simply a formal evaluation of the situation surrounding an incident. It is an integral part of establishing command at any incident and is an integral component of the management of an MCI. The initial size-up, as well as ongoing size-ups, are key in ensuring that both the operational personnel and the IC have a high level of **situational awareness**. This will keep personnel out of danger and help keep them aware of the hazards that they are likely to encounter on an incident scene. It is vital that EMS responders maintain a good operational picture and situational awareness at all times when operating on any emergency scene.

During the initial and ongoing size-ups, you must keep in mind the three main priorities of all emergency services operations:

● Life safety
● Incident stabilization
● Property conservation

Life Safety

Life safety is always the top priority in response to any incident. If you arrive first on the scene of a high-impact incident, you must observe and protect all rescuers, including yourself, from hazards. Then and only then will you attend to patients who are in immediately life-threatening situations. At this point, keep in mind that the needs of the many usually outweigh the needs of the few. If you commit to caring for the first patient you encounter, you may neglect ten other critical patients lying nearby—some of whom may be more salvageable than the first one you came across.

If you are the IC, remember that responsibility for triage belongs to the **triage officer**. At a small-scale incident, the IC may end up triaging some patients. Even so, the triage officer assumes the main responsibility for sorting patients into categories based on the severity of their injuries.

Depending on the scope of the incident and local protocols, you and your partner will most likely fill the roles of incident commander and triage officer if you are the first public safety unit on the scene. These designations will remain in place at least until other units arrive.

Never forget the importance of establishing command early in an incident.

Incident Stabilization

While attending to the first priority, life safety, all response personnel should also keep in mind the second priority, incident stabilization. To achieve this goal, quickly identify whether the situation is an open incident or a closed incident. An **open incident**, also known as an *uncontained incident*, has the potential to generate more patients at any time. A fire that traps people inside an office building is an example. You may find only a few patients when you arrive on scene. However, other patients, including firefighters injured during incident operations, may soon appear. Consequently, the IC must anticipate the need for additional resources. Whenever you find yourself in command of an open incident, remember this point: It is better to call too many resources than too few; you can always send them home.

In the case of a **closed incident**, or *contained incident*, the injuries have usually already occurred by the time you arrive on scene. An example might be a multiple-vehicle collision. However, even a so-called closed incident carries the potential for additional hazards such as an undetected gas leak, a distraught family member who rushes into traffic, or further injury to patients wandering about the scene and, of course, injuries to responders during the course of incident operations. As a result, it makes sense for an IC to expend effort in stabilizing an incident. Preventing further injuries, either of patients or of rescue personnel, helps to ensure smoother and more successful management of an MCI.

Property Conservation

As with any other call, the third priority of an IC is conservation of property. At no time during an operation should rescue personnel damage property unless it is absolutely necessary for achieving the first two priorities: life safety and incident stabilization. Property conservation should include protection of the environment where operations are staged.

Most MCIs are "won or lost" in the first 10 minutes. Without the establishment of incident command, emergency personnel may begin to "freelance." They may fail to prioritize patients, underestimate the severity of the incident, or delay requesting additional resources. Successful handing of any MCI involves coordination of all key personnel, whether 2 people or 20.

Singular versus Unified Command

Most agencies have a single person who is the agency's highest-ranking official. That person carries the authority to administer the agency in full on a day-to-day basis, without question. However, in the case of nearly all evolving incidents, command is established by the first-arriving public safety official. This will generally be the way things work at all smaller-scale incidents with limited jurisdictional issues. This type of command is called **singular command**, and it usually works out well for all concerned. Singular command incidents usually have a smaller scope than an MCI and usually do not involve outside agencies. For example, a traffic collision may involve the local fire department, EMS, and police department. Prior to the incident, the three agencies involved might have agreed that the fire department will assume overall command of this type of incident, thus creating a singular command situation.

In many incidents, however, a singular command will not be feasible because of overlapping responsibilities or jurisdictions. Instead, a **unified command** will be established. Examples of incidents in which unified command is used include terrorist attacks, explosions, sniper or hostage situations, and large-scale natural disasters. In each of these examples, the managers from several agencies, such as law enforcement, fire, and EMS at multiple jurisdictional levels of government (local, state, and federal), will coordinate their activities and share command responsibilities for the overall incident while also maintaining control of their respective agencies.

In establishing a unified command, the managers of the respective agencies and jurisdictions try to achieve balanced decision making. Together, they identify and access the appropriate agencies or specialized organizations that might be needed at the scene, such as the American Red Cross, the local health department, or public works. They also create divisions of labor on the basis of reasonable and accepted spans of control.

Finally, the incident commander determines the need for an information officer to interact with the media as well as a liaison officer to deal with all the agencies and organizations that will undoubtedly respond to any incident of significance. At any complex incident that in time will involve multiple agencies and may well be multijurisdictional in nature, the issue of command will be complicated. The decision to remain in a singular command structure or to move to a unified command structure will depend greatly on the scope and nature of the incident and may well be dictated by legislation—as is usually the case in incidents known to be or suspected to be related to terrorism—or the decision may be dictated by a preexisting disaster plan. (The importance of planning will be discussed later in this chapter.)

When an incident is of such a magnitude that the incident commander deems it necessary, he may direct that an **incident command post (ICP)** be established on or near the incident scene. The ICP provides a place where representatives and officers from the various agencies involved in the incident can meet with one another and make relevant decisions. Because an ICP may operate continuously for days or weeks, the site for the ICP should be selected carefully. Access to telephones, restrooms, and shelters should be taken into account. Also, the command post should be close enough to the scene that officers can easily monitor scene operations but far enough away so that they are outside the direct operational area. Persons operating on the scene, members of the media, and bystanders should not have routine access to the ICP.

Identifying a Staging Area

Identification of a staging area goes hand in hand with the scene assessment. At MCIs involving hazardous materials or structural fires, for example, you must note wind speed and direction. The IC must ensure that the staging area and ICP lie well beyond the reach of any fumes, smoke, water, chemicals, or other hazardous materials.

Once you establish command of an MCI, you should also designate both a primary and a secondary staging area. In picking a primary site, keep in mind the main purpose of a staging area: organization of resources in one place for quick and easy deployment throughout the incident. Position the primary staging area as close to the scene as possible without compromising the safety of the responders and resources placed in staging. Make sure the site has good access and exit points to ensure the flow of emergency vehicles.

If required, the secondary staging area should ideally be located in a different area from the primary staging area. This will provide the IC with a contingency plan in case the primary staging area becomes unusable. Conditions that may force a change in staging areas include altered traffic patterns, shifts in wind direction, or restricted access due to the deployment of fire hoses or other special equipment.

Incident Communications

Communications forms the cornerstone of the IMS. Once command is established, the IC has a responsibility to relay this information to dispatch. Then, as soon as possible, the IC should transmit a preliminary report that includes the following data: type of incident, approximate number of patients by priority, request for additional resources, staging instructions, and a plan of action. If a fixed incident command post has been set up, the IC should communicate the location of this site as well.

Once an MCI has been declared, further communications should be moved to a secondary, or tactical, channel. The IC must be able to supply the information necessary to coordinate resources. That is the whole purpose of the IMS. Use of a secondary channel will also prevent an IC from interfering with the communications by other jurisdictions and agencies or from overwhelming the primary EMS channel. Communications and interoperability issues are generally cited as the main reasons for problems in both exercises of disaster plans and in actual incidents.

When you act as an IC, remember that communications will involve units from different jurisdictions and perhaps different districts. One of the foundations of any incident management is the use of a common terminology. When communicating, you should eliminate all radio codes and use only plain English. A radio code may have different meanings in different places. As an IC, you must eliminate any unnecessary confusion in an already complicated situation. In fact, it may be preferable to avoid radio codes even in routine operations. Then there will be no need to even think about switching to plain English when you assume command of an MCI.

Resource Utilization

Few EMS departments have the resources to handle an MCI without outside help. Regardless of the nature of an incident, most units will need additional ambulances, personnel, equipment, and medical supplies. In many cases, they will also require specialized equipment and perhaps the help of public or private agencies.

The primary role of an IC is the strategic deployment of all necessary resources at an incident. Development of a strategy means setting goals and determining the tactics needed to

accomplish these goals. Because of the complicated nature of an MCI, the IC must continually assess the effectiveness of a given strategy or plan.

To ensure flexibility, an IC should radio a brief progress report to the dispatcher approximately every 10 minutes until the incident has been stabilized. The report should state established goals, tactics, and resources being used to meet these goals, and any progress or lack of progress. This forces an IC to monitor an operation, to adapt tactics or resources to changing circumstances, and to eliminate ineffective tactics entirely. Subordinates should deliver similar reports to the IC so he can properly evaluate the overall operation.

Command Procedures

Several procedures help an IC manage an MCI. First and foremost, all personnel must be able to recognize the IC and the ICP once it is established. At smaller, single-agency events, everyone may know the IC simply by his voice over the radio. However, at medium or large-scale incidents, such recognition is often impossible. As a result, the IMS calls for the IC and other officers to wear special reflective vests (Figure 3-5 ●). The vests can be color coded to functional areas and may have the officer's title on the front and back. Such vests should be worn whenever IMS is used, even at smaller incidents. By making a basic set of vests available on every response unit—especially for command and triage—personnel will get in the habit of wearing and/or recognizing the vests prior to a major incident.

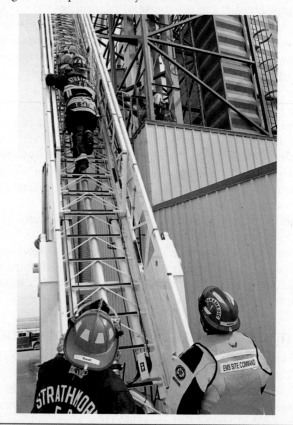

● **Figure 3-5** Using a command vest at a multiple-casualty incident makes it easier to identify personnel. The incident commander directs the response and coordinates resources. (© *Kevin Link*)

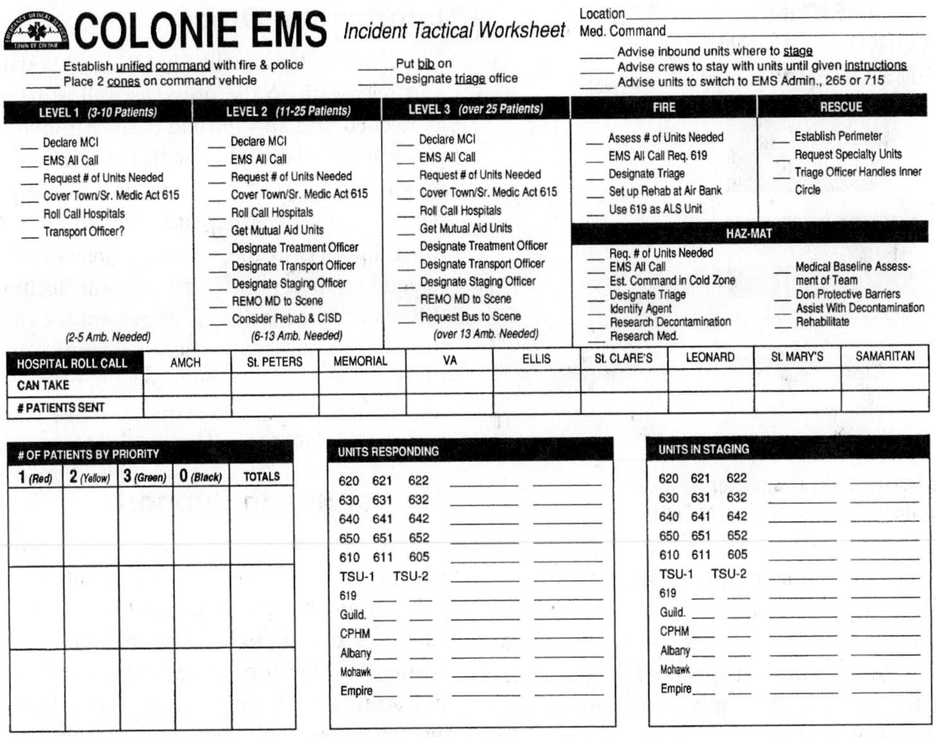

COLONIE EMS *Incident Tactical Worksheet*

Location _____
Med. Command _____

___ Establish unified command with fire & police
___ Place 2 cones on command vehicle
___ Put bib on
___ Designate triage office
___ Advise inbound units where to stage
___ Advise crews to stay with units until given instructions
___ Advise units to switch to EMS Admin., 265 or 715

LEVEL 1 (3-10 Patients)	LEVEL 2 (11-25 Patients)	LEVEL 3 (over 25 Patients)	FIRE	RESCUE
__ Declare MCI	__ Declare MCI	__ Declare MCI	__ Assess # of Units Needed	__ Establish Perimeter
__ EMS All Call	__ EMS All Call	__ EMS All Call	__ EMS All Call Req. 619	__ Request Specialty Units
__ Request # of Units Needed	__ Request # of Units Needed	__ Request # of Units Needed	__ Designate Triage	__ Triage Officer Handles Inner Circle
__ Cover Town/Sr. Medic Act 615	__ Cover Town/Sr. Medic Act 615	__ Cover Town/Sr. Medic Act 615	__ Set up Rehab at Air Bank	
__ Roll Call Hospitals	__ Roll Call Hospitals	__ Roll Call Hospitals	__ Use 619 as ALS Unit	
__ Transport Officer?	__ Get Mutual Aid Units	__ Get Mutual Aid Units		

HAZ-MAT

__ Req. # of Units Needed		__ Medical Baseline Assessment of Team
__ EMS All Call		__ Don Protective Barriers
__ Est. Command in Cold Zone		__ Assist With Decontamination
__ Designate Triage		__ Rehabilitate
__ Identify Agent		
__ Research Decontamination		
__ Research Med.		

LEVEL 2 (continued): __ Designate Treatment Officer, __ Designate Transport Officer, __ Designate Staging Officer, __ REMO MD to Scene, __ Consider Rehab & CISD

LEVEL 3 (continued): __ Designate Treatment Officer, __ Designate Transport Officer, __ Designate Staging Officer, __ REMO MD to Scene, __ Request Bus to Scene

(2-5 Amb. Needed)   (6-13 Amb. Needed)   (over 13 Amb. Needed)

HOSPITAL ROLL CALL	AMCH	St. PETERS	MEMORIAL	VA	ELLIS	St. CLARE'S	LEONARD	St. MARY'S	SAMARITAN
CAN TAKE									
# PATIENTS SENT									

 # OF PATIENTS BY PRIORITY

1 (Red)	2 (Yellow)	3 (Green)	0 (Black)	TOTALS

UNITS RESPONDING

620 621 622 ____
630 631 632 ____
640 641 642 ____
650 651 652 ____
610 611 605 ____
TSU-1 TSU-2
619
Guild. ___ ___ ___
CPHM ___ ___ ___
Albany ___ ___ ___
Mohawk ___ ___ ___
Empire ___ ___ ___

UNITS IN STAGING

620 621 622 ____
630 631 632 ____
640 641 642 ____
650 651 652 ____
610 611 605 ____
TSU-1 TSU-2
619
Guild. ___ ___ ___
CPHM ___ ___ ___
Albany ___ ___ ___
Mohawk ___ ___ ___
Empire ___ ___ ___

● **Figure 3-6** An incident tactical worksheet from the Town of Colonie (New York) EMS.

An IC can also benefit from the use of a worksheet or clipboard, two useful tools for tracking decisions and actions (Figure 3-6 ●). An IMS worksheet should include basic information on the incident, a small area to sketch the scene, and a checklist of important items to remember. It might also include a section to record the on-scene units and personnel, their assignments, and relevant patient information, particularly transport data. Many commercial products are currently available for this purpose, including programs for generating worksheets by computer.

You will find a worksheet especially useful when transferring command, as often happens when higher-ranking officers arrive on scene. Command is transferred only face to face, with the current IC conducting a short but complete briefing on the incident status. A higher-ranking officer does not become IC simply by his arrival; a briefing must take place. The worksheet serves as an outline for the briefing.

Termination of Command

As the incident progresses, resources will be reassigned or released. For example, an IC who transfers command to a higher-ranking officer may become an aide to the new IC or be assigned to a totally new IMS role. Eventually resources will be **demobilized**, or released for use elsewhere in the EMS system. Once the incident has progressed to the point at which the IMS is no longer needed, command should be terminated. A final progress report should be delivered to the communications center. All units will then return to routine rules of operation.

The point at which command terminates depends on the incident. Some high-impact incidents, such as natural disasters or terrorist events, may last for weeks. However, not all agencies may have a significant presence for the long term. EMS may have a strong initial response, for example, but may simply have a single ambulance stand by for the long term. Other agencies may be released entirely from the incident if their services are no longer needed.

SUPPORT OF INCIDENT COMMAND

As noted earlier, incident command—the C in C-FLOP—is supported by four sections or functional areas:

- Finance/administration
- Logistics
- Operations
- Planning

Each section has a place within the IMS and is headed by a **section chief**. All these areas have functions that will in some way, shape, or form be fulfilled in every emergency response, even in a day-to-day-type response. However, all four areas may not be formally established at every incident. At small- or medium-sized incidents, for example, operations may be the only section implemented. At large-scale or long-term incidents, the IMS may activate the areas of finance/administration, logistics, and planning. Depending on the type of incident and the structure of command, these sections may not be filled with EMS personnel. However, they may help coordinate some EMS activities.

In addition, several important officers may report directly to the incident commander. These officers handle information, safety, outside liaisons, and mental health support. Together they are known as the **command staff**. The combination of

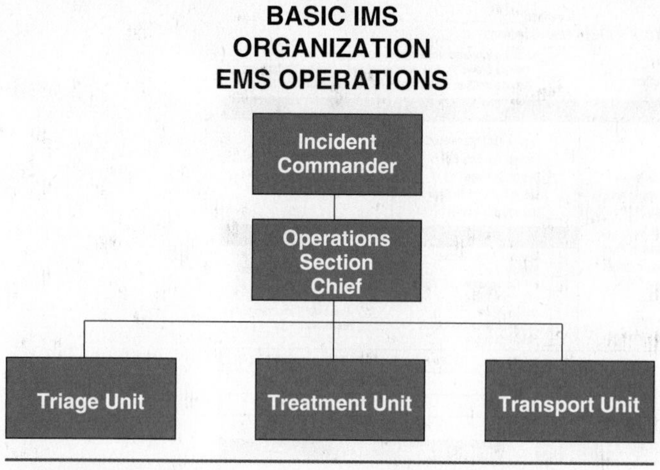

BASIC IMS ORGANIZATION EMS OPERATIONS

● **Figure 3-7** Basic Incident Management System organization for a small- to medium-sized incident.

command staff and section chiefs comprises and carries out what are called **staff functions**.

As a paramedic, it is more important for you to know how the IMS works than to be an expert in specific job functions. Figure 3-7 ● and the following sections give you a quick overview of the basic elements of the IMS.

Command Staff

The establishment and role of command have already been described. However, the command staff can play an important role in supporting the incident commander, particularly at major incidents or disasters. Therefore, you should be familiar with the roles of the following command staff officers.

Safety Officer

The **safety officer (SO)** may hold the most important role at an MCI. This person or, in some cases, team of people monitors all on-scene actions and ensures that they do not create any potentially harmful conditions. Because almost anything that happens at an incident is potentially harmful, the SO assumes an enormous responsibility. Some of the areas that must be monitored for safety compliance include infection control, use of personal protective equipment, crowd control, lifting of patients and equipment, and quality of scene lighting. Under the IMS, the SO has the authority to stop any action that is deemed an immediate life threat with no further action needed. In other words, the SO may at any time terminate any operations at the incident on his authority alone. This authority must be seen as an absolute if the safety of the incident is to be ensured.

Liaison Officer

The **liaison officer (LO)** coordinates all incident operations that involve outside agencies. These agencies may include other emergency services, disaster support networks, private industry representatives, government agencies, and more. As the title implies, the LO makes sure these outside agencies are connected with the appropriate functional areas within the IMS. This ensures, based on requests and reports from the incident commander, that specialized resources are deployed effectively.

Information Officer

The **information officer (IO)** collects data about the incident and releases it to the press, as well as to other agencies, on an as-needed and appropriate basis. Although you may not have a preexisting relationship with the media in your community, a major incident will put your unit in the public spotlight. Your department's image depends on favorable exposure in the media. More important, the safety and reassurance of the public may depend on their receiving timely and accurate information about the event. As a result, it is important for an IMS to have an effective IO. In any large-scale, high-impact incident where a large press presence can be expected, appointment of a specific public information officer (PIO) may also be made; in that instance, the PIO would report to the IO for coordination of information flow.

Mental Health Support

A large incident has the capacity to overwhelm resources and tax personnel, both physically and mentally. Thus, it is important to continually rotate personnel in and out of the event to allow adequate rest. Personnel should be evaluated periodically to ensure that they are not exhibiting signs or symptoms of excessive stress or abnormal stress reactions. Persons exhibiting abnormal stress should be removed from service. Critical incident stress management is no longer recommended. Instead, support and mental health personnel should provide "psychological first aid." This entails simply providing for the rescuer's immediate needs (food, water, rest)—not attempting to provide therapy or forcing personnel to talk.

All EMS agencies should have a licensed mental health professional affiliated with the organization. For large-scale events, it would be prudent to have this person respond and assist in screening personnel for excessive stress. The mental health professional must understand the work and the culture and be able to screen personnel who are showing maladaptive stress reactions and refer them to competent mental health personnel for additional evaluation and care.

The following general guidelines are recommended for organizational response to stressful events.

Small Incidents The mental health needs of those involved in small incidents, including those that result in the death of colleagues, should be handled by competent mental health personnel, as follows:

● Psychological first aid should be provided.

● Debriefing and defusing should not be provided.

● Mental health personnel should screen affected personnel for up to two months following the incident for abnormal responses to stress.

● Personnel not adapting normally should be referred to competent personnel for accepted forms of therapy.

Major Incidents/Disasters The stress of major events can be mitigated by several strategies:

● Proper use of the IMS

● Rotating personnel in and out of the disaster scene

● Providing psychological first aid

- Not providing debriefing or defusing
- Constant surveillance of personnel by competent mental health personnel for signs of stress
- Postincident surveillance of involved personnel by competent mental health personnel

Finance/Administration

The **finance/administration section** rarely operates on small-scale incidents, even though financial considerations are obviously important in all day-to-day incidents. However, on large-scale or long-term incidents, the finance/administration staff supports command by assuming responsibility for all accounting and administrative activities. This section keeps personnel and time records. It also estimates costs, pays claims, and handles procurement of items required at the incident. These functions are usually performed by the jurisdictional government where the incident has occurred. The need for accuracy in the work of this unit cannot be overstressed, because a large-scale response may be eligible for reimbursements from federal or other disaster funding sources. Such reimbursements will depend directly on the ability of the agencies involved to document expenses, particularly those that are above and beyond normal operational expenditures.

Logistics

The **logistics section** supports incident operations. One of its most critical functions is operating the **medical supply unit**. This unit coordinates procurement and distribution of equipment and supplies at an MCI. Depending on the structure of the IMS used, other units may also be established by the logistics section. The **facilities unit**, for example, selects and maintains areas used for command and rehabilitation. It makes sure that adequate food, water, restrooms, lighting, power, and so on are available to support incident operations. Other units might be set up to manage field communications, on-scene medical care for workers, and other functions.

Operations

Whatever work needs to be performed at an incident takes place under the **operations section**. This section carries out tactical objectives, directs front-end activities, participates in planning, modifies the action plan, maintains discipline, and accounts for personnel. In short, the operations section gets the job done.

As will be explained later in the chapter, the operations section may have many **branches**, which are functional levels based on primary roles or geographic locations. Branches organized by role might include sections within the various jurisdictions at an incident: EMS, rescue, fire, law enforcement, and so on. Branches based on geography might include operations at various locations. The IMS structure used at the 1993 bombing of the World Trade Center, for example, assigned a branch of operations to each building in the complex.

Planning/Intelligence

The **planning/intelligence section** provides past, present, and future information about an incident. The planning section helps formulate the overall incident action plan (IAP) and oversees changes in that plan. It collects information such as weather reports, documents incident actions, and develops contingency plans. It ensures that written standard operating procedures (SOPs) for **mutual aid agreements** that govern sharing of departmental resources are activated or fulfilled.

The planning/intelligence section operates according to the principle of "anything that can go wrong will go wrong." The staff uses past incidents to anticipate trouble that might arise at the current incident. The section then acts accordingly. When the command and operations sections must change tactics, the planning section stands ready to provide the necessary strategic support.

DIVISION OF OPERATIONS FUNCTIONS

As already noted, getting organized quickly and early is essential to the success of any IMS operation. There are several ways to divide functions at an incident. The choice of organization depends on the scope of an incident and its associated strategic goals, the structure of your department, the implementation of singular or unified command, and so on.

If you are an incident commander, one of your jobs will be to organize line functions—that is, operations—in the most effective manner. To do this, you should become familiar with the basic functional levels within the IMS.

Branches

The incident commander or the comanagers of a unified command incident may choose to establish any number of branches. As mentioned, these branches may be organized by primary role or by geography. Branches are supervised by branch directors, who report to the section chief for that particular functional area. The EMS branch director supervises all operations involved with patient care and transportation. Figure 3-8 ● shows the functional levels within a typical EMS branch. Depending on the system and the scope and magnitude of the incident, rescue may be an independent branch or it may report to the director of the EMS or fire branch.

Groups and Divisions

Branches may be further organized into groups and divisions—working areas of an incident where specific job tasks are accomplished. Groups are based on function, whereas divisions are based on geography. As an example, think of triage as a group and the responders working on the third floor of a multiple-floor incident as a division. Groups and divisions are managed by supervisors who, in turn, report to the branch director.

Units

Groups and divisions can be broken into even more task-specific groups known as units. They are supervised by unit leaders, who report to the supervisor of a group or division.

IMS EMS BRANCH

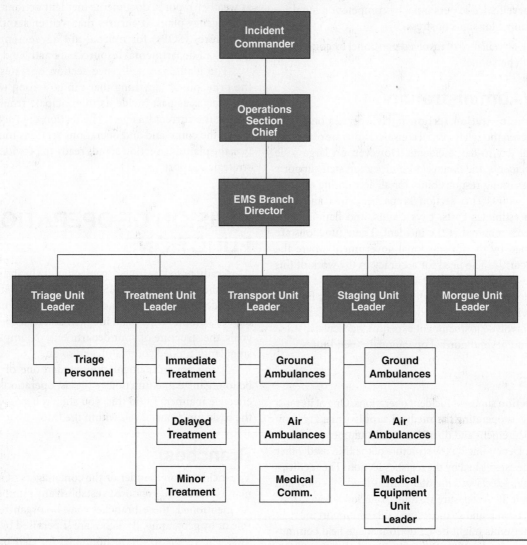

- **Figure 3-8** Example of branches that may operate during a major incident.

Sectors

Depending on the type of IMS used in your area, you may hear the term **sector** used. A sector is an interchangeable name for a branch, group, or division. However, it does not designate a functional or geographic area. Although there is no formal name for individuals who supervise a sector, they are often called sector officers.

FUNCTIONAL GROUPS WITH AN EMS BRANCH

The IMS operates under the so-called toolbox theory: Do not remove a tool from the toolbox unless you actually need to use it. The flexibility of IMS is founded on the ability to implement only the areas of IMS that are needed at an incident. This theory holds for all areas of IMS, including branches, groups, sectors, divisions, and specific areas where EMS operates. At many EMS incidents, the basic IMS organization—triage, treatment, and transport (review Figure 3-7)—will be all the "tools" you need.

Triage

As you have read, **triage** is the act of sorting patients based on the severity of their injuries. The objective of emergency medical services at an MCI is to do the most good for the most people. For this reason, you need to determine which patients need immediate care to live, which patients will live despite delays in care, and which patients will die despite receiving medical care.

Because triage will drive subsequent incident operations, it is one of the first functions performed at an MCI. As a result, all personnel should be trained in triage techniques and all response units should carry triage equipment. The **triage group supervisor** may act independently or may supervise the triage group or triage sector.

Primary and Secondary Triage

Triage occurs in phases. **Primary triage** takes place early in the incident, when you first contact patients. The action provides a basic categorization of sustained injuries. It must be done quickly and efficiently so that command can determine on-site treatment needs and resources. Universally recognized triage categories include the following:

Category	Color	Priority
Immediate	Red	Priority-1 (P-1)
Delayed	Yellow	Priority-2 (P-2)
Minimal	Green	Priority-3 (P-3)
Expectant	Black	Priority-0 (P-0)

The category names have the following meanings: *Immediate* means the patient should receive immediate treatment; *delayed* means the patient's treatment may safely be delayed; *minimal* means the patient requires minimal or no treatment; *expectant* means the patient is expected to die or is deceased.

Secondary triage is ongoing and takes place throughout the incident as patients are collected, moved to treatment areas, given appropriate medical care, and, finally, transported off scene. A patient's condition may change over time, requiring you to upgrade or downgrade his triage category.

The START System

The most widely used triage system is **START**, an acronym for **S**imple **T**riage **a**nd **R**apid **T**ransport.[2-4] The system was developed at Hoag Memorial Hospital in Newport Beach, California. START's easy-to-use procedures allow for rapid sorting of patients into the categories listed earlier. START does not require a specific diagnosis on the part of the responder. Instead, it focuses on these areas (Figure 3-9 ●):

- Ability to walk
- Respiratory effort
- Pulses/perfusions
- Neurologic status

CONTENT REVIEW

► Signs in START

- Can get up and walk
- Open airway; respirations over 30/minute
- Radial pulse
- Follows commands

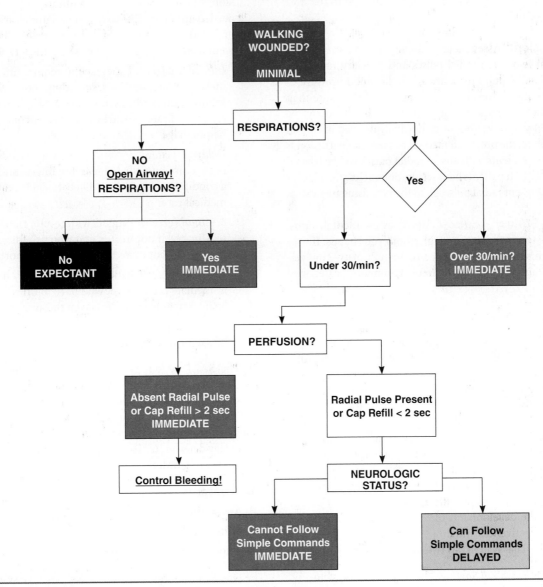

START TRIAGE SYSTEM

● **Figure 3-9**   Operation of the START system, the most widely used triage system.

Ability to Walk   You initiate the START system by asking patients who can walk to get up and come to you. Any patients who can complete these acts, despite their injuries, will be categorized Priority-3 or "green." Either you or another member of the triage group should place the appropriate tag on these patients. Because patients who can walk will walk, you should make every effort to confine them to one site. There is already enough confusion at an MCI without having the "walking wounded" wandering around the scene.

Respiratory Effort   Next, you begin to triage the nonwalking patients. Remember to keep the focus on tagging patients. Your only treatment effort should be directed toward correction of airway problems and severe bleeding.

Begin by assessing breathing effort. If patients are not breathing, open their airways manually. Categorize those patients who start to breathe spontaneously as Priority-1 or "red." Tag those who fail to respond as Priority-0 or "black." For those patients who are breathing, quickly assess their respiratory rates. Patients with respirations above 30 per minute should be tagged "red." If respirations are less than 30 per minute, go to the next assessment step.

Pulse/Perfusion   Assessment of circulatory status can be accomplished in two ways: radial pulses and capillary refill. The presence of a radial pulse indicates a systolic blood pressure of at least 90 mmHg. However, delayed capillary refill (more than 2 seconds) is a poor indicator of perfusion in adults. It can be compromised by cold weather or be normally delayed in certain people. Therefore, the preferred method of assessing perfusion is the radial pulse. Patients with absent radial pulses will be triaged Priority-1 or "red." If patients have respirations of less than 30 per minute *and* a present radial pulse, go to the next assessment step.

Neurologic Status   You now quickly assess mental status. Use this quick test. Ask patients to grip both your hands. If they can perform this simple task, categorize them Priority-2 or "yellow." If they cannot follow such simple commands, categorize them Priority-1 or "red."

The SALT System

In 2006, the Centers for Disease Control and Prevention (CDC) established and funded a working group to review the scientific literature on the various mass-casualty triage systems in use. The goal was to identify and recommend a mass-casualty triage system that could be adopted as a standard for the United States. This consensus group reviewed the major and minor triage systems in use and found little scientific support for any of these. The group then looked at the best practices of each system and created a proposed national triage system called **SALT** (**sort–assess–lifesaving interventions–treatment/transport**) **triage.**[5, 6] SALT is not age specific and can be used for all age groups. Since the development of SALT, several studies have looked at the effectiveness and utility of this triage scheme.

The SALT triage system has two phases (Figure 3-10 ●):

● **Step 1—SORT: Global Sorting.** The SALT triage system begins with a global sorting of patients in order to prioritize them for individual assessment. First, patients should be asked to walk to a designated area. Those able to walk are given the lowest priority (3rd) for individual assessment. Those who remain after the first group have walked away are asked to wave (or follow a similar command) or be observed for purposeful movement. Those who do not move (e.g., remain still) and those with obvious life threats (e.g., uncontrolled hemorrhage) are made the highest priority (1st) and should be assessed first. Those who could wave, yet who were unable to walk away are given the intermediate (2nd) priority. In summary, step 1 should result in the following categorization:

  ○ *Priority 1:* Still/obvious life threat
  ○ *Priority 2:* Wave/purposeful movement
  ○ *Priority 3:* Walk

● **Step 2—Assess: Individual Assessment.** During step 2, the first prority is to complete individual assessment of all victims to determine who needs lifesaving procedures (e.g., opening an airway, controlling major hemorrhage, decompressing a tension pneumothorax, or providing a needed antidote). Lifesaving interventions are to be completed before assigning a triage category. The SALT system uses five triage categories (Figure 3-11 ●):

  ○ *Immediate (red).* Patients who require immediate lifesaving interventions, including those who do not follow commands, do not have a peripheral pulse, are in respiratory distress, or have uncontrolled hemorrhage

  ○ *Delayed (yellow).* Patients who have injuries that do not require immediate lifesaving interventions, yet have a condition or conditions likely to deteriorate without medical care

  ○ *Minimal (green).* Patients with minor injuries that are self-limited if not treated and who can tolerate a delay in care without increasing their risk of mortality

  ○ *Expectant (gray).* Patients who would fall into the immediate category yet who have injuries that are felt to be incompatible wth life (given the available resources)

  ○ *Dead (black).* Patients who remain nonbreathing after lifesaving interventions

The SALT system is dynamic; triage assignment can be changed based on changing patient condition, scene resources, and scene safety. After patients categorized as immediate have been cared for, those categorized as expectant, dead, or minimal should be reassessed, as some patients may improve, whereas others may deteriorate. Treatment/transport should be provided in the following order:

1. Immediate
2. Delayed
3. Minimal
4. Expectant (if resources permit)

The effectiveness and utility of the SALT triage system remains to be seen. Unfortunately, until a national (or international)

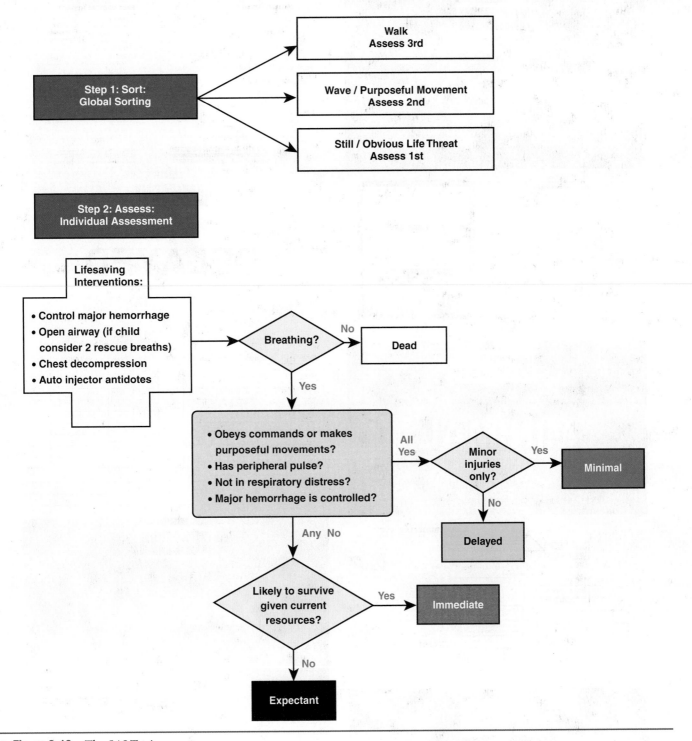

● **Figure 3-10** The SALT triage system.

triage system is developed, paramedics may need to be familiar with more than one triage system.

The JumpSTART System

The JumpSTART Pediatric MCI Triage Tool is an objective tool developed specifically for the triage of children in the multicasualty/disaster setting and was designed to parallel the structure of the START system, the adult MCI triage tool most commonly used in the United States.[7] The JumpSTART system takes into consideration the anatomic and physiologic differences found in children. The objectives of JumpSTART are:

1. To optimize the primary triage of injured children in the MCI setting

2. To enhance the effectiveness of resource allocation for all MCI victims

3. To reduce the emotional burden on triage personnel who may have to make rapid life-or-death decisions about injured children in chaotic circumstances

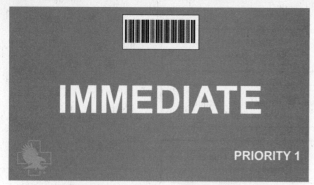

IMMEDIATE

PRIORITY 1

PATIENT DETAILS

Name: _____

ID / Call Sign: _____

SSN#: [ ][ ][ ] [ ][ ] [ ][ ][ ][ ]

○ Male   ○ Female   DOB / Age: _____

Chief Complaint: _____

Mechanism of Injury: _____

PAST MEDICAL HISTORY

○ Unknown   ○ Cardiac
○ No Past History ○ Cancer
○ COPD or Asthma ○ Diabetes
○ CVA/Stroke   ○ Seizures
○ Hypertension
○ Other
_____

○ Medications   ○ Unknown
_____
_____
_____

○ Allergies   ○ No Known Allergies
_____
_____

NORTH AMERICAN RESCUE®
www.NARescue.com • 1-888-689-6277

NAR T2 Tag® (Triage & Treatment Tag)
PN: 20-0033   NSN: 6515-01-537-4163
©2008 North American Rescue® LLC. All rights reserved.

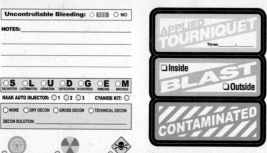

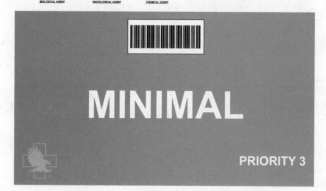

DELAYED

PRIORITY 2

MINIMAL

PRIORITY 3

Time	Treatment / Intervention	BP	Pulse	Resp	Loc / AVPU	SaO₂
_____	_____	/				
_____	_____	/				
_____	_____	/				
_____	_____	/				
_____	_____	/				
_____	_____	/				
_____	_____	/				
_____	_____	/				

NOTES: _____

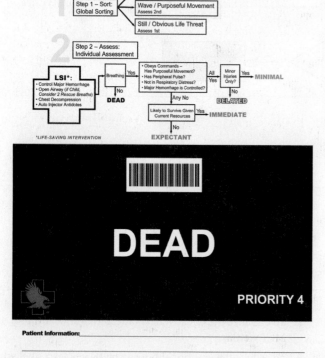

EXPECTANT

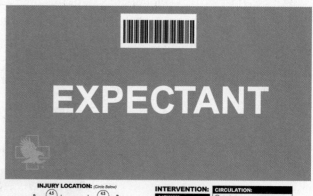

DEAD

PRIORITY 4

Patient Information: _____

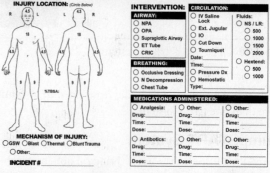

● **Figure 3-11**   Triage tags for use with the SALT triage system.

50 ● **Chapter 3**   Multiple-Casualty Incidents and Incident Management

JumpSTART provides an objective framework that helps to ensure that injured children are triaged by responders using their heads instead of their hearts, thus reducing overtriage that might siphon resources from other patients who need them more and result in physical and emotional trauma to children from unnecessary painful procedures and separation from loved ones. Undertriage is addressed by recognizing the key differences between adult and pediatric physiology and using appropriate pediatric physiologic parameters at decision points (Figure 3-12 ●). The JumpSTART system readily integrates with the START system (Figure 3-13 ●).

JumpSTART Pediatric MCI Triage

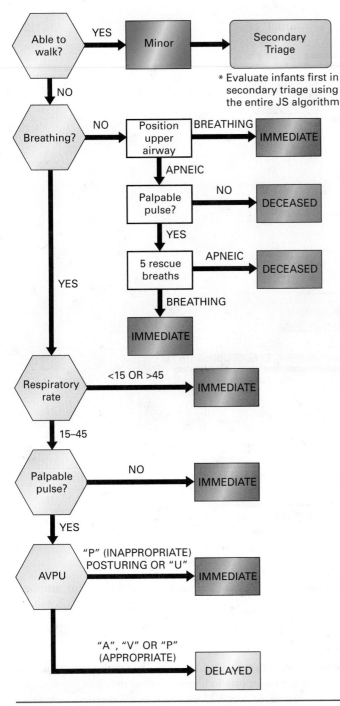

● **Figure 3-12** The JumpSTART pediatric triage system.

Triage Tagging/Labeling

As already mentioned, you should attach a color-coded tag to each patient that you have triaged. Tagging offers these advantages:

- Alerts care providers to patient priorities—that is, provides organization of treatment
- Prevents retriage of the same patient
- Serves as a tracking system during transport and/or treatment

Commercial tags are available, such as the METTAG (Figure 3-14 ●) or the SALT tag. However, you can also use colored surveyor's tape. Each has its advantages and disadvantages. Tags provide tear-off strips that help you count patients in each triage category. Tags also make it easier to track patients, record treatment information, and indicate a patient's location in a transportation accident. However, tags can be damaged in wet weather, and tear-off strips can make it difficult to change patient categories. Surveyor's tape costs less money but does not allow you to count patients during triage. Also, black tape cannot easily be seen at night.

Some systems combine the use of tags and tape. Others use tags only when immediate transport is unavailable and/or when patients need to be sorted into separate treatment areas. Whatever method of tagging you use, it must meet these two criteria:

- Be easy to use
- Provide rapid visual identification of priorities

The Need for Speed

As stated on several occasions, you must not become committed to one-on-one patient care during triage. However, that does not mean that you do nothing. Simple care, such as opening airways and applying direct pressure on profuse bleeding, can save lives early in an incident. As a result, the triage officer should carry certain medical equipment: infection control supplies, oral airways, and trauma dressings. Other essential items for the triage officer include tags or tape, a portable radio to communicate with the incident commander, a command vest, and a flashlight (at night).

Ideally, it will take you less than 30 seconds to triage each patient. However, that means it will take you 5 minutes to triage 10 patients, more than 20 minutes to triage 40 patients, and so on. As a result, other personnel will often assist the triage officer in MCIs with a large number of patients. The simple decision to add personnel can dramatically reduce triage time and speed treatment and transport. Triage personnel can act individually or be assigned to units. Either way, they report to the triage officer, who in turn relays necessary information to the IC. After completing the task of triage, personnel can be reassigned to other units, such as treatment.

Morgue

You should collect patients who are triaged "black" or expectant (Priority-0) in an area away from treatment. Access to this area, known as the **morgue**, should be controlled so that bystanders or the media cannot enter it. In determining the disposition of the deceased, you will need to work closely with the medical examiner, coroner, law enforcement, and other appropriate agencies. (If possible, delay dealing further with the deceased

Combined START/JumpSTART Triage Algorithm

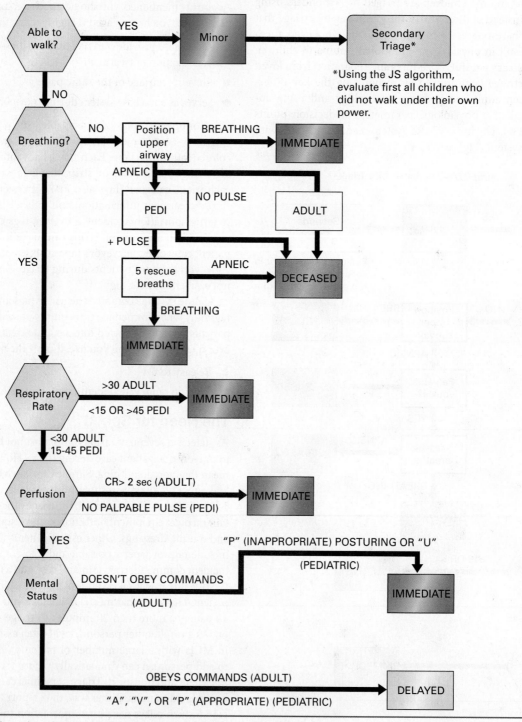

● **Figure 3-13** Algorithm showing integration of the START and JumpSTART triage systems.

who have been gathered in the morgue area until a decision and plan for the disposition of their bodies can be determined.)

Once a morgue is established, it will be supervised by a **morgue officer**. This person may report to the triage officer or the treatment officer. In many cases, these supervisors will assist in selecting and securing an area for the morgue.

Keep in mind the importance of having a preexisting plan for managing situations with large numbers of fatalities. Special facilities may be required to care for the victims. In addition,

responders may require the support of counselors or members of the clergy.

Treatment

When the number of patients exceeds the number of ambulances available for transportation, you will need to collect patients into treatment areas (Figure 3-15 ●). The **treatment group supervisor** controls all actions in the treatment group/sector. The responders

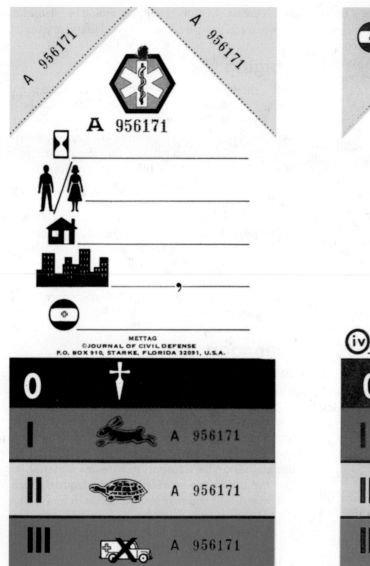

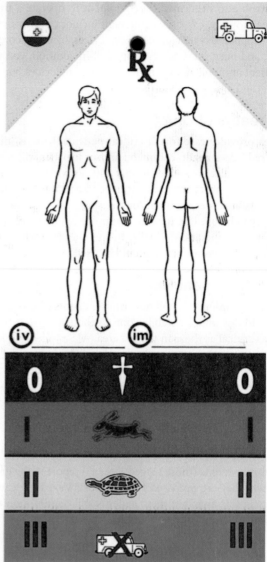

● **Figure 3-14** The METTAG. (© *Journal of Civil Defense*)

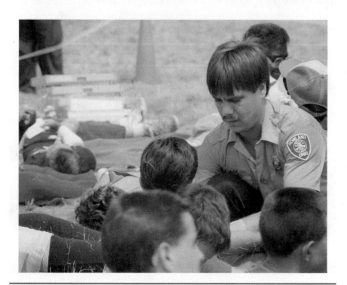

● **Figure 3-15** Treatment area at a multiple-casualty incident.

who carry patients to the treatment area should be organized into teams of four to prevent lifting injuries. As patients arrive in the treatment area, you should conduct or oversee secondary triage to determine if their status has changed. Patients should then be separated into functional treatment areas based on their category:

● START Triage system:
  ○ Red (Immediate, P-1)
  ○ Yellow (Delayed, P-2)
  ○ Green (Minimal, P-3)
  ○ Black (Expectant, P-0)
● SALT Triage system:
  ○ Red (Immediate)
  ○ Yellow (Delayed)
  ○ Green (Minimal)
  ○ Gray (Expectant)
  ○ Black (Dead)

You will also need medical equipment to operate a treatment area properly. Essential equipment includes airway maintenance supplies, oxygen and delivery devices, bleeding control supplies, and burn management supplies. In addition, you will need patient immobilization and transportation devices, such as stretchers and long spine boards.

Red Treatment Unit

This area provides care for all critical patients—that is, those tagged "red." As a result, command and/or logistics will assign the bulk of medical resources to this unit. Providers with ALS skills usually report to the red treatment area so they can stabilize patients and prepare them for transport. Because medical resources can be used up quickly, a supply system is necessary to support this operation. Finally, this is the place where any on-scene physicians or nurses should be used.

Yellow Treatment Unit

Teams of responders carry all noncritical patients (those tagged "yellow") to this unit for stabilization. Although these patients are not as critical as those in the red area, ALS procedures may still be necessary. A patient with an isolated femur fracture, for example, will probably be categorized yellow. Although this patient does not require immediate intervention or transport, he may still require an intravenous line and eventual surgical intervention.

Green Treatment Unit

Ambulatory patients (those tagged "green") report to the green area, where they are prepared for transport. Very little care is necessary in this area, but these patients still require monitoring in case their conditions deteriorate. In such instances, they will be retriaged and moved to the appropriate treatment area.

Supervision of Treatment Units

Each of the preceding units is supervised by a **treatment unit leader** who reports to the treatment group supervisor. The leader's job requires extreme flexibility to ensure that patients receive adequate care. Patient conditions can change and responders, equipment, or supplies may not be available in the subarea. As a result, communications must be carefully coordinated. The treatment group supervisor must be apprised of activities in each subarea. He must also help coordinate operations with other functional areas, particularly command, triage, and transport.

On-Scene Physicians

At some high-impact or long-term incidents, physicians may be used on scene to support EMS. Physicians may use their advanced medical knowledge and skills in several ways at an MCI. For example, they may be better able to make difficult triage decisions, to perform advanced triage and treatment in the treatment area, or to perform emergency surgery to extricate a patient as a last resort. Physicians also provide direct supervision and medical direction over paramedics in the treatment area, removing the need to operate under standing orders or

radio contact. A contingency plan should be established outlining when and how physicians respond to and operate at an MCI.

Staging

Ambulances may be the most precious resource at a multiple-casualty incident. As a result, ambulances must be staged as they arrive to allow proper access to the scene and, equally important, egress with the patients. If ambulances arrive before they are needed to treat patients, they should be kept in a **staging area** that is supervised by a **staging officer**. This area may be a roadway, a parking lot, or some other site where the units can wait until they are deployed by command (Figure 3-16 ●).

Depending on local protocols, drivers or crew members will be required to wait with the vehicles until they are needed for transport. A staging pool keeps personnel from "freelancing" and ensures their availability for quick deployment. It also prevents premature commitment of resources. If ambulances are required for immediate transport, the staging area can serve as a loading area for patients.

Transport Unit

The **transportation unit supervisor** coordinates operations with the staging officer and the treatment supervisor. His job is to get patients into the ambulances and routed to hospitals. If you are assigned to this role, you will need to be flexible in determining the order in which patients are packaged and loaded. You may, for example, elect to place two critical patients in one ambulance for transport to a trauma center. If you decide that the ambulance provider cannot adequately care for two critical patients, you may instead decide to transport one critical and one noncritical patient. You may also take into account the facilities at a given hospital and avoid overwhelming its resources with critical patients.

The routing of patients to hospitals is as important as getting them into the ambulances. Early in the incident, your communications center should contact local hospitals and determine how many patients in each triage category they can handle. You must take this information into account. You must also consider

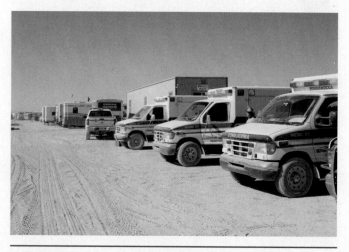

● **Figure 3-16** The staging area is an important component of any large MCI. (© *Dr. Bryan E. Bledsoe*)

any specialties that a hospital may have, such as trauma centers, burn units, and neurologic teams. Keep in mind, too, that many patients may have left the scene before the arrival of EMS and transported themselves to the closest hospital. Depending on the scope and nature of the incident, you may have to factor in such self-transport as well.

As you might suspect from this discussion, a Transportation Supervisor needs to implement some type of tracking system or destination log. Ideally, the tracking sheet or log will include the following data:

- Triage tag number
- Triage priority
- Patient's age, gender, and major injuries
- Transporting unit
- Hospital destination
- Departure time
- Patient's name, if possible

The tracking sheet not only helps to organize activities at an MCI, but it also proves invaluable in reconstructing the incident at a later time. In addition, this record will help document on-scene patient care.

Extrication/Rescue Unit

Depending on your system, extrication or *rescue* may be a branch or a group. If this operation is considered an EMS function, it will be a group (sector) under the EMS branch. If it is a fire department function, it may be under the fire branch. If the rescue is extensive or long term, the operation may be separated into its own branch within the IMS.

In general, the extrication/rescue group removes patients from entanglements at the incident and arranges for them to be carried to treatment areas. The operation has many facets and may require specialized personnel and equipment. During extended operations, treatment personnel will need to work in this area and begin patient care prior to removal.

Depending on the circumstances, personnel operating in this area will need personal protective equipment, including helmets, eye protection, gloves, breathing apparatus, and/or protective clothing (Figure 3-17 ●). Some rescue tools may also require specific support materials, such as gasoline, electricity, or compressed air. Extrication/rescue is a very dangerous area, and all efforts should be taken to ensure that operations are well supervised and safe.

Rehabilitation (Rehab) Unit

At extended operations, a special rehabilitation (rehab) area should be established to support on-scene responders. Arrangements should be made with logistics to ensure the necessary food, water, and medical monitoring supplies.

Ideally, rescuers should regularly rotate through a dedicated rehab area away from the incident. The site should provide thermal control and shelter from fumes, crowds, and the media. In this environment, rescuers can rest and hydrate themselves. Medical personnel operating in this area will take the vital signs

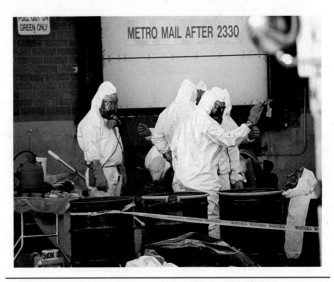

● **Figure 3-17**   A hazardous materials team may be involved in the extrication and rescue phases of some multiple-casualty incidents. Here, a hazmat team prepares to enter the Brentwood mail facility on October 25, 2001, following an anthrax contamination. (© *AP Images/Ron Thomas*)

of rescuers and watch for signs of fatigue or incident stress. A predetermined threshold should be established so that rescuers with abnormal vitals are removed from the operation. This is especially important when working in extremely hot or cold conditions.

Provision should also be made for the availability of a **rapid intervention team**. If possible, an ambulance and crew should be dedicated to stand by outside the staging area. The incident commander can then contact the unit if a rescuer becomes ill or injured. Unfortunately, the demands of a large-scale MCI sometimes prevent implementation of this aspect of the IMS.

Communications

This chapter has already covered communications issues such as size-up, progress reports, frequency use, and more. However, it cannot be said too often: *Communication forms the cornerstone of the Incident Management System.* Therefore, it will be helpful to review some basic rules of communications within the system's EMS branch.

First, when communicating, think about what you are going to say before you say it. Does the message really need to be transmitted over the radio? Remember that the frequencies at an MCI will already be congested with messages. As a result, you should try to prevent as much unnecessary radio traffic as possible.

Second, key up your radio before transmitting. Wait 1 second after pressing the button to speak. This allows your radio to begin transmitting effectively and all other radios to begin listening before you begin your message. Keep in mind that missed messages mean missed chances at increased coordination and efficiency.

Third, acknowledge each message you receive with feedback to ensure that you understood it. For example, the message "Staging from Transport, please send two ambulances to pick up patients" should not be acknowledged with "Staging received."

It should be answered with "Staging received two ambulances to pick up patients."

Other rules include points already covered in the chapter: the use of plain English instead of radio codes; the need for a common radio channel between command, groups (sectors), divisions, and units; face-to-face communications when appropriate; and respect for the lines of communication established by the IMS. In other words, report to the person you are supposeod to report to at all times.

EMS Communications Officer

At large-scale incidents, the Incident Management System may provide for an **EMS communications officer**. This position may also be known as the *EMS COM* or the *MED COM*. This person works closely with the transportation unit supervisor to notify hospitals of incoming patients. A dedicated radio channel works best for this purpose, although use of cellular phones is common for this function. The EMS COM will not deliver complete patient reports, which would increase the communications traffic. Instead, he will transmit the basic information collected by the transportation unit supervisor, such as the number of Priority-1 or red patients en route to a hospital and the expected arrival time.

Alternative Means of Communication

Remember that your primary radio system may not always work at an MCI. Disasters can knock out radio towers and power. Frequencies can be overwhelmed. Telephone lines can be down. Radio batteries can fail. As a result, alternative means of communication should be included in every MCI preplan and should be practiced regularly. You might use cellular phones, mobile data terminals, alphanumeric pagers, fax machines, or other technology to overcome the failure of your primary radio system. When all else fails, runners can be used to hand-deliver messages around the incident scene. Although this method has obvious limitations, it may be your last resort—so know how to use it.

DISASTER MANAGEMENT

Disasters can alter the operating procedures routinely used at high-impact events. For example, disasters can damage a region's infrastructure, preventing the operation of railroads, hospitals, radio systems, and so on. If a disaster occurs in your jurisdiction, you will be a victim as much as a responder, which is why outside assistance is often required. As a rule, **disaster management** occurs in four stages: mitigation, planning, response, and recovery.

Mitigation

Mitigation involves the prevention or limiting of disasters in the first place. For example, the public safety community tries to prevent people from building houses on floodplains or from putting up structures that are unable to withstand the impact of natural phenomena or terrorist attacks. In addition, most communities today have early-warning systems to alert people to weather emergencies, such as hurricanes and tornadoes, or to geological emergencies, such as volcanic eruptions or earthquakes.

Planning

As already indicated, planning is integral to the successful management of all high-impact emergencies. Every community, including your own, should take part in a hazard analysis and then rate these hazards according to their likelihood. For more on this analysis, see the section on preplanning later in this chapter.

Depending on your hazard analysis, devise relocation plans and/or evacuation procedures, as needed. When possible, every effort should be made to keep people in their natural social groupings. That is, provide home-based relocation instead of removing people to hospitals and clinics when they are not injured. If you must evacuate people, use whatever means you have to spread the message frequently and with urgency. Alert people to the nature of the disaster, its estimated time of impact, and description of its expected severity. Advise people of safe routes out of the area and the appropriate destinations for people who must leave an area.

Critical to any successful disaster plan will be provision for an efficient communications system in case the primary system fails. Decide, for example, where a central communications center might be established for people needing help. Set up guidelines on the use of radios by all EMS personnel. Make arrangements for portable radios and recorders as necessary.

Response

In a disaster, there is a great disparity between the casualties and resources. The event overwhelms the natural order and causes a great loss of property and/or life. As a result, a disaster almost always requires outside assistance and alternative operating plans. In general, you will follow the guidelines set up by the Incident Management System.

Recovery

Recovery involves the return of your department, your jurisdiction, and your community to normal as soon as possible. Actions taken will vary with the nature of the disaster and/or the disaster plan under which you operate. You may be involved with the reunion of families, follow-up care, and support of the personnel charged with handling potential hazards such as collapsed buildings or highways.

MEETING THE CHALLENGE OF MULTIPLE-CASUALTY INCIDENTS

As implied in the preceding sections, you will never be more challenged in your EMS career than when you respond to an MCI. The routine actions that you do every day will suddenly become more difficult or, in some cases, impossible because of the stress or complexities of the incident. For this reason, you should anticipate various problems and work to overcome them.

Common Problems

Things can, do, and most assuredly will go wrong at MCIs and disasters. One way to avert or minimize complications is to anticipate them. As the saying goes, "Forewarned is forearmed." Studies of past incidents have revealed the following common problems, any one of which can hinder the success of a rescue operation:

- Lack of recognizable EMS command in the field
- Failure to provide adequate widespread notification of an event
- Failure to provide proper triage
- Lack of rapid initial stabilization of patients
- Failure to move, collect, and organize patients rapidly into a treatment area
- Overly time-consuming patient care
- Premature transportation of patients
- Improper or inefficient use of in-field personnel
- Improper distribution of patients to medical facilities
- Failure to establish an accurate patient-tracking system
- Inability to communicate with on-scene units, regional EMS agencies, or other personnel
- Lack of command vests for all IMS officers or supervisors
- Lack of adequate training and/or practice of rescuers at an MCI
- Lack of drills among regional agencies involved in the IMS
- Lack of proper community assessment, preplanning, and contingency plans

Preplanning, Drills, and Critiques

As we have mentioned several times, planning for an MCI or disaster makes response much smoother. Anticipate any problems that may occur and work toward removing them. Anything that can be planned in advance should be planned in advance.

The first step involves a complete assessment of the potential hazards, both natural and man-made, that could occur in your area. If you live in Kansas, for example, you might not worry about hurricanes, but tornadoes are a very real possibility. Sites of potential incidents in almost any community include chemical or nuclear plants, factories or mines, schools, jails, sporting arenas, entertainment centers, railroads, and airports.

Once you have completed the assessment, your agency should develop a plan that outlines the SOPs and protocols for potential incidents. You will not, of course, be able to plan

for every possible scenario. If you develop 100 preplans, for example, you can expect to be summoned to scenario 101 or 102—that is, the unscripted event. For this reason, you must develop contingency plans for worst-case scenarios. For example, how would you communicate with ambulances if something or someone knocked out the dispatch center? What would you do if the local hospital suddenly became unusable because of chemical contamination?

After you have completed a preplan, test it. Start small. Tabletop drills, for example, are a good place to begin. Once you have worked out the wrinkles, distribute the plan to everyone in your department, the surrounding departments, local police, fire departments, hospitals—in short, to anyone who could be involved in the IMS in your area. Use the plan to ensure that the necessary mutual aid agreements are in place and that the appropriate personnel within the IMS know about these agreements.

Then make sure that all personnel who could show up at an MCI have received proper training in use of the IMS. As you have learned, the first responders on the scene will often determine the course of an event. Run or take part in drills so that you can gain practice in MCI operations and large-scale use of the IMS. Again, start small. Use local drills within your department to help personnel become familiar with the system. Then, aim for large-scale drills that involve outside agencies.

Finally, never say "It will never happen here." Experience has proven time and again that multiple-casualty incidents and disasters can occur almost anywhere and at any time. Make it part of your professional training to be ready to act as an incident commander, the person charged with establishing and organizing the IMS (Figure 3-18 ●).

Disaster Mental Health Services

The emotional well-being of both rescuers and victims is an important concern in any MCI. In the past, critical incident stress

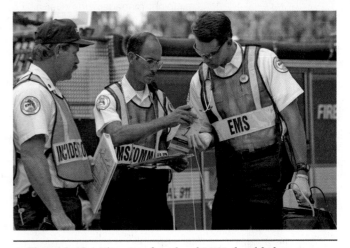

● **Figure 3-18** Planning for a local MCI should always include review of past similar MCI events. Make it part of your professional training to be ready to act as an incident commander. (© Craig Jackson/In the Dark Photography)

management (CISM) was recommended for use in emergency services. However, recent evidence has clearly shown that CISM and critical incident stress debriefing do not appear to mitigate the effects of traumatic stress and, in fact, may interfere with the normal grieving and healing process.[8, 9]

However, an important role remains for competent mental health personnel in any MCI. Mental health personnel should be available on scene to provide psychological first aid for those affected by the event, including emergency personnel.[10] This requires no special training or certification and provides no psychological intervention but rather involves just meeting basic human needs. It includes:

- Listening
- Conveying compassion
- Assessing needs

- Ensuring that basic physical needs are met
- Not forcing personnel to talk
- Providing or mobilizing company from family or significant others
- Encouraging, but not forcing, social support
- Protecting from additional harm

Competent mental health personnel can also begin to screen both rescuers and victims for abnormal signs and symptoms associated with traumatic stress. Often, these symptoms take up to two months to develop. Because of this, mental health personnel should remain available and work with emergency personnel to identify anyone who may not be recovering normally from the event. Persons so affected may be referred for additional counseling or other mental health care.

SUMMARY

Every paramedic should be thoroughly familiar with IMS procedures and should follow these procedures at every multiple-patient, multiple-unit response from the smallest incident to the largest incident. Keep in mind the saying "We play as we practice." If you do, you will be prepared for the MCI or disaster that puts the emergency medical system to its biggest tests.

YOU MAKE THE CALL

At 05:15 hours on a dark and dreary Wednesday morning, the Hall County Sheriff's Office dispatch center receives a single call from a cellular phone reporting smoke coming from the back side of the Lone Pines Motel. The caller reports that he sees thick smoke in the area and smells something burning. The dispatcher immediately dispatches the Hall County Fire and Sheriff's Departments and your EMS agency. Hall County EMS responds with one ALS ambulance, one BLS ambulance, and the on-duty field supervisor in his ALS chase car (Figure 3-19 ●).

You arrive in the ALS ambulance. You do a windshield survey and observe heavy fire and smoke coming from the rear portion of the building; several motel guests are now leaving their rooms. The night manager runs over and says that there are at least 20 people in those rooms in that part of the motel.

1. What two roles in the Incident Management System will you and your partner fill, as you are first on scene?

2. How would you size up the incident?

3. What additional resources would you anticipate, and what instructions would you provide for them?

4. How would you use the Incident Management System to organize this incident?

5. What would your initial radio report sound like in this incident?

See Suggested Responses at the back of this book.

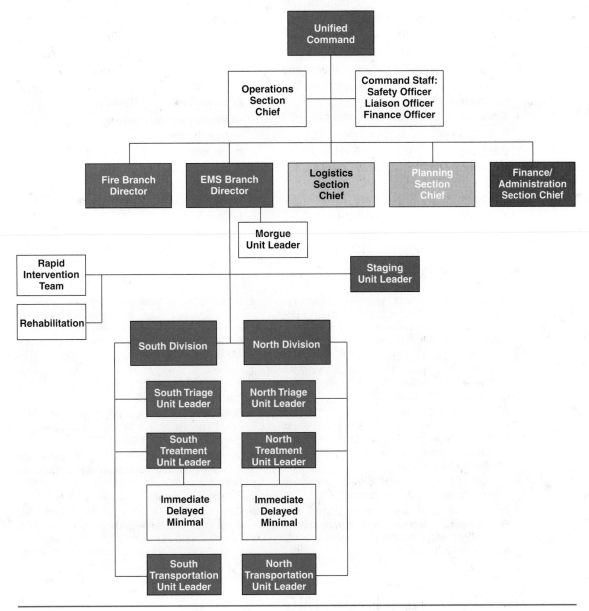

LONE PINES MOTEL
INCIDENT MANAGEMENT SYSTEM

● **Figure 3-19** Sample command structure for a multiple-casualty incident at a motel.

REVIEW QUESTIONS

1. A management program designed for controlling, directing, and coordinating emergency response resources is an ICS or a(n) _____.
   a. MCI
   b. IMS
   c. ISC
   d. PAR

2. When the Incident Management System is expanded or the scene is large, the incident commander sets up a _____.
   a. control tower
   b. command post
   c. treatment area
   d. operational area

3. In managing an MCI, which of the following is *not* one of the three main priorities?
   a. life safety
   b. incident stabilization
   c. property conservation
   d. cost outlay evaluation

4. In the case of a(n) _____ incident, the injuries have usually already occurred by the time you arrive on scene.
   a. open
   b. uncontained
   c. closed
   d. controlled

5. To ensure flexibility, an incident commander should radio a brief progress report approximately every _____ minutes until the incident has been stabilized.
   a. 5
   b. 10
   c. 15
   d. 20

6. This person monitors all on-scene actions and ensures that they do not create any potentially harmful conditions.
   a. section chief
   b. safety officer
   c. liaison officer
   d. information officer

7. Because _____ will drive subsequent operations, it is generally one of the first functions performed at an MCI.
   a. triage
   b. survey
   c. priority
   d. assessment

8. During triage, patients with respirations above 30 per minute should be tagged _____.
   a. red
   b. green
   c. black
   d. yellow

9. _____ involves the return of your department, your jurisdiction, and your community to normal as soon as possible.
   a. Planning
   b. Response
   c. Recovery
   d. Mitigation

10. Command is transferred only _____.
   a. face to face
   b. via telephone
   c. over the radio
   d. in written documentation

See Answers to Review Questions at the back of this book.

 ## REFERENCES

1. Department of Homeland Security. Homeland Security Presidential Directive 5: Management of Domestic Incidents. [Available at http://www.fas.org/irp/offdocs/nspd/hspd-5.html]

2. Kahn, C. A., C. H. Schultz, K. T. Miller, and C. L. Anderson. "Does START Triage Work? An Outcomes Assessment after a Disaster." *Ann Emerg Med* 54 (2008): 424–430.

3. Hong, R., P. R. Sierzenski, M. Bollinger, C. C. Durie, and R. E. O'Connor. "Does the Simple Triage and Rapid Treatment Method Appropriately Triage Patients Based upon Injury Severity Score?" *Am J Disaster Med* 3 (2008): 265–271.

4. Gebhart, M. E. and R. Pence. "START Triage: Does It Work?" *Disaster Manag Response* 5 (2007): 68–73.

5. Deluhery, M. R., B. Lerner, R. G. Pirallo, and R. B. Schwartz. "Paramedic Accuracy Using SALT Triage after a Brief Initial Training." *Prehosp Emerg Care* 15(4) (2011): 526–532.

6. Lerner, E. B., R. B. Schwartz, P. L. Coule, et al. "Mass Casualty Triage: An Evaluation of the Data and Development of a Proposed National Guideline." *Disaster Med Public Health Prep* 2 Suppl 1 (2008): S25–S34.

7. Romig L. E. "Pediatric Triage. A System to Jump-START Your Triage of Young Patients at MCIs." *JEMS* 27 (2002): 52–58.

8. Bledsoe, B. E. "Critical Incident Stress Management (CISM): Benefit or Risk for Emergency Services?" *Prehosp Emerg Care* 7 (2003): 272–279.

9. Macnab, A. J., J. A. Russell, J. P. Lowe, and F. Gagnon. "Critical Incident Stress Intervention after Loss of an Air Ambulance: Two-Year Follow-Up." *Prehosp Disaster Med* 14 (1999): 8–12.

10. Everly, G. S., Jr., D. J. Barnett, N. L. Sperry, and J. M. Links. "The Use of Psychological First Aid (PFA) Training among Nurses to Enhance Population Resiliency." *Int J Emerg Ment Health* 12 (2010): 2131.

FURTHER READING

Molino, L. N., Sr. *Emergency Incident Management Systems: Fundamentals and Applications*. Hoboken, NJ: John Wiley and Sons, 2006.

National Incident Management System (NIMS). Washington, DC: U.S. Department of Homeland Security, 2004. NIMS information also available from the Department of Homeland Security website: *http://www.dhs.gov* (keyword: NIMS).

NFPA 1500. *Standard on Fire Department Occupational Safety and Health*. 1995 ed. Quincy, MA: National Fire Protection Association.

NFPA 1561. *Standard on Fire Department Incident Management System*. 1995 ed. Quincy, MA: National Fire Protection Association.

NFPA 1600. *Recommended Practices for Disaster Management*. 1995 ed. Quincy, MA: National Fire Protection Association.

4

Rescue Awareness and Operations

Bryan Bledsoe, DO, FACEP, FAAEM, EMT-P

STANDARD
EMS Operations (Vehicle Extrication)

COMPETENCY
Applies knowledge of operational roles and responsibilities to ensure patient, public, and personnel safety.

OBJECTIVES

Terminal Performance Objective
After reading this chapter, you should be able to effectively perform the expected functions of EMS personnel in a rescue situation.

Enabling Objectives
To accomplish the terminal performance objective, you should be able to:

1. Define key terms introduced in this chapter.

2. Describe the concept of rescue awareness training with respect to the role of paramedics in rescue situations.

3. Describe the protective equipment needed by rescue and EMS personnel for a variety of rescue responses.

4. Describe equipment and measures used to protect patients in rescue situations.

5. Describe considerations in safety procedures in the approach to rescue situations.

6. Describe the goals and tasks of each of the seven phases of a rescue situation.

7. Describe the principles and practices related to surface water rescues.

8. Describe special considerations and hazards for moving water rescues.

9. Describe the principles and practices related to hazardous atmosphere rescues.

10. Describe the principles and practices related to highway operations and vehicle rescues.

11. Describe the principles and practices related to hazardous terrain rescues.

12. Describe considerations for extended care of patients in rescue situations.

KEY TERMS

active rescue zone, p. 70

disentanglement, p. 67

eddies, p. 74

extrication, p. 69

heat escape lessening position (HELP), p. 72

recirculating currents, p. 72

scrambling, p. 84

scree, p. 84

short haul, p. 87

strainers, p. 73

A call comes into Fire Unit 1204, a volunteer-operated paramedic ambulance, to assist an injured person in a rural state park approximately 15 miles from the station. You hear the call over your radio and respond promptly, along with another volunteer.

Because of the distance and the winding roadways leading to the park, it takes nearly 30 minutes to arrive on scene. At the park entrance, one of the rangers informs you that a rock climber fell while trying to rappel down a popular cliff to meet his climbing partner on a rock ledge. Using a four-wheel-drive vehicle, the ranger takes you to the trail leading to the patient. Because the portable radio will not reach dispatch from the park, your partner stays with the ambulance.

From a vantage point along the trail, you spot the patient through binoculars. You see a young man lying on a rock ledge, about 55 feet below the trail. The climber's partner waves frantically to catch your attention, but seems unharmed. The cliff above the ledge is nearly vertical with a smooth rock face. You quickly determine the need for a high-angle rescue team and possibly a helicopter for rescue and medical evacuation.

You relay the size-up information to the ambulance. Your partner, in turn, calls dispatch and requests the necessary resources. Dispatch arranges for two members of a regional high-angle rescue team to fly with the helicopter, which has been placed on standby.

On arrival, rangers lead the team to the emergency site. The two specially trained paramedics quickly confer with you, size up the situation, and ensure scene and personal safety. They then prepare their equipment for descent and access to the patient.

When the first rescuer rappels to the ledge, the uninjured climber blurts out: "I don't know what happened. He's such a good climber. Did you see all those leaves and pebbles near the anchor? I think he must have slipped while setting up his rappel. He's breathing but hasn't really moved since landing. A hiker saw the fall and called the ranger station with her cell phone—but that was so long ago. Please help—he's my best friend!"

To avoid having two patients, the rescuer directs the uninjured climber to "tie in" at a safe spot on the ledge. Because of the significant mechanism of injury, she performs a primary assessment on the patient, followed by a rapid secondary assessment. Her assessment reveals an unresponsive patient with multiple fractures. Nonetheless, his blood pressure and pulse appear stable at this time.

Because of the heavy forest canopy, rescuers decide not to do a short haul with the helicopter. While the other high-angle rescuer rigs the ropes and rescue system, the paramedic immobilizes the patient and establishes an IV of normal saline solution. Because she anticipates a prolonged removal time, the paramedic collects some of the patient history from the uninjured climber and begins the detailed physical exam. She starts a second IV, administers fentanyl, cleans and dresses all wounds, and splints all fractures.

It takes approximately 25 minutes for the team to rig the rescue and haul the patient off the ledge in a Stokes basket stretcher. Although badly shaken, the uninjured climber is hoisted to the top and turned over to your care. Meanwhile, the high-angle team carries the patient to the helicopter, which is waiting in a clearing about 200 yards down the trail. He is then flown to the nearest trauma unit for treatment. About 1 hour later, a violent thunderstorm hits the area. Without use of the high-angle team, the patient might still be lying unprotected on the ledge.

INTRODUCTION

EMS personnel usually have no trouble reaching their patients—that is, unless they are pinned beneath a vehicle, trapped in a collapsed building, or injured climbing a rock face or crawling into a cave. When people get injured or stranded in such situations, often somebody must first rescue the patients before emergency medical care can even begin.

So what does *rescue* mean? According to the dictionary, it is "the act of delivering from danger or imprisonment." In the case of EMS, rescue means extricating and/or disentangling the victims who will become your patients. Without rescue, there are no patients.

ROLE OF THE PARAMEDIC

Rescue is a patient-driven event, and EMS is a patient-driven profession. However, not all EMS crews have the training to perform rescues. In most cases, it is simply not practical to train every paramedic in the detailed knowledge or operational skills necessary for each rescue specialty (Figure 4-1 ●). It is possible, though, to instruct paramedics in the concept of rescue and to train them to what is known as an "awareness level." Awareness training imparts enough knowledge about rescue operations to EMS personnel that they can recognize hazards and realize the need for additional expertise at the scene. Failing to train paramedics in rescue awareness will eventually end in the injury or death of EMS personnel, patients, or both.

Rescue involves a combination of medical and mechanical skills with the correct amount of each applied at the appropriate time. Think of the medics who serve in the military. All armies throughout the world train and deploy medical people into combat. Even if the medics do not fire a weapon, they have enough military and medical training to treat patients in a combat situation. It's the same with the paramedics who serve on high-angle teams, SCUBA teams, and other specialized rescue units. If a rescue unit does not have medical training, your unit provides the balance.

In any rescue situation, treatment begins at the site of the incident. If the patient can be accessed in any way, treatment may in fact start before the patient is actually released from entrapment. Once medical care begins, it continues throughout the incident. The trick is to balance the medical and mechanical rescue skills to ensure that the patient obtains effective and timely extraction. Teams must work together to provide a well-coordinated effort to meet the patient's medical and physical needs.

The role of EMS in a rescue operation varies from area to area. Some localities, for example, may require additional training beyond the awareness level. In general, however, all paramedics should have the proper training and personal protective equipment (PPE) to allow them to access the patient, provide assessment, and establish incident command.

As first responders, paramedics should understand the hazards associated with various environments, such as extreme heat or cold, potentially toxic atmospheres, and unstable structures. They should also be able to recognize when it is safe and unsafe to access the patient or attempt a rescue. If you deem an environment safe and if you have the training to effect a rescue, you should at least participate in the rescue under the guidance of individuals with additional expertise. You should also understand the rescue process so that you can decide when various treatments are indicated or contraindicated. In the climbing accident in the case study, for example, you would direct all parties not to move the patient until he was immobilized.

Because the field of rescue entails so many specialties, a single chapter cannot provide a step-by-step list of procedures and equipment for all the various scenarios you may encounter. Although practice scenarios can be found in related course materials, this chapter focuses on considerations that apply to most rescue situations. It discusses rescuer PPE and safety, presents the seven general phases of a rescue operation, and provides an "awareness level" of rescue operations in the following environments:

- *Surface water*—for example, "low head" dams, flat water, moving water
- *Hazardous atmospheres*—for example, confined spaces, trenches, hazmat incidents
- *Highway operations*—for example, unstable vehicles, hazardous cargoes, volatile fuels
- *Hazardous terrains*—for example, high-angle cliffs, off-road wilderness areas

PROTECTIVE EQUIPMENT

The use of personal and patient safety equipment is paramount in any rescue situation. To prepare for a rescue response, you must develop a PPE cache. Without the appropriate protective gear, you will jeopardize both your own safety and the safety of the patient. Some of the equipment listed in the following

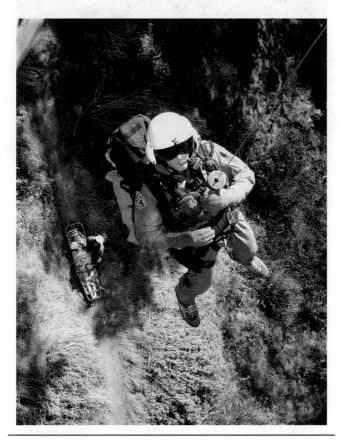

● **Figure 4-1**   Rescue is a dangerous activity and safety is the number-one priority. It is impossible for an individual paramedic to be highly trained in all types of rescue. Instead, specialized rescue teams should be used. *(© Jeff Forster)*

sections has application in many rescue situations. Other pieces of gear are appropriate to specific environments or conditions.

Rescuer Protection

In all rescue environments, EMS personnel should wear highly visible clothing so they can be spotted easily. Ideally, PPE should fit the situation, but gear can be adapted, if necessary. For example, your PPE may not completely prevent exposure to infectious disease. Nonetheless, it minimizes the risk of infection (Figure 4-2 ●). In fact, most PPE has not been specifically designed for EMS use. Instead, it has been borrowed from other fields, such as firefighting, mountaineering, caving, occupational safety, and more.

The use of adapted gear has resulted from the lack of a national uniform reporting system to identify risk-related exposures for EMS personnel. Future risk management and PPE design should be driven by such data. As a *minimum*, you should have the following equipment available:

- *Helmets.* The best helmets have a four-point, nonelastic suspension system (Figure 4-3 ●). Most of the four-point suspension helmets are designed to withstand a greater impact than the two-point system found in hard hats worn at construction sites. Avoid helmets with nonremovable "duck bills" in the back—this will compromise your ability to wear the helmet in tight spaces. A compact firefighting helmet that meets National Fire Protection Association standards is adequate for most vehicle and structural applications. Climbing helmets work better for confined space and technical rescues, while padded rafting or kayaking helmets are more appropriate for water rescues.

- *Eye protection.* Two essential pieces of eye gear are goggles, which should be vented to prevent fogging, and industrial safety glasses. These should be approved by the American National Standards Institute (ANSI). Do not rely on the face shields found in fire helmets. They usually provide inadequate eye protection.

- *Hearing protection.* From a purely technical standpoint, high-quality earmuffs provide the best hearing protection. However, you must take into account other factors such as practicality, convenience, availability, and environmental

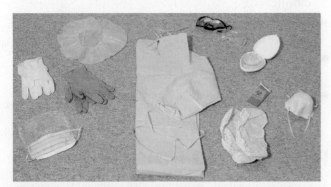

● **Figure 4-2** Your personal protective equipment helps to minimize the risk of exposure to infectious diseases. For more specialized operations, such as water rescues, you need more specialized equipment.

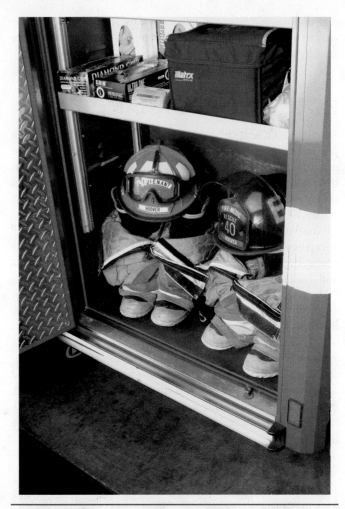

● **Figure 4-3** The quantity of safety and rescue equipment that can be carried on a standard ambulance is limited. However, helmets should be among the minimum types of rescue gear aboard each unit.

considerations. In high-noise areas, for example, you might use the multi-baffled rubber earplugs used by the military or the spongelike disposable earplugs.

- *Respiratory protection.* Surgical masks or commercial dust masks prove adequate for most occasions. These should be carried routinely on all EMS units.

- *Gloves.* Leather gloves usually protect against cuts and punctures. They allow free movement of the fingers and ample dexterity. As a rule, heavy, gauntlet-style gloves are too awkward for most rescue work.

- *Foot protection.* As a rule, the best general boots for EMS work are high-top, steel-toed, and/or shank boots with a coarse lug sole to provide traction and prevent slipping. For rescue operations, lace-up boots offer greater stability and better ankle support by limiting the range of motion. They also do not come off as easily as pull-on boots when walking through deep mud. Insulation may be useful in some colder working environments.

- *Flame/flash protection.* Every service should have a standard operating procedure (SOP) calling for the use of flame/flash protection whenever the potential for fire exists.

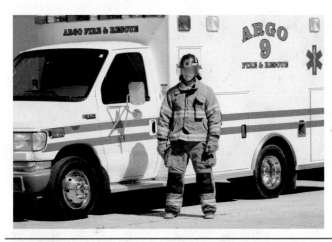

● **Figure 4-4** Full protective gear, including turnout gear, eye protection, helmet, and gloves.

Turnout gear, coveralls, or jumpsuits all offer some arm and leg protection and help prevent damage to your uniform (Figure 4-4 ●). They also have the added advantage of being quick and easy to don. For protection against the sharp, jagged metal or glass found at many motor vehicle crashes or structural collapses, turnout gear generally works best. For limited flash protection, use gear made from Nomex®, PBI®, or flame-retardant cotton. For high visibility, pick bright colors such as orange or lime and reflective trim or symbols. Some services, for example, have an SOP calling for highly visible gear and/or orange safety vests to be worn during all highway operations—both day and night. Insulated gear or jumpsuits are helpful in cold environments, but they can also increase heat stress during heavy work or in situations where high ambient temperatures prevail.

● *Personal flotation devices (PFDs).* If your service includes areas where water emergencies can result, your unit should carry PFDs that meet the U.S. Coast Guard standards for flotation. They should be worn whenever operating on or around water. The Type III PFD is preferred for rescue work. You should also attach a knife, strobe light, and whistle to the PFD in such a way that they are easily accessible.

● *Lighting.* Depending on the type and location of the rescue, you might also consider portable lighting. Many rescuers carry at least a flashlight or, better yet, a headlamp that can be attached to a helmet for hands-free operation. Consider the long-burning headlamps commonly worn by mountaineers and found through catalogs, the Internet, or climbing/camping stores.

● *Hazmat suits or self-contained breathing apparatus (SCBA).* These items should only be made available to personnel who have been trained to use them. Most services or regions have special hazmat units to provide the highly specialized support required at rescue situations involving toxic substances. (For a discussion of hazmat training and equipment, see Chapter 5.)

● *Extended, remote, or wilderness protection.* If your unit provides service to a remote or wilderness area, you might need to hike into—or even be air transported into—a rugged environment. In such cases, you would be advised to have a backcountry survival pack as part of your gear. This backpack should be preloaded with PPE for inclement weather (cold, rain, snow, wind), provisions for personal drinking water (iodine tablets/water filter), snacks for a few hours (energy gels or bars), temporary shelter (tent/tarp/bivouac ["bivy"] sack), a butane lighter, and some redundancy in lighting in case of a light source failure.

CONTENT REVIEW

► Checklist for Backcountry Survival Pack

- PPE for inclement weather
- Provisions for drinking water
- Snacks for a few hours
- Temporary shelter
- Butane lighter
- Redundant light sources

Patient Protection

Many of the considerations for rescuer safety also apply to patients, with several significant differences. A patient protective equipment cache should include at least the following items:

● *Helmets.* Patients usually do not require the same heavy-duty helmets as rescuers. As a result, the less expensive, construction-style hard hats often provide adequate protection against minor hazards. However, if you anticipate greater danger, as in climbing or caving rescues, outfit patients with the same high-grade helmets as rescuers would use in the same or similar environments.

● *Eye protection.* Vented goggles, held in place by elastic bands, are ideal. They are not as easily dislodged as safety glasses. You might also use workshop face shields.

● *Hearing and respiratory protection.* Apply the same considerations for hearing and respiratory protection as you would for yourself. Earplugs are usually adequate.

● *Protective blankets.* You should have a variety of protective blankets to shield patients from debris, fire, or weather. Inexpensive vinyl tarps do a good job of protecting patients from water, weather, and most debris. Aluminized rescue blankets protect from fire, heat, or glass dust. Commercially available wool blankets provide excellent insulation from the cold. Plastic shielding (the kind used by landscapers) and plastic trash bags of many sizes and weights are also very useful. One 55-gallon-drum liner is large enough to cover a single patient. It can serve as a disposable blanket, poncho, vapor barrier, or, in a wilderness situation, bivy sack.

● *Protective shielding.* Circumstances may call for protective equipment that is more substantial than blankets or plastic sheets. All rescue teams should be trained to use backboards and other commonly found equipment as shields to protect patients from fire, weather, falling rock or debris, glass, or other sharp-edged objects. Shields specifically designed for a Stokes basket should be available. Keep in mind that a device that shields a patient from debris or the elements may also limit rescuers' access to the patient. The more securely you package a patient, the more difficult it will be for you to monitor him. As patient care becomes more complicated, changing patient conditions may be overlooked.

SAFETY PROCEDURES

As you already know, safety—your own and that of your crew—is your first priority. Yet in rescue situations, a number of factors prod you to take action: your own desire to access the patient for treatment, the urging of people to "do something," the patient's cries for help, the presence of media, frustration at rescuers' lack of medical experience, and more. However, one mistake can spell disaster for you, your crew, and/or the entrapped victim. One way to curb "heroics" is by establishing rescue SOPs, determining crew assignments, and, above all else, preplanning scenarios well in advance of actual rescues.

Rescue SOPs

Standard operating procedures are the nuts and bolts of effective EMS practice. At rescue situations, all teams should have written safety procedures familiar to everyone. Contents should include sections on all types of anticipated rescues. Each section should specify required safety equipment, required or prohibited actions, and any rescue-specific modifications in assignments. SOPs should include a statement requiring that a safety officer be present and an explanation of that person's relationship to incident command. Ideally, the safety officer should be someone with the knowledge and authority to intervene in unsafe situations. This person makes the "go/no go" decision in the operation. (For more on the role of safety officers, see Chapter 3.)

Crew Assignments

In addition to SOPs, an EMS unit must anticipate crew assignments and special needs *before* the rescue operation. This task can be done through personnel screening, careful preplanning, and regular practice of any dangerous rescue techniques that members of your unit may be trained to perform (Figure 4-5 ●).

Search-and-rescue planners often use personnel screening to determine the participants in the rescue process. Programs exist to identify the physical capabilities of crew members. Findings of these programs could have a significant impact on personnel assignments. In addition, psychological testing is recommended. It may even be desirable to screen for specific traits, such as phobias. For example, a rescuer's inordinate fear of heights or small spaces should be taken into account when assigning duties.

Preplanning

As stressed in Chapter 3, one of the most critical factors in promoting safety and operational success is preplanning. Preplanning starts with the identification of potential rescue locations, structures, or activities within your area. Effective preplanning then evaluates the specific training and equipment needed to manage each of these events. The preplan also generates ideas on efficient use of existing resources and anticipates the need for additional equipment, rescuers, and/or expertise.

Because of the intensity and length of many rescue operations, provisions must be made for the maintenance and rotation of rescue personnel. Plans should be made for "standby" or staging sites that offer protection from the weather. Sites

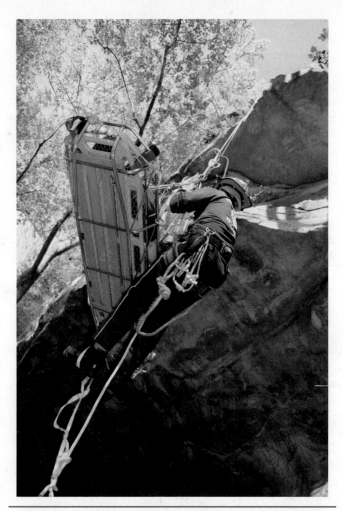

● **Figure 4-5** Dangerous rescue techniques, such as vertical rescue, should be frequently practiced to ensure the utmost safety during actual rescue situations.

should be away from the immediate operations area and secure from bystanders and the media. Personnel should be rotated at controlled intervals. Predetermined policies should be set regarding food and hydration of crews. On-scene diets should be high in complex carbohydrates and low in sugars and fats. Fluid replacement should consist of diluted (at least 50 percent) electrolyte solutions, such as those found in sports drinks. The classic coffee-and-donuts regimen should be avoided altogether.

The preplanning should be the basis of a broader regional emergency rescue plan, to be tested and modified in practice exercises. When possible, other specialized rescue agencies, such as high-angle teams, should take part in the exercises. These "test run" scenarios will give you and other members of your unit ample opportunity to utilize the incident management system (IMS) as it applies to rescue situations.

RESCUE OPERATIONS

As already mentioned, there are several types of rescue operations, each of which includes technically difficult procedures, very specialized equipment, or both. *They should be attempted only by personnel with special training and experience in these areas.* Some of these special rescue operations will be examined later in the chapter. First, however, you need to be aware of the general approach to most rescue situations.

As in any other EMS incident, rescue operations go through phases. Although specific procedures vary from area to area and from rescue to rescue, most calls will go through seven general phases: arrival and size-up, hazard control, patient access, medical treatment, **disentanglement**, patient packaging, and removal/transport.

Phase 1: Arrival and Size-Up

Size-up begins with the dispatcher's call and subsequent arrival at the scene (Figure 4-6 ●). Although the dispatcher's message may indicate a rescue situation, you must still understand the environment and potential risks. On arrival, you or another paramedic must quickly establish medical command and appoint a triage officer. You must also conduct a rapid scene size-up, determine the number of patients, and notify dispatch of the magnitude of the event. Now is the time to implement the IMS, any mutual-aid agreements, and the procedures for contacting off-duty personnel or backup advanced life support (ALS) units.

Prompt recognition of a rescue situation and identification of the specific type of rescue are essential. You may be summoned to a structural collapse, vehicle rollover, or climbing accident. Each of these situations holds out the potential for entrapment and the need for specialized crews and equipment. Often, you must make a quick risk-versus-benefit analysis based on the conditions found on arrival. Be careful not to overestimate your capability to handle a rescue situation. As indicated, individual acts of courage may be called for, but safety comes first. If in doubt, err on the side of safety.

In calling for backup, follow this precaution: "Don't undersell overkill." Remember that it is always easier to send back a rescue crew than to rectify a personal tragedy caused by too few rescuers or hasty heroics. Also keep in mind the realistic time needed to access and evacuate an entrapped patient. Make use of the IMS to shave off valuable response minutes in what may be a life-threatening situation.

Phase 2: Hazard Control

On-scene hazards must be identified with speed and clarity (Figure 4-7 ●). You must often deal with these hazards before even attempting to reach the patient. To do otherwise would place you and other personnel at risk. Control as many of the hazards as possible, but do not attempt to manage any condition beyond your training or skills. Some situations, for example, involve chemical spills, radiation, gas leaks, explosives, or other dangerous substances. You will need to employ a hazmat team and confine your actions to a safe area. (For more on setting up zones at a hazmat scene, see Chapter 5.) Electric wires hold a "double threat" for fire and shock.

The very environment in which you stand can be risk filled. Look around to determine the possibility of lightning, avalanches, rock slides, cave-ins, and so on. Manage and minimize the risks from uncontrollable hazards as soon as possible to avoid other injuries. Ensure that all personnel, for example, wear appropriate PPE. Never forget the dangers of traffic. EMS providers have been killed at highway crash sites by drunks attracted to the bright lights striking crew members in nonreflective gear. The following are some other potential hazards that

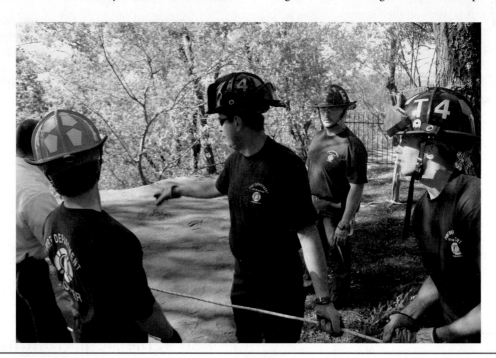

● **Figure 4-6** The first phase of a rescue operation is arrival and scene size-up. If the scene assessment reveals any hazards, efforts must be taken to control them, the second step of a rescue operation.

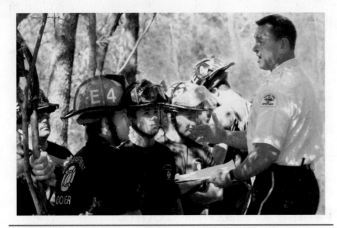

● **Figure 4-7** The second phase of a rescue operation is hazard control. Hazards must be quickly identified and dealt with.

you may encounter. As you skim this list, keep in mind that these are only a sampling of the conditions you may encounter.

- Poisonous or caustic substances
- Biological agents or germ-infected materials
- Swiftly moving currents, floating debris, or water contaminated with toxic agents
- Confined spaces such as vessels, trenches, mines, or caves
- Extreme heights or icy rock faces, especially in mountainous situations
- Possible psychological instability, as is often experienced in hostage crises, urban violence, mass hysteria, or individual emotional trauma on either the part of the patient or the crew (Recall the need for preassessment of crew members.)

Phase 3: Patient Access

After controlling hazards, you will then attempt to gain access to the patient or patients (Figure 4-8 ●). Begin by formulating a plan. Determine the best method to gain access and deploy the

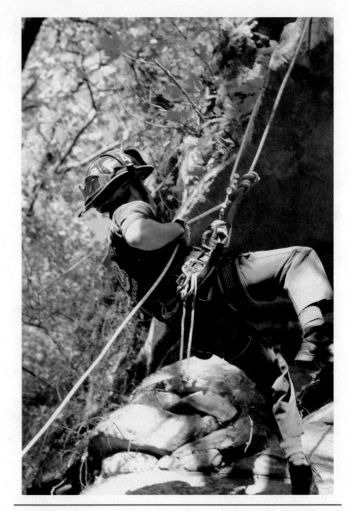

● **Figure 4-8** The third phase of a rescue operation is gaining access to the patient. In specialized rescues, such as vertical rescue, this can be a long process.

necessary personnel. Make sure that you take steps to stabilize the physical location of the patient. For example, look for threats of structural collapse, cave-ins, or vehicle rollovers.

Access triggers the technical beginning of the rescue. While gaining access, you must use appropriate safety equipment and procedures. This is the point when you and/or the incident commander and safety officer must honestly evaluate the training and skills needed to access the patient. Untrained, poorly equipped, or inexperienced rescue personnel must not put their safety and the safety of others at risk by attempting foolhardy, heroic rescues.

During the access phase, key medical, technical, and command personnel must confer with the safety officer on the strategy they will use to accomplish the rescue. To ensure that everyone understands and supports the rescue plan, a formal briefing should be held for rescue personnel before the operation begins. Even with well-trained personnel and adequate equipment, rescue efforts can be poorly executed because team members do not understand the "big picture" or they do not know what is expected of each member of the team.

Phase 4: Medical Treatment

After devising a rescue plan, medical personnel can begin to make patient contact. Remember: No personnel should enter an area to provide patient care unless they are physically fit, protected from hazards, and have the technical skills to reach, manage, and remove patients safely. The interests of both rescuer and patient may be served by a first responder with expertise in the type of rescue required. However, if a first responder does not have the required fitness or skills, he may end up needing to be rescued because of some hasty, ill-advised effort to treat the patient.

In general, a paramedic has three responsibilities during this phase of the rescue operation:

- Initiation of patient assessment and care as soon as possible
- Maintenance of patient care procedures during disentanglement
- Accompaniment of the patient during removal and transport

Again, whether or not you actually fulfill each of these responsibilities depends on the medical expertise of the special rescue team. Recall, for example, the opening case study, in which a trained high-angle paramedic accessed *and* treated the patient.

If you are treating the patient, take these actions if the conditions allow. Quickly conduct a primary assessment (mental status, ABCs, and C-spine status) on each patient (Figure 4-9 ●). The next critical steps include rapid secondary assessment for the patient with a significant mechanism of injury, detailed physical exam, and medically oriented recommendations to the evacuation team.

Because a long time may elapse before transport, a patient's condition may change dramatically during disentanglement and removal. As a result, you should perform patient assessment with two goals in mind. First, identify and care for existing patient problems. Second, anticipate changing patient conditions, and determine the assistance and equipment needed to cope with those changes.

Continually evaluate risks to both rescuers and the patient. In many situations, the best overall patient care requires rapid stabilization and immediate removal. A final positive patient outcome may depend on initial sacrifice of definitive patient care so that the patient and rescuers can be removed from imminent danger. Examples of such situations might include:

- Injured, stranded high-rise window cleaners; workers on water, radio, or TV towers; high-rise construction workers
- Workers or bystanders involved in a trench cave-in
- Persons stranded in swift-running, rising water
- Patients entrapped in vehicles with an associated fire
- Patients overcome by life-threatening atmospheres
- Victims entrapped with unstable and/or volatile hazardous materials

In such cases, rapid transport of a nonstabilized patient to a safer location may be justified by the risk of injury to the rescuers and exposure of the patient to even greater complications. Rapid movement might be required even though the transport will aggravate existing patient injuries. Generally, management for the entrapped patient has the same foundation as all emergency care. Steps include:

- Primary assessment of the MS-ABCs
- Management of life-threatening airway, breathing, and circulation problems
- Immobilization of the spine
- Splinting of major fractures
- Packaging with consideration to patient injuries, **extrication** requirements, and environmental conditions
- Ongoing reassessment during the transport phase

Specifics of patient management during a rescue often follow the same or similar protocols to those used "on the street." However, some specifics may be, or should be, significantly different. Differences result mainly from the lengthy time periods often required to access, disentangle, and/or evacuate the patient. EMS personnel are trained in rapid stabilization and transport, particularly with trauma patients. However, during a rescue mission, the desire to achieve speedy transport may be impossible to fulfill. As a result, you must be able to "shift gears" mentally to an extended care situation. (For some background on time-related changes in treatment, see the discussion of distance in Chapter 7, on rural EMS.)

In addition to extended field time, you must be prepared to provide more in-depth psychological support for rescue patients than might otherwise be required. This is especially true in situations in which a patient has already been entrapped for a considerable amount of time. Establish a solid rapport with the patient, striking up a constant and reassuring conversation. In quieting the fears of rescue patients, keep in mind the following tips:

- Learn and use the patient's name.
- Be sure that the patient knows your name and knows that you will not abandon him.
- Be sure that other team members know and use the patient's correct name. The term "it" should never be substituted for the patient's name in any prehospital setting.
- Avoid negative or fearful comments regarding the operation, the causes of the operation, or the patient's condition within earshot of the patient.

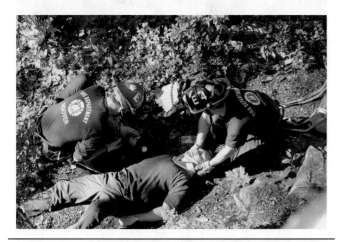

● **Figure 4-9** The fourth phase in a rescue operation is patient treatment. Assessment and care may need to be modified, depending on the on-scene environment and any special hazards.

CONTENT REVIEW

▶ Goals of Rescue
Assessment

• Identify and care for
existing patient problems
• Anticipate changing patient
conditions and determine
in advance the assistance
and equipment needed

• Explain all delays to
the patient and identify
steps that will be taken
to remedy the situation.

• Ask special rescue teams
to explain any technical
aspects of the operation
that could frighten the
patient or affect the
patient's condition.

Translate these operations into clear, simple terms for
the patient.

• Do not lie to the patient. If something may hurt during
rapid movement, acknowledge it. If the patient suspects an
unstable environment, acknowledge that too. However, be
sure to explain what will be done to mitigate the situation
(i.e., the pain or the unstable environment).

• Above all else, stay calm and act every bit the professional.
If you do not know the answer to a question, find
somebody who does. Remember: Rescues are driven by
patient needs.

Phase 5: Disentanglement

Disentanglement involves the actual release from the cause of
entrapment, such as the dashboard of a wrecked automobile, a
concrete slab from a structural collapse, or the blocked entry
to a cave. This phase may be the most technical and time-
consuming portion of the rescue (Figure 4-10 ●). If assigned
to patient care during this phase of the rescue, you have three
responsibilities:

• Personal and professional confidence in the technical
expertise and gear needed to function effectively in the
active rescue zone, sometimes referred to as the "hot zone"
or "inner circle"

• Readiness to provide prolonged patient care, that is,
medical support of technical efforts

• Ability to call for and/or use special rescue resources

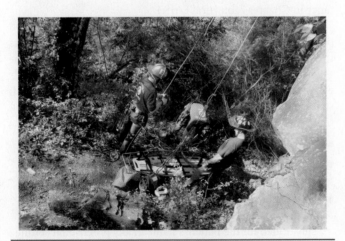

● **Figure 4-10** The fifth phase in a rescue operation is
disentanglement. It can be prolonged, as in the case of auto
entrapment.

If you or another member of the rescue team cannot fulfill
these requirements, reassess available rescue personnel and call
for backup. Disentanglement is not a task for persons who are
claustrophobic—extrication may involve crawling into a tight
space. Disentanglement is also not a task for the squeamish—in
some cases, an amputation may be required.

Methods used to disentangle the patient must be constantly
analyzed on a risk-to-benefit basis. You and/or other members of
the rescue team must balance the patient's medical needs with such
concerns as the time it will take to perform treatment, the safety
of the environment, and so on. If a patient has a severely crushed
extremity and it will take an inordinate amount of time to release
the extremity, the patient may in fact bleed to death without an
amputation. This is only one of the hard treatment decisions that
may be faced during the disentanglement phase of the operation.

Phase 6: Patient Packaging

After disentanglement, a patient must be appropriately packaged
to ensure that all medical needs are addressed (Figure 4-11 ●).
You must consider such things as the means of egress—for example, a litter carry through the woods versus walking a patient
out. You must also factor time based on the patient's medical
conditions—for example, rapid extrication techniques versus

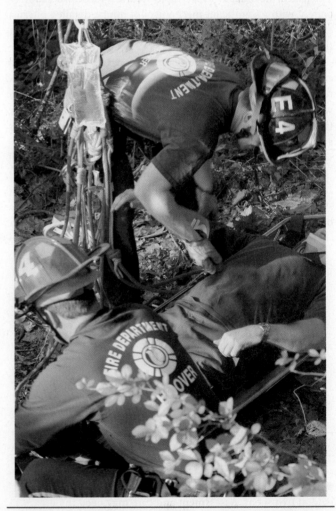

● **Figure 4-11** The sixth phase in a rescue operation is
packaging of the patient.

application of a Kendrick extrication device (KED). Some forms of patient packaging can be more complex than others, depending on the specialized rescue techniques required to extricate the patient—for example, being lifted out of a hole in a Stokes basket by a ladder truck, being vertically hauled through a manhole in a Sked stretcher, and so on. In situations in which the patient may be vertical or suspended in a Stokes basket, it is paramount that the rescuer know how to properly package the patient to prevent additional injury.

Phase 7: Removal/Transport

Removal of the patient may be one of the most difficult tasks to accomplish (Figure 4-12a ●) or it may be as easy as placing the person on a stretcher and wheeling the stretcher to a nearby ambulance. Activities involved in the removal of a patient will require the coordinated effort of all personnel. Transportation to a medical facility should be planned well in advance, especially if you anticipate any delays. Decisions regarding patient transport—whether by ground vehicle (Figure 4-12b ●), by aircraft, or by physical carry-out—should be coordinated based on advice from medical direction. En route to the hospital, perform the reassessment, repeating vitals every 5 minutes for an unstable patient and every 15 minutes for a stable patient. Update the patient's condition and administer additional therapy per medical direction.

SURFACE WATER RESCUES

As previously mentioned, there are a number of different categories of rescue operations in which you may apply the principles and practices described thus far in the chapter. Water emergencies are among the most common. Because people are attracted to water in such great numbers and for such a wide variety of activities, accidents can take many different forms.

Most water rescues are resolved without the involvement of EMS personnel—for example, bystanders jump into a pool to pull out a struggling swimmer or other boaters rescue someone whose canoe has overturned. However, some water emergencies require that the rescuers have special training and equipment. In such cases, the temperature and dynamics of flat or moving water place both the victim and the rescuer at high risk of entrapment. Although all the possible scenarios for water rescue training cannot be supplied in a single section of a chapter, the following are some general concepts and methods to raise your "water rescue awareness."

General Background

Water rescues may involve many kinds of water bodies: pools, rivers, streams, lakes, canals, flooded gravel pits, or even the ocean. Some communities also have drainage systems that remain dry until flash floods turn them into raging rivers.

Most people who get injured or drown in these bodies of water do not intend to get into trouble. But one or more factors conspire to create an emergency: The weather changes, swimmers underestimate the water's power, nonswimmers neglect to wear a PFD and fall in, people develop a muscle stitch or cramp

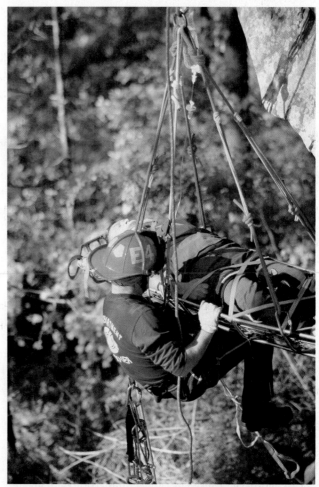

(a)

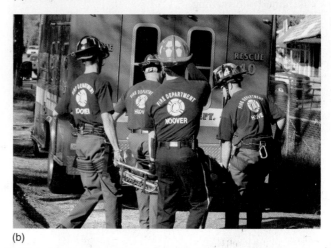

(b)

● **Figure 4-12** The seventh and final phase in a rescue operation is (a) removal and (b) transport of the patient. This can be by helicopter or by ground ambulance, depending on the situation and the condition of the patient.

while in the water, submerged debris knocks waders off their feet, boats collide, and more.

Nearly all incidents in and around water are preventable. It is important for you to become familiar with safe aquatic practices. First and foremost, know how to swim and make swimming part of your physical exercise. Second, remember that even the strongest swimmer can get into trouble. Therefore, always carry PFDs aboard your unit and always wear a PFD whenever you are around water or ice (Figure 4-13 ●). (Make sure your crew does the same.) Third, you might consider taking a basic water rescue course.

Water Temperature

Because the human body temperature is normally 98.6°F (37°C), almost any body of water is colder and will cause heat loss. Water temperature in smaller bodies of water varies widely with the seasons and the amount of runoff. Yet, even on warm days, water temperature can be quite cold in most places. As a result, water temperature and heat loss figure in the demise of most victims and ill-equipped rescuers.

As implied, immersion can rapidly lead to hypothermia, a condition discussed in Volume 5, Chapter 12. As a rule, people cannot maintain body heat in water that is less than 92°F (33°C). The colder the water, the faster the loss of heat. In fact, water causes heat loss 25 times faster than the air. Immersion in 35°F (1.6°C) water for 15 to 20 minutes is likely to kill a person.[1,2] Factors contributing to the demise of a hypothermic patient include:

● Incapacitation and an inability to self-rescue

● Inability to follow simple directions

● Inability to grasp a line or flotation device

● Laryngospasm (caused by sudden immersion) and greater likelihood of drowning

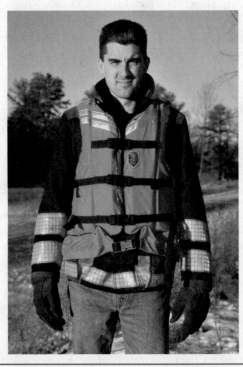

● **Figure 4-13** A personal flotation device (PFD) is mandatory equipment for any water-related rescue.

A number of actions can delay the onset of hypothermia in water rescues. The use of PFDs slows heat loss and reduces the energy required for flotation. If people suddenly become submerged, they can also assume the **heat escape lessening position (HELP)**. This position involves floating with the head out of water and the body in a fetal tuck. Researchers estimate that someone who has practiced with HELP can reduce heat loss by almost 60 percent, as compared to the heat expended when treading water. If a group of victims find themselves in the water, researchers also suggest huddling together. This technique not only prevents heat loss, but also provides a better target (more visibility) for members of a rescue team.

Basic Rescue Techniques

Basic rescue techniques vary with the dynamics of the water; rescue in moving water will differ from rescue in nonmoving (flat) water. If your unit responds to frozen bodies of water, you may also add techniques for ice rescue and include the proper cold-water-entry dry suits as part of your PPE cache (Figure 4-14 ●). Also keep in mind that a PFD is useless if it is not worn. Therefore, all EMS personnel should put one on, even for shore-based rescues.

The water rescue model is reach–throw–row–go. All paramedics should be trained in reach-and-throw techniques. If, at first, you are unable to talk the patient into a self-rescue, then reach with a pole or long rescue device. If this is not effective or if the victim is too far out, try throwing a flotation device. All paramedics should become proficient with a water-throw bag for shore-based operations. Remember: Boat-based techniques require specialized rescue training. Water entry ("go") is used only as the last resort—and is an action best left to specialized water rescuers.

Moving Water

By far the most dangerous water rescues involve water that is moving. Competency at handling the power and dynamics of swift-water rescues comes only with extensive training and experience. The force of moving water can be very deceptive. The hydraulics of moving water change with a number of variables, including water depth, velocity, obstructions to flow, changing tides, and more. Only specially trained rescuers can readily recognize these factors.

To train for swift-water entry, rescuers must develop a proficiency in many specialized skills. In preparation for technical rope rescues, they must master the skills required for high-angle rope rescues. They must also become well practiced in such skills as crossing moving bodies of water, defensive swimming, use of throw bags and boogy boards, shore-based swimming, boat-based rescue techniques, management of water-specific emergencies, and the capability to package the patient with water-related injuries.

Four swift-water rescue scenarios present a special challenge and danger to rescuers. They are recirculating currents ("drowning machines"), strainers, foot/extremity pins, and dams or hydroelectric intakes.

Recirculating Currents

Recirculating currents result from water flowing over a uniform obstruction such as a large rock or low head dam. The

it very difficult to escape. The resulting rescue can be extremely hazardous, even for specially trained rescuers.

Strainers

When moving water flows through obstructions such as downed trees, grating, or wire mesh, an unequal force is created on the two sides of the so-called **strainers** (Figure 4-16 ●). Currents can literally force a patient up against a strainer, making it difficult to remove him because of the power of the current. In some cases, the current might be flowing into a drainage pipe under the surface, which is in turn covered by a rebar (metal) grate. Victims can get sucked into the grate and then pinned against it.

This, too, can be a hazardous rescue. If you get stuck floating downstream and see the potential of getting pinned against a strainer, attempt to swim over the object. Whatever you do, do not put your feet on the bottom of the river—your feet could get stuck or, even worse, you could get swept off your feet and slammed into the obstruction.

Foot/Extremity Pins

For the sake of safety, keep this point in mind: It is always unsafe to walk in fast-moving water over knee depth because of the danger of entrapping a foot or extremity. When this occurs, the weight and force of the water can knock you below the surface of the water. To remove the foot or extremity, it must be extracted the same way it went in. Water currents often make this extremely difficult. Again, this is a hazardous rescue because of the need to work below the surface in already dangerous water conditions.

Dams/Hydroelectric Intakes

Yet another dangerous situation involves dams and hydroelectric intakes, such as those often found along rivers. The height of the dam is no indication of the degree of hazard. As already indicated, low head dams can create powerful drowning machines. As a result, assume that all dams have the ability to form recirculating currents. Hydroelectric intakes, however, serve as dangerous strainers with all the accompanying hazards.

Self-Rescue Techniques

Some water survival techniques, such as wearing PFDs and the use of HELP, have already been mentioned. However, if you suddenly fall in swift-running water (or flat for that matter), keep these suggestions in mind:

- Cover your mouth and nose during entry.
- Protect your head and, if possible, keep your face out of the water.
- Do not attempt to stand up in moving water.
- Float on your back, with your feet pointed downstream.
- Steer with your feet, and point your head toward the nearest shore at a 45-degree angle or continue to float downstream until you come to an area where the water slows enough for you to swim to the edge.

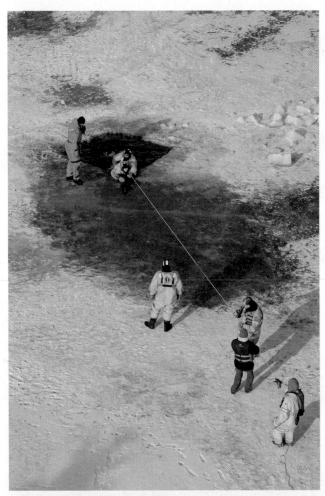

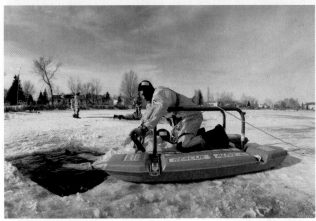

● **Figure 4-14** Safe ice rescue requires proper equipment and protective clothing. *(© Kevin Link)*

movement of currents can literally create what is known as a "drowning machine" (Figure 4-15 ●).

On first appearance, recirculating currents can look very tame. Anglers, for example, often fish on the downstream portion of a low head dam, casting their lines into the recirculating waters. This is a good place to catch fish because they can often be seen just below the dam. But think about it. If fish with their natural ability to swim get stuck in the recirculating currents, imagine what would happen to humans if they got too close to the dam. Once caught in the recirculating currents, people find

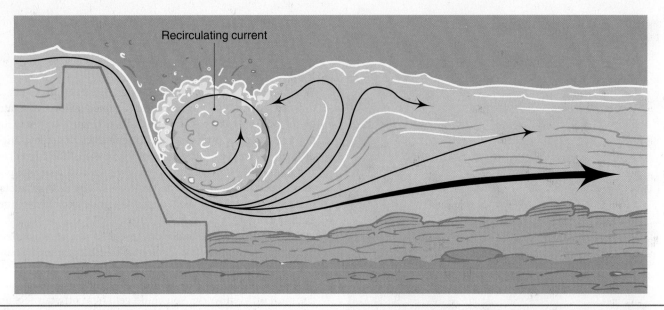

● **Figure 4-15** When water flows over a large uniform object, it can create a hydraulic trap or hole with a recirculating current that moves against the river's flow and can trap people.

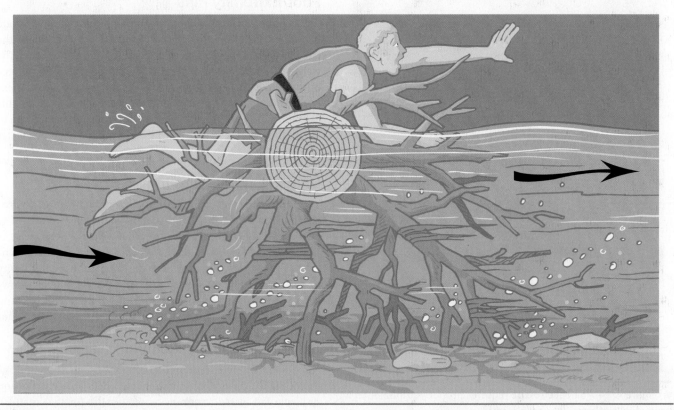

● **Figure 4-16** Strainers are objects that allow water to flow through them but that will trap other objects—and people.

- If the water turns a bend, remember that the outside of the curve moves faster that the inside of the curve.
- Look for large objects, such as rocks, that can block the water and cause recirculating currents or strainers.
- Learn to identify **eddies**—water that flows around especially large objects and, for a time, flows upstream around the downside of the obstruction. These back currents move more slowly and can actually sweep you toward the edge—and safety.

- Above all else, take precautions not to fall into the water in the first place. Remember: Reach–throw–row–go, with "go" being the absolutely last resort.

Flat Water

The greatest problem with flat water is that it looks so calm. However, a large proportion of drowning or near-drowning incidents take place in flat or slow-moving water (Figure 4-17 ●). Some of the factors in these deaths were mentioned earlier.

In a significant number of cases, alcohol plays a role in the incident. Nearly 50 percent of boating fatalities, for example, result from alcohol intoxication or impairment. As a result, many states have enacted tough laws to restrict the operation of boats while under the influence of alcohol, which impairs the ability to think, reason, and survive in an alcohol-related water incident.[3]

Factors Affecting Survival

A number of factors help determine the demise or survival of a patient. A person's "survivability profile" is affected by age, posture, lung volume, water temperature, and more. Two especially important factors include the presence of PFDs and what is known as the "cold-protective response."

Personal Flotation Devices

Many recreational water users associate "life preservers" with rough water or people who cannot swim. However, PFDs should be essential items for all water-related activities. One study, for example, linked nearly 89 percent of all boating fatalities to the lack of a PFD. This fact is a reminder of why you should don a PFD whenever you approach water.

Every system should have a strict SOP mandating the use of PFDs for all EMS personnel. Even services in arid regions can be involved in water rescues. They can be called to swimming pool incidents or river-rafting accidents. In some places, especially in the Southwest, they can respond to flash-flooding in canyons that can trap or kill hikers or "canyoneers." The same flash flooding can overload drainage systems, creating hazardous conditions for the public and rescuers alike.

CONTENT REVIEW

► Factors Affecting Survival
- Age
- Posture
- Lung volume
- Water temperature
- Use of PFDs

Cold-Protective Response

Brain cells deprived of oxygen will normally begin to die in as little as 4 to 8 minutes. Keeping the head above water, as in the HELP and self-rescue techniques discussed earlier, ensures that the person can breathe and keep the brain supplied with oxygen. Additionally, although cold water can cause death from hypothermia, cold water can also trigger a protective response known as the "mammalian diving reflex." This is how it works: When the face of a human, or any mammal, is plunged into cold water less than 68°F (20°C), the parasympathetic nervous system is stimulated. The heart rate rapidly decreases to a bradycardic rhythm. Meanwhile, blood pressure drops and vasoconstriction occurs throughout the body. Blood is shunted from less vital organs to the heart and brain, temporarily delivering life-sustaining oxygen. As a general rule, the colder the water, the more oxygen is diverted.

UNINTENTIONAL DROWNING

- Every day, approximately ten people die from unintentional drowning.
- Drowning is the second leading cause of unintentional injury death for children ages 1-14.
- Drowning is the fifth leading cause of unintentional injury death for all age groups.

All Unintentional Drowning, 2007

Natural Water	43.0%
Swimming Pool	18.6%
Unspecified	13.9%
Bathtub	10.4%
Boating	9.2%
Other	4.9%

A Few Prevention Tips

- Children should be given formal swimming lessons. Even when they have had these lessons, they should be under constant, careful adult supervision in or around water.
- Avoid drinking alcohol.
- Use life jackets when boating.
- Be aware of drop offs and hidden obstacles in natural water.
- Watch for dangerous waves and signs of rip currents.
- Know local weather conditions before boating and swimming.

● **Figure 4-17** Unintentional drowning. From "Drowning Risks in Natural Water Settings," Centers for Disease Control and Prevention. http://www.cdc.gov/Features/dsDrowningRisks/.

Two factors, then, can significantly delay death when a person is in cold water: the length of time the person is able to keep his head above water and the mammalian diving reflex once the person's face becomes submerged. Some patients have been resuscitated after 45 minutes underwater. The record is 66 minutes for a patient rescued in Salt Lake, Utah, on June 10, 1989. As a rule, the reflex is more pronounced in children than in adults.

Location of Submerged Victims

Because of protective physiologic responses, rescuers must make every effort to locate submerged victims. Interview witnesses to establish a relative location. Ask each witness, for example, to locate an object across the water to form a line. Repeat this process with each witness. Use the point of convergence among lines to target the most accurate "last seen" location. Start searching from this point and fan out in larger and larger circles, forming a radius equal to the depth of the water.

Rescue versus Body Recovery

A number of conditions determine when a rescue turns into a body recovery. Some factors are length of time submerged, any known or suspected trauma, age and physical condition of the victim, water temperature and environmental conditions, and estimated time for rescue or removal.

Once a patient is recovered, you should attempt resuscitation on any hypothermic and/or pulseless, nonbreathing patient who has been submerged in cold water. (Some experts advise providing resuscitation to every drowning patient, regardless of water temperature, even those who have been in the water for some time.) A patient must be rewarmed before an accurate assessment can be made. Remember: Water-rescue patients are "never dead until they are warm and dead." (For more on drowning and near-drowning, see Volume 5, Chapter 12.)

In-Water Patient Immobilization

In flat water where you are able to safely stand, it is important that you know how to perform in-water immobilization (Figure 4-18 ●). Cervical spine injuries are associated with trauma (e.g., diving) rather than simple submersion.[4] In general, the procedure mirrors the application of a long board, with the following modifications:

- *Phase One: In-Water Spinal Immobilization*
  1. Apply the head-splint technique. (There are other techniques, but they do not work as well because of the use of PFDs by the rescuers.)
  2. Approach the patient from the side.
  3. Move the patient's arms over the head.
  4. Hold the patient's head in place by using the patient's arms as a "splint."
  5. If the patient was found in a face-down position, perform steps 1 through 4, then rotate the patient toward the rescuer in a face-up position.

6. Ensure an open airway.
7. Maintain this position until a cervical collar is applied.

- *Phase Two: Rigid Cervical Collar Application*
  1. A second rescuer determines the proper collar size.
  2. This second rescuer then holds the open collar under the victim's neck.
  3. The primary rescuer maintains immobilization and a patent airway.
  4. The second rescuer brings the collar up to the back of the patient's neck and the primary rescuer allows the second rescuer to bring the collar around the patient's neck while the primary rescuer maintains the airway.
  5. The second rescuer secures the fastener on the collar while the primary rescuer maintains the airway.
  6. The second rescuer secures the patient's hands at the waist of the patient.

- *Phase Three: Backboarding and Extrication from the Water*
  1. Secure the necessary personnel—two rescuers in the water and additional rescuers at the water's edge—and the correct equipment. Rescuers are strongly urged to use a floating backboard for water rescue.
  2. Submerge the board under the patient's waist.
  3. Never lift the patient to the board. Instead, allow the board to float up to the victim. (If the board does not float, lift it gently to the victim.)
  4. Secure the patient with straps, cravats, or other devices.
  5. Move the patient to an extrication point along the shore or boat.
  6. Always extricate the patient head first, so the body weight does not compress possible spinal trauma.
  7. If possible, avoid extrication of the patient through surf, because the board could capsize and dump the patient back into the water. Consider using bystanders who can swim as a breakwall behind the patient.
  8. Maintain airway management during extrication.

HAZARDOUS ATMOSPHERE RESCUES

Confined-space rescues present any number of potentially fatal threats, but one of the most serious is an oxygen-deficient environment. At first glance, most confined spaces appear relatively safe. As a result, you might mistakenly think that rescue procedures will be easier and/or less time-consuming and dangerous than they really are. Here is where rescue awareness comes in. According to the National Institute for Occupational Safety

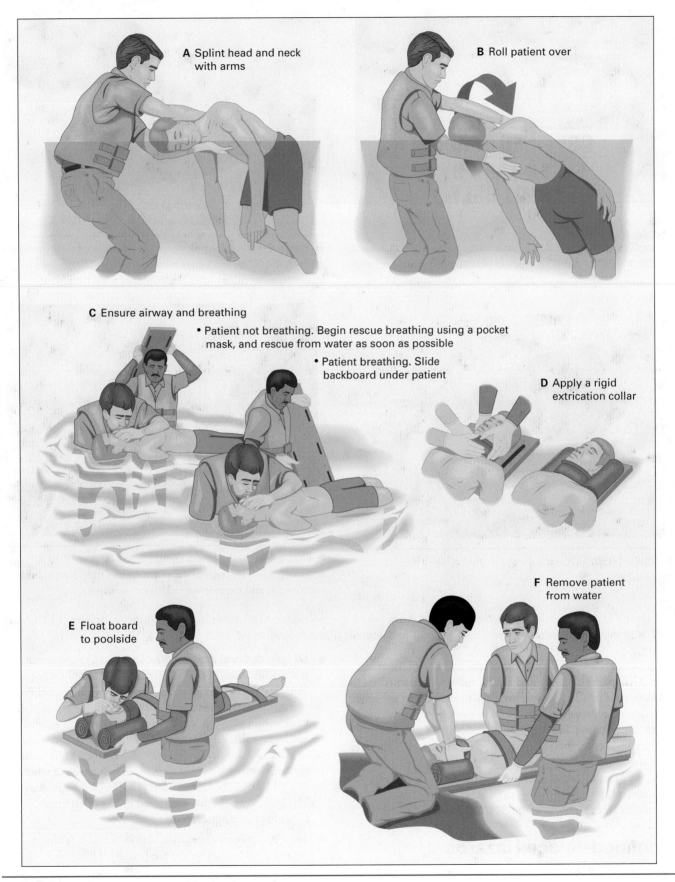

A Splint head and neck with arms

B Roll patient over

C Ensure airway and breathing

- Patient not breathing. Begin rescue breathing using a pocket mask, and rescue from water as soon as possible
- Patient breathing. Slide backboard under patient

D Apply a rigid extrication collar

E Float board to poolside

F Remove patient from water

● **Figure 4-18** Water rescue, possible spinal injury.

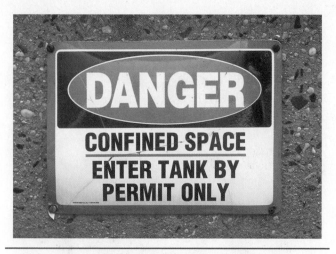

● **Figure 4-19a** Look for clues to potentially hazardous atmospheres and confined spaces, such as warning signs.

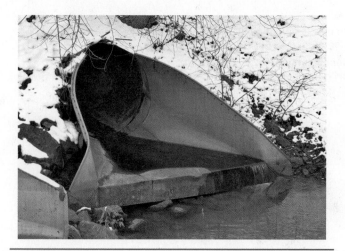

● **Figure 4-19b** Treat a culvert for what it is— a dangerous confined space.

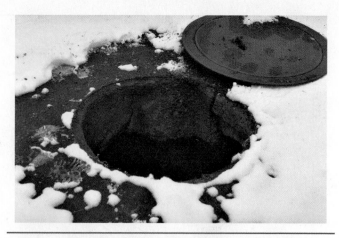

● **Figure 4-19c** Manholes provide access to underground utility vaults. The vault may have a limited or hazardous atmosphere and may offer the potential for entrapment.

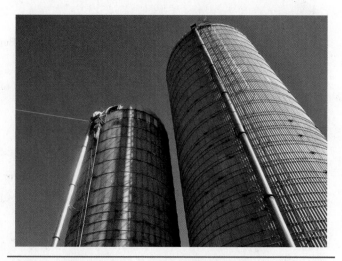

● **Figure 4-19d** Rescuers should never be permitted to enter confined spaces, such as silos, unless they have training, equipment, and experience in this environment.

and Health (NIOSH), nearly 60 percent of all fatalities associated with confined spaces are people attempting to rescue a victim.

Although "confined space" can have a variety of interpretations, Occupational Safety and Health Administration (OSHA) regulation CFR 1910.146 interprets the term to mean any space with limited access/egress that is not designed for human occupancy or habitation. In other words, confined spaces are not safe for people to enter for any sustained period of time. Examples of confined spaces are transport or storage tanks, grain bins and silos, wells and cisterns, manholes and pumping stations, drainage culverts, pits, hoppers, underground vaults, and mine or cave shafts (Figures 4-19a through 4-19d ●).

Confined-Space Hazards

As already mentioned, confined spaces present a wide range of hazards. You may confront one or more of these hazards in any given confined-space rescue. As a first responder, it is your responsibility to identify these hazards as soon as possible, both for purposes of scene safety and for summoning the

necessary support. Some of the most common risks include the following:

● *Oxygen-deficient atmospheres.* Untrained rescuers may not readily think of oxygen deficiency. It simply is not a "visible" threat. Special entry teams know otherwise. Before going into a confined space, they monitor the atmosphere to determine the following: oxygen concentration, levels of hydrogen sulfide, explosive limits, flammable atmosphere, or toxic contaminants. They are also aware that increases in oxygen content for any reasons—such as a gust of wind— can give atmospheric monitoring meters a false reading. The bottom line is this: Confined spaces often mean hazardous atmospheres.

● *Toxic or explosive chemicals.* Many chemicals found in confined spaces can be toxic, especially if inhaled (Figure 4-20 ●). Some of the poisonous fumes contain gases that displace oxygen in the red blood cells. Other chemicals are highly explosive. Dangerous chemical gases commonly found in confined spaces include hydrogen sulfide (H_2S), carbon dioxide (CO_2), carbon monoxide (CO), exceptionally

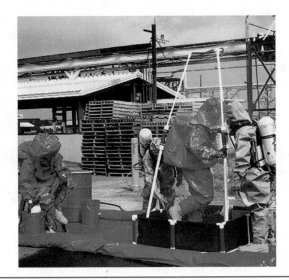

● **Figure 4-20** Rescuers exposed to toxic or hazardous materials will need to go through decontamination.

low or high oxygen concentrations, chlorine (Cl_2), ammonia (NH_3), and nitrogen dioxide (NO_2).

● *Engulfment.* Some confined spaces contain physical substances—grain, coal, sand, and so on—that can literally bury a patient or a rescuer who falls into the space. Dust from these materials can also create a highly explosive atmosphere.

● *Machinery entrapment.* Confined spaces come with all sorts of machinery or equipment that can entrap a person. Augers or screws can also entrap a victim.

● *Electricity.* Confined spaces often contain motors or materials management equipment powered by electricity. In addition to the risk of shock or electrocution, these machines may contain stored energy. To ensure safe entry, rescue crews will have to take a number of steps. First, it may be necessary to blank out the flow of all power into the site. Second, stored energy should be dissipated, and all machinery should be shut down following lock-out/tag-out procedures. (After you shut off the equipment, lock off the switch and place a tag on the switch stating why it is shut off to prevent inadvertently tripping the switch.) Third, the space may need to be ventilated to ensure against oxygen deficiency or explosive dust particles. Remember: It takes only one spark to trigger an explosion.

● *Structural concerns.* Structure supports and shapes further complicate confined-space rescues. Some confined spaces have I-beams that can cause injury due to limited light and height. Other confined spaces have noncylindrical shapes that present difficult extrication problems. Confined spaces can be shaped in the form of Ls, Ts, Xs, and any combination thereof. Because of limited access, rescuers may find it difficult or even impossible to use standard self-contained breathing apparatus. They may have to resort to supplied air breathing apparatus (i.e., oxygen lines). They may also need to be lowered into the space with a full-body harness or other system to make retrieval easier in case something goes wrong.

Confined-Space Protections in the Workplace

Fortunately, state and federal laws require most industries to develop a confined-space rescue program. This means that employers must provide a training program for all employees who work in or around confined spaces. These employees may be called on to perform on-site rescues and may indeed be an important part of the emergency response.

OSHA also requires a permit process before workers may enter a confined space such as a trench. In addition, most industries must fulfill strict requirements such as ongoing atmospheric monitoring, posted warnings, and work-site permits with detailed data on hazard management. The area must be made safe and workers must don PPE. Retrieval devices must also be in place whenever workers enter the spaces. Nonpermitted sites are the most likely locations for emergencies because of the oxygen deficiencies that result from inadequate atmospheric monitoring.

The types of confined-space emergencies most commonly encountered in the workplace include falls, medical emergencies (often hazmat related), oxygen deficiencies or asphyxia, explosions, and entrapment. You should never allow rescuers into a confined space unless they have the training, equipment, and experience specific to the particular environment involved. You will almost always summon outside specialized agencies for support.

Cave-Ins and Structural Collapses

As earthquakes in California have proven, it can be very dramatic to watch rescues from cave-ins or structural collapses. But it does not take an earthquake to produce this type of confined-space emergency. Collapsed trenches or cave-ins can occur in almost any community. In fact, most trench collapses occur in trenches less than 12 feet deep and 6 feet wide, particularly in trenches that do not comply with OSHA regulations (Figure 4-21 ●).

To understand the medical magnitude of a collapsed trench, consider these facts. A typical cubic foot of soil weighs 100 pounds.

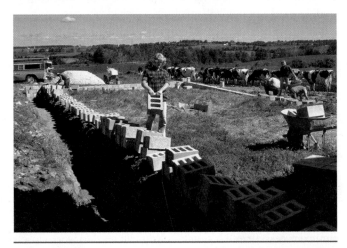

● **Figure 4-21** If trenches do not comply with OSHA regulations, the possibility of collapse is increased. (© *Michal Heron*)

As a result, just 2 feet of soil on top of a worker's chest or back, which could have a surface area of 4 to 5 square feet, would weigh between 800 and 1,000 pounds. People are literally buried alive. Unless uncovered quickly, they suffer death by asphyxiation.

Reasons for Collapses/Cave-Ins

Trenches collapse or cave-in for a number of reasons. The most common reasons include:

- Contractors disregard safety regulations, either out of negligence or out of efforts to save money. (Federal law requires either shoring or a trench box for excavations deeper than 5 feet. Anything less is an invitation to trouble.)
- The lip of one or both sides of the trench caves in.
- The wall shears away or falls in entirely.
- The "spoil pile," or dirt removed from the hole, is placed too close to the edge of the trench.
- Water seepage, ground vibrations, intersecting trenches, or previously disturbed soil weaken the structural integrity.

Rescue from Trenches/Cave-Ins

If a collapse has caused burial, a secondary collapse is likely. Therefore, your initial actions should be geared toward safety. Secure the scene, establish command, secure a perimeter, and immediately summon a team specializing in trench rescue. While waiting for the team to arrive, do not allow entry in the area surrounding the trench or cave-in. Safe access can take place only when proper shoring is in place.

HIGHWAY OPERATIONS AND VEHICLE RESCUES

As you already know, the most common rescue situations encountered by EMS personnel involve motor vehicle collisions. These incidents generally go through the phases covered at the start of this chapter. However, certain modifications must be made to meet the special hazards associated with traffic control and the extrication of patients from wrecked vehicles.

Hazards in Highway Operations

To prepare for highway rescues, you must size up the scene, identify all hazards, and ensure scene safety—that is, control any potentially dangerous situations. In the case of highway operations, this means reducing traffic-related hazards and identifying hazards related to the vehicle crash itself.

Traffic Hazards

Traffic flow is the largest single hazard associated with EMS highway operations. You may have to respond to incidents on roads with limited access and to incidents on highways with unlimited access. In either situation, you will need to work closely with police to avoid unnecessary congestion as well as other injuries. Remember that traffic backups impede the flow both to and from the scene.

An even bigger personal danger results from the risk of vehicles hitting EMS apparatus or personnel. Studies have shown that drivers who are tired, drunk, or drugged actually drive right into the emergency lights. Spectators can worsen the situation by getting out of their cars to watch or even "help."

At this point in your career, you probably already know some of the things you can do to reduce traffic hazards. Here are a few tried-and-tested techniques:

- *Staging.* Staging is always critical at any multiple-casualty incident, but it takes on added importance on limited-access roads or highways. Always consider staging emergency vehicles away from the scene. Then have command bring the vehicles in whenever there is an appropriate place and/or assignment for the crews. The staging area should be within a minute or two of the scene, ideally in a large parking lot or less congested area. Some situations simply cannot accommodate the entire response at once.

- *Positioning of apparatus.* When apparatus does arrive, ensure that it causes the minimum reduction of traffic flow. As much as possible, apparatus should be positioned to protect the scene. The ambulance loading area should *NOT* be directly exposed to traffic. Also, *DO NOT* rely solely on ambulance lights to warn traffic away. These lights are often obstructed when medics open the doors for loading.

- *Emergency lighting.* Use only a minimum of warning lights to alert traffic of a hazard and to define the actual size of your vehicle. Too many lights can confuse or blind drivers, causing additional collisions. Experts strongly advise that you turn off all headlights when parked at the scene and rely instead on amber scene lighting.

- *Redirection of traffic.* Be sure traffic cones and flares are placed early in the incident. If the police are not already on scene, this is your responsibility. As a first responder, you must redirect traffic away from the collision and away from all emergency workers. In other words, you need to create a safety zone. Make sure that you do not place lighted flares too near any sources of fuel or brush; otherwise, you risk an explosion or fire. Once you light the flares, allow them to burn out. *DO NOT* try to extinguish them. Attempting to pick up a flare can cause a very severe thermal burn.

- *High visibility.* As already mentioned, all rescuers should be dressed in highly visible clothing. Because many EMS, police, and fire agencies wear dark-colored uniforms, you should don a brightly colored turnout coat or vest with reflective tape. You can apply the tape at the scene.

Other Hazards

Other hazards besides traffic control exist at highway operations. In some communities, paramedics receive training to manage these hazards. In other communities, they receive "awareness training" and learn to summon specialized rescue personnel. Regardless of the procedure in your service area, you must be able to recognize all nontraffic hazards (Figure 4-22 ●).

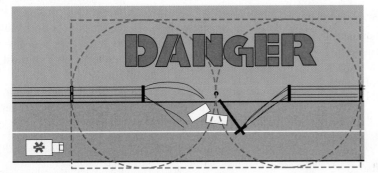

Downed Lines

In accidents involving downed electrical wires and damaged utility poles, the danger zone should extend beyond each intact pole for a full span and to the sides for the distance that the severed wires can reach. Stay out of the danger zone until the utility company has deactivated the wires, or until trained rescuers have moved and anchored them.

● **Figure 4-22** Establish a danger zone in motor vehicle collisions involving electrical hazards.

Otherwise, you risk injuring yourself, your crew, the patient, or even passing motorists. Some of these nontraffic hazards include:

- *Fire and fuel.* Fuel spilled at the scene increases the chances of fire. Be very careful whenever you smell or see pools of liquid at a collision. Keep in mind that bystanders who are smoking can cause a bigger problem than the original crash if they flick lighted ashes into a fuel leak. *DO NOT* drive your emergency vehicle over a fuel spill or—worse yet—park on one. Remember that all automobiles manufactured since the 1970s have catalytic converters. They run at a temperature of around 1,200°F—hot enough to heat fuel to the point of ignition. Be especially careful when a vehicle has gone off the road into dry grass or brush. The debris can be just as dangerous as spilled fuel, especially when brought into contact with a blazing hot catalytic converter.

- *Alternative fuel systems.* Be equally cautious of vehicles powered by alternative fuel systems. High-pressure tanks, especially if filled with natural gas, are extremely volatile. Even vehicles powered by electricity can be dangerous. The storage cells possess the energy to spark, flash, and more.

- *Hybrid and electric vehicles.* Hybrid and electric vehicles pose a particular danger for rescuers. These vehicles have high-voltage systems that can be a risk for rescuers unfamiliar with the vehicles.

- *Sharp objects.* Automobile collisions mean lots of sharp objects, including glass, metal, plastic, and fiberglass. Be sure to wear appropriate protective gear, such as heavy leather gloves and eyewear.

- *Electric power.* Contact with downed power lines or underground electrical feeds can be lethal. If a vehicle is in contact with electrical lines, consider it to be "charged" and call the power company immediately. In most newer communities, electrical lines run underground. However, a vehicle can still run into a transformer or an electrical feed box. As a result, make sure you look under the car and all around it during your scene size-up. *DO NOT* touch a vehicle until you have ruled out all electrical hazards.

- *Energy-absorbing bumpers.* The bumpers on many vehicles come with pistons and are designed to withstand a slow-speed collision. The intent is to limit front- or rear-end damage. Sometimes, however, these bumpers become "loaded" in the crushed position and do not immediately

bounce back out. When exposed to fire or even just tapped by rescue workers, the pistons can suddenly unload their stored energy. Some bumpers have been thrown a hundred feet from the vehicle when they unload. As a result, you must examine bumpers for loading. If you discover a loaded bumper, stay away from it unless you are specially trained to deal with this hazard.

- *Supplemental restraint systems (SRS)/air bags.* Air bags also have the potential to release stored energy. If they have not deployed during the collision, they may do so during the middle of an extrication. As a result, these devices must be deactivated prior to disentanglement. Auto manufacturers can provide information about power removal or power dissipation for their particular brand of SRS. Also, keep in mind that many new model vehicles come equipped with side impact bags.

- *Hazardous cargoes.* An incredible amount of hazardous material travels across the highways of North America. You will learn much more about the role of EMS in highway crashes involving hazmat in Chapter 5. For your personal safety, suspect hazmat at any scene involving commercial vehicles.

- *Rolling vehicles.* As you already know, you must size up the position of a vehicle whenever you arrive at the scene of a collision. Do not overlook the subtle situations that can occur at any collision. You might arrive on the scene and see the vehicle on all four wheels and consider it stable. Then someone from your crew jumps into the rear seat to stabilize the patient's neck manually. Suddenly the vehicle starts rolling down the street. This situation is not only embarrassing—it is dangerous! As a result, always check that the transmission is in park. Make sure the parking brake is on, the ignition is off, and any key rings with remote ignition starters are removed.

- *Unstable vehicles.* Motor vehicles can land in all kinds of unstable positions. They can roll onto a side or the roof. They can stop on an incline or unstable terrain. They can be suspended over a cliff or river. They can come to rest on a patch of ice or an on-site spill or leak. In such situations, you need to request the necessary stabilization crews or equipment. You should also know how to apply proper techniques for temporary stabilization, using ropes, chocks, or a come-along. Under no circumstances should you allow rescuers to access the patient until the vehicle is stabilized.

Auto Anatomy

Motor vehicle collisions present EMS personnel with the most common access and/or extrication problems. As a result, you must know some basic information about automobile construction or "anatomy." Obviously, vehicles can differ greatly, both in terms of manufacture and design. However, most recent automobiles have certain features in common that can guide you in simple access situations.

Basic Constructions

Vehicles can have either a unibody or a frame construction. Most automobiles today have a unibody design, whereas older vehicles and lightweight trucks have a frame construction. For unibody vehicles to maintain their integrity, all of the following features must remain intact: roof posts, floor, firewall, truck support, and windshield.

Both types of construction have roofs and roof supports. The support posts are lettered from front to back. The first post, which supports the roof at the windshield, is called the "A" post. The next post is the "B" post. The third post, found in sedans or station wagons, is the "C" post. Station wagons have an additional rear post, known as the "D" post.

If you remove the plastic molding on the posts, the remaining steel can be easily cut with a hacksaw. Application of power steering fluid helps reduce the heat produced by cutting. In the case of a unibody design, remember that cutting a post will interrupt the vehicle's construction.

Firewall and Engine Compartment

The firewall separates the engine compartment and the occupant compartment. Frequently, the firewall can collapse on a patient's legs during a high-speed, head-on collision. Sometimes, a patient's feet may go through the firewall. Movement at other parts of the vehicle, such as cutting a rocker panel or roof support post, can place additional pressure on the feet.

The engine compartment usually contains the battery. This can cause a fire hazard; therefore, many rescue teams cut the battery cables to eliminate this risk. Before disconnecting the power, it is a good idea to move back electric seats and lower power windows. Otherwise, you might needlessly complicate the extrication.

Glass

Vehicles have two types of glass: safety glass and tempered glass. Safety glass is made from three layers of fused materials: glass–plastic laminate–glass. It is found in windshields and designed to stay intact when shattered or broken. However, safety glass can still produce glass dust or fracture into long shards. These materials can easily get into a patient's eyes, nose, or mouth and/or create cuts. As a result, be sure to cover a patient whenever you remove this type of glass.

Tempered glass has a high tensile strength. However, it does not stay intact when shattered or broken. It fractures into many small beads of glass, all of which can cause injuries and cuts.

Doors

The doors of most newer vehicles contain a reinforcing bar to protect the occupant in side-impact collisions. They also have a case-hardened steel "Nader" pin. Named for consumer advocate Ralph Nader, these pins help keep the doors from blowing open and ejecting the occupants. If the Nader pin has been engaged, it will be difficult to pry open the door. You must first disengage the latch or use hydraulic jaws.

Before attempting to assist a patient through a door, you should be trained in proper extrication techniques. In general you should follow these steps:

- Try all four doors first—a door is usually the easiest means of access.
- Otherwise, gain access through the window farthest away from the patient(s).
- Alternatively, use simple hand tools to peel back the outer sheet of metal on the door, exposing the lock mechanism. Unlock the lock and pry the cams from around the Nader pin. Then pry out the door.

These steps can be highly useful in situations in which the patient must be promptly removed from the vehicle or the vehicle rescue team is delayed for some reason. Before removing a patient, keep in mind the earlier points about deactivating or dissipating front and/or side air bags.

Rescue Strategies

In managing highway operations or vehicle rescues, you should use the following general strategies:

- *Initial scene size-up.* Establish command, call for appropriate backup, then locate and triage the patients. Triage may be delayed until hazards are controlled.
- *Control hazards.* This topic has already been covered. But always remember this point: Traffic can be your worst enemy at a collision.
- *Assess the degree of entrapment and fastest means of extrication.* Try all doors. If they cannot be opened, decide whether it is advisable and/or necessary to break glass. Although you may not have the training or responsibility to use extrication equipment, you should observe its use so you know what technical skills are available should you need them (Figure 4-23 ●). Be aware of the considerations and techniques for door removal, roof removal, dashboard or firewall rollup, and construction of a new door.
- *Establish circles of operation.* Set up two circles of operation early in the incident. The inner circle is the area where the actual rescue takes place. Limit the number of workers in this area to team members operating rescue tools and/or charged with actual patient care. If two different units must work in the inner circle (e.g., a fire department extrication crew and an EMS crew), you will need to maintain a good working balance between the crews to avoid "over-rescuing." The outer circle is where staging takes place. Hold all additional equipment and personnel in this area until they are assigned a duty.

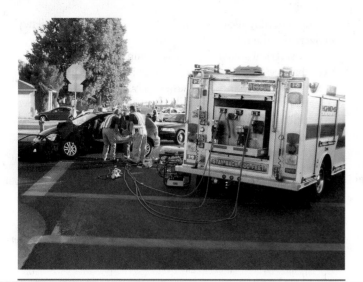

● **Figure 4-23** Modern extrication equipment is essential for a fast, efficient rescue. Paramedic skill in using these devices will depend on local protocols and the location of extrication units. *(© Pat Songer)*

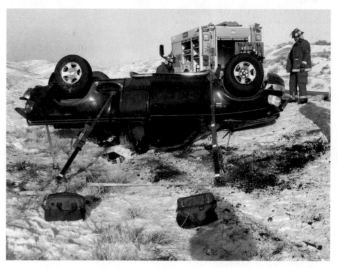

● **Figure 4-24** Vehicle stabilization equipment must be used to protect rescuers during extrication operations. *(© Pat Songer)*

● ***Treatment, packaging, removal.*** As a rule, the role of EMS personnel in vehicle stabilization and removal is that of patient care provider. Once specialized rescue personnel assure you that the vehicle is stable and the scene is safe to enter, you may approach the patient, initiate assessment, and administer emergency care. Patient care always precedes removal from the vehicle unless delay would endanger the life of the patient, EMS personnel, or other rescuers. Again, work with rescuers in any way possible to minimize risk, both to the patient and to on-scene personnel. You should be well practiced in the application of long spine boards for

rapid removal of the patient through the doors or vertical extrication through removed roofs.

Rescue Skills Practice

Depending on local protocols, you should practice or observe the use of the rescue skills and equipment needed for initial vehicle stabilization (Figure 4-24 ●). Some of the common tools used for vehicle stabilization can be found in Table 4–1.

You should also make a point of practicing and/or observing the various disentanglement or extrication skills commonly

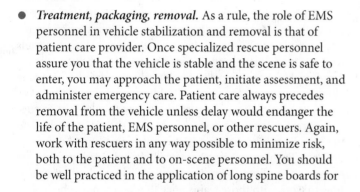

TABLE 4–1 | Vehicle Stabilization Equipment

Type	Description and Use
Air bag	Synthetic bag, available in various shapes and sizes, that, when inflated, has great lifting capability
Come-along	Ratcheting cable device used to pull in a straight direction
Cribbing	4- × 4-inch or 2- × 4-inch blocks of hardwood cut to approximately 18-inch-long sections
Hydraulic cutter	Hydraulic power tool used to cut metal
Hydraulic ram	Hydraulic power tool used to push or pull in a straight direction
Hydraulic spreader	Hydraulic power tool used to open, spread, or separate items such as vehicle doors
Jack	Manual device used much as a ram would be used
Step chock	Set of several 2- × 6-inch blocks of hardwood cut to varying lengths and secured together to form "steps"
Wedge	4- × 4-inch piece of cribbing tapered to an edge on one end
Winch	Powered cable reel, usually electrically or hydraulically driven and mounted to a truck, which is used for pulling

used with vehicle rescues, many of which have already been mentioned. Know how to gain access using hand tools through nondeformed doors, deformed doors, safety and tempered glass, trunks, and floors. Become familiar with the use of heavy hydraulic equipment employed by special rescue teams in your area and take part in practice scenarios to build agency cooperation. Again, preplan and prepare so that you are ready when this all-too-common type of rescue occurs.

Hybrid Vehicles

Hybrid automobiles, also called hybrid electric vehicles (HEVs), are becoming increasingly popular. HEVs contain both an electric motor and an internal combustion motor (Figure 4-25 ●). A large array of batteries powers the electric motor, while the internal combustion motor is powered by gasoline or diesel fuel.

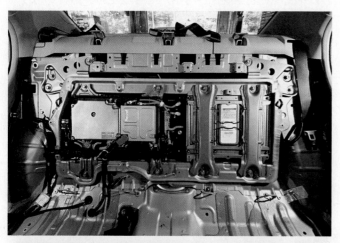

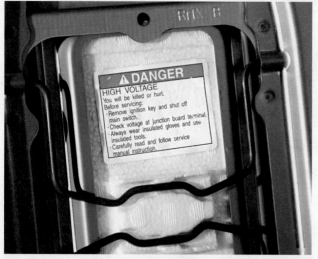

● **Figure 4-25** Modern hybrid electrical vehicle (HEV). These vehicles have a high-voltage electrical system that poses a particular hazard to rescuers.

This combination allows significantly increased fuel efficiency and decreases the release of pollutants.

The electrical system of HEVs contains a high-voltage and a 12-volt battery. The high-voltage component poses a particular risk for rescue personnel. The easiest way to inactivate the high-voltage component is to simply turn off the vehicle and remove the key from the ignition. This prevents electric current from flowing into the cables from the motor or high-voltage battery, and turns off power to the air bags and the seat belt pretensioners. To ensure rescuer safety, it is recommended that the 12-volt battery also be disconnected to further isolate the electrical system.

Because battery locations vary by vehicle type, rescuers should be familiar with the popular HEV vehicle types on the market.

HAZARDOUS TERRAIN RESCUES

In recent years, outdoor activities—mountain climbing, rock climbing, ice climbing, mountain biking, cross-country skiing, snowboarding, and hiking—have drawn more and more people into rugged areas. Inevitably, accidents happen, and they happen in places that can be difficult to reach. You do not have to live in the wilderness to take part in a hazardous terrain rescue. For example, a mountain biker can get injured along the trails that run along many power lines or a rock climber can get injured on an outcropping in a relatively populated area. Some climbers even scale the sides of buildings!

As a paramedic, you must know how to take part in rugged terrain rescues. At a minimum, you should know how to perform litter evacuations without causing additional injury to patients. Even more important, you should develop a "rescue awareness" so that you know when to call specialized teams and how to work with those teams once they arrive on scene.

Types of Hazardous Terrain

In general, there are three types of hazardous terrain: steep slope or "low-angle" terrain, vertical or "high-angle" terrain, and flat terrain with obstructions. Low-angle terrains typically can be accessed by walking or scrambling—climbing over boulders or rocks using both hands and feet. Footing can be difficult, and it may be hazardous to carry a litter, even with multiple people. As a result, low-angle teams use ropes to counteract gravity and/or may set a rope to act as a hand line. Any error can result in a fall or tumble. Depending on the presence of boulders, brush, downed trees, and so on, injuries can be quite serious.

High-angle terrain usually involves a cliff, gorge, side of a building, or terrain so steep that hands must be used when scaling it. Crews depend on rope and/or aerial apparatus for access and litter movement. Errors are likely to cause serious, life-threatening injuries. In many cases, falls can be fatal.

Flat terrain with obstructions includes trails, paths, or creek beds. Obstructions can take many forms such as downed trees, rocks, slippery leaves or pine needles, and scree—the loose pebbles or rock debris that can form on the slopes or bases of mountains.

Although this is the least hazardous type of rugged terrain, it is still possible to slip while carrying a patient, causing injury.

Patient Access in Hazardous Terrain

Unless you have been trained in high-angle or low-angle rescue, patient access and removal should be left to specialized teams. Even if you have the skills to perform the rescue, you will, in all likelihood, need additional resources to provide the necessary balance of technical and medical support for the patient.

High-Angle Rescues

High-angle, or vertical, rescuers must constantly contend with the effects of gravity. Any organization that could be assigned a vertical technical rescue must have extensive initial training, additional advanced training, frequently supervised practice sessions, and top-of-the-line equipment (Figure 4-26a ●). Each member of a high-angle team must have complete competency in knot tying, use of ladders and/or ropes to ascend and descend a steep face, ability to rig a hauling system, and the skills for packaging a patient for evacuation by litter and rope. Some of the specialized terms that you will hear high-angle rescuers use include:

- *Aid*—using means other than hands, feet, and body to get up a vertical face, such as in "aided ascent"

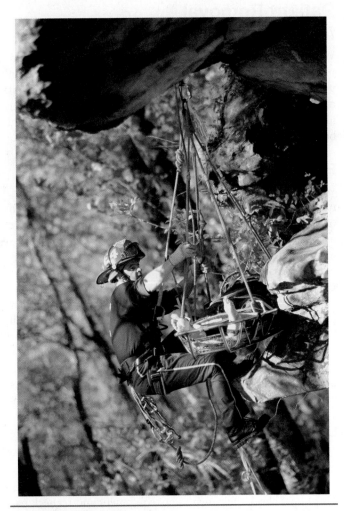

● **Figure 4-26a** High-angle rescue is dangerous and difficult. It should be deferred to persons trained and experienced in high-angle rescue techniques.

- *Anchor*—technique for securing rescuers to a vertical face; an anchor may be rope or a combination of rope and other special hardware or "gear"
- *Belay*—procedure for safeguarding a climber's progress by controlling a rope attached to an anchor (The person controlling the rope is sometimes also called the belay.)
- *Rappel*—to descend by sliding down a fixed double rope, using the correct anchor, harness, and gear

Low-Angle Rescues

Many EMS systems have trained their paramedics in the skills of low-angle rescue or "off-the-road" rescue. Like high-angle rescues, crews require rope, harnesses, hardware, and the necessary safety systems (Figure 4-26b ●). A rescue is considered a low-angle rescue up to 40°, except if the face is overly smooth. Then a high-angle team will be better able to handle the more technical access and evacuation.

Each member of a low-angle crew must know how to assemble a hasty harness tied from 2-inch tubular webbing (or don a climbing harness), rappel and ascend by rope, package a patient in a litter, and rig a simple hauling system to assist the litter team up the embankment. Teams must also know how to set up a hasty rope slide to assist with balance and footing on rough terrain. Although low-angle rescues involve less technical skill than high-angle rescues, they still require ongoing practice and proper equipment.

Patient Packaging for Rough Terrain

Packaging a patient is a critical aspect of any hazardous terrain rescue. The Stokes basket stretcher is the standard litter for rough terrain evacuation (Figures 4-27a ● and 4-27b ●). It provides a rigid frame for patient protection and is easy to carry with an adequate number of personnel. Alternative spinal immobilizers can be used in a Stokes basket, such as the KED, "halfback" backboard (extrication/rescue vest), or the Sked®. As a last resort, the Stokes itself can be used as a spinal immobilizer.

Stokes baskets come in wire and tubular, as well as plastic, styles. The older "military-style" wire mesh Stokes basket will

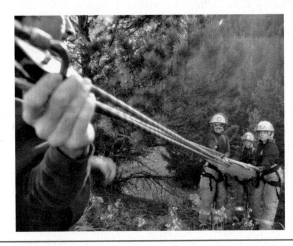

● **Figure 4-26b** Low-angle situations are not the same as high-angle situations. Therefore, many EMS agencies have trained their paramedics in the skills of low-angle rescue.

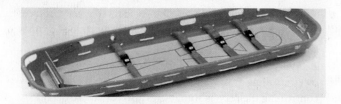

● **Figure 4-27a**   A basket stretcher.

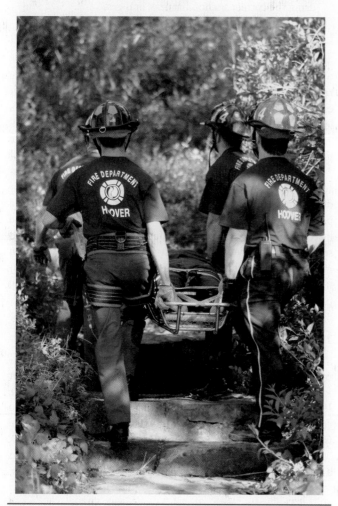

● **Figure 4-27b**   A basket stretcher is often used to carry patients over rough terrain.

not accept a backboard. Newer models, however, offer several advantages:

● Generally greater strength
● Less expense per unit
● Better air/water flow through the basket
● Better flotation, an important concern in water rescues

Plastic basket stretchers are usually weaker than their wire mesh counterparts. They are often rated for only 300 to 600 pounds. However, they tend to offer better patient protection. In general, Stokes baskets with plastic bottoms and steel frames are best. These versatile units can also be slid in snow, when necessary.

Most Stokes baskets, regardless of their style, are not equipped with adequate restraints. As a result, they will require additional strapping or lacing for rough terrain evacuation

and/or extrication. A plastic litter shield can be used to protect the patient from dust and objects that may fall on the person's face. When moving across flat terrain, lace the patient into the Stokes basket to limit movement. When using a Stokes basket for high-angle or low-angle evacuation, take the following additional steps:

● Apply a harness to the patient.
● Apply leg stirrups to the patient.
● Secure the patient to a litter to prevent movement.
● Tie the tail of one litter line to the patient's harness.
● Use a helmet or litter shield to protect the patient.
● Administer fluids (IV or orally).
● Allow accessibility for taking blood pressure, performing suction, and assessing distal perfusion.
● Ensure adequate padding—a crucial consideration.
● Consider use of a patient heating/cooling system, especially for prolonged evacuations.
● Provide for an airway clearing system via a gravity "tip line," if necessary.

Patient Removal from Hazardous Terrain

When removing the patient from hazardous terrain, a nontechnical/nonrope evacuation is usually faster. In other words, when possible, walk the patient out. Remember: Carrying a patient on a litter over flat ground can be a strenuous task even under ideal conditions. As the terrain becomes rougher, the litter carry becomes more demanding.

Flat, Rough Terrain

When removing a patient in a litter from flat, rough terrain, make sure you have enough litter carriers to "leapfrog" ahead of each other to save time and to rotate rescuers. An adequate number of litter bearers would be two—or, better yet, three—teams of six. Litter bearers on each carry should be approximately the same height.

Several devices exist to ease the difficulty of a litter carry. For example, litter bearers can run webbing straps over the litter rails, across their shoulders, and into their free hands. This will help distribute the weight across the bearers' backs. Another helpful device is the litter wheel. It attaches to the bottom of a Stokes basket frame and takes most of the weight of the litter. Bearers must keep the litter balanced and control its motion. As you might suspect, the litter wheel works best over flatter terrain.

Low-Angle/High-Angle Evacuation

As already mentioned, low-angle and high-angle evacuations require specialized knowledge and skills. Before beginning patient removal, rescuers must ensure that all anchors are secure. They must check their own safety equipment and recheck patient packaging. They must also have the necessary lowering and hauling systems in place, again doing the recommended safety checks.

Materials, especially ropes, should never be used if there is any question of their safety. If you see a frayed rope or any stressed or damaged equipment, do not hesitate to point it out to the rescuers in a polite, but professional manner. Also, because hauling sometimes requires many "helpers," you may be asked to assist. Make sure you understand all directions given by the rescuers. Evacuation is a team effort.

Some high-angle units, especially fire departments, make use of aerial apparatus such as tower-ladders or bucket trucks to assist in the removal of a patient in a Stokes basket. These units are usually employed in structural environments, but can be adapted to hazardous terrain if there is room for a truck.

When using aerial apparatus, it is necessary to provide a litter belay during movement to a bucket. Litters, of course, must then be attached correctly to the bucket. Use of aerial ladders can be difficult because upper sections are usually not wide enough to slot the litter. The litter must always be properly belayed if being slid down the ladder. Finally, ladders or other aerial apparatus should *not* be used as a crane to move a litter. They are neither designed nor rated for this work. Serious stress can cause accidents resulting in patient death.

Use of Helicopters

Helicopters can be useful in hazardous terrain rescues, especially when hospitals lie at a distant location (see Chapter 2). You must understand the capabilities of local helicopter systems and know who provides helicopter rescue in your region. Be aware of the difference in mission, crew training, and capabilities of helicopters that do air medical care versus helicopters that do rescue. You should be familiar with the advantages, disadvantages, and local restrictions for each of the following practices or techniques *before* you summon a helicopter from the field:

- Boarding and deboarding practices
- Restrictions on carrying noncrew members
- Use of cable winches for rescues
- Weight restrictions
- Restrictions on hovering rescues
- Use of **short hauls** or sling loads of equipment and/or personnel, as opposed to the more dangerous rappel-based rescues

Packaging/Evacuation Practice

Depending on local protocols, you should practice the packaging and evacuation techniques expected of EMS personnel in your region (Figure 4-28 ●). You should familiarize yourself with the specific types of basket stretchers and litters available to your unit and the proper packaging, immobilization, and restraint techniques for use with each type. You should also practice with other equipment used for rough-terrain rescues, including the Sked and appropriate half-spine devices.

Practice or observe the skills required for low-angle and high-angle rescues. When possible, take part in exercises with the rescue units that you would summon to perform these evacuations. By fully understanding the capabilities of the rescue

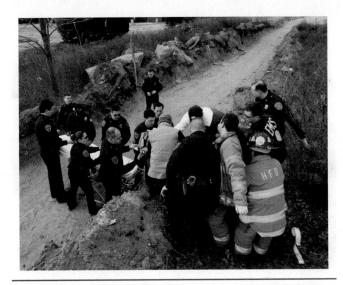

● **Figure 4-28** Patient removal over rough terrain requires adequate planning and personnel. *(© Craig Jackson/In The Dark Photography)*

response teams in your area, you will circumvent any "turf" issues. You will also know how to work together whenever a multijurisdictional event occurs.

Extended Care Assessment and Environmental Issues

As you learned in Volume 5, Chapter 12, environmental emergencies can present their own special challenges. For rescue operations, at least some personnel should have formal training in managing patients whose injuries have been aggravated by prolonged lack of treatment, often under extreme conditions. If SOPs do not already exist, procedures adopted from wilderness medical research will prove useful. Position papers written by the Wilderness Medical Society or the National Association for Search and Rescue can serve as guidelines for protocols.

Regardless of the source, you will discover that many protocols for extended care vary substantially from standard EMS procedures. If your agency anticipates involvement in some of the rescue situations described in this chapter, you should consider protocols that at least address the following areas:

- Long-term hydration management
- Repositioning of dislocations
- Cleansing and care of wounds
- Removal of impaled objects
- Nonpharmacological pain management—using proper splinting, distracting the patient by talking or asking questions, scratching or creating sensory stimuli when doing painful procedures
- Pharmacological pain management—utilizing pharmacological agents with isolated trauma, such as amputation or fracture, or with multiple trauma, such as crushing or pinning of more than an extremity
- Assessment and care of head and spinal injuries
- Management of hypothermia or hyperthermia

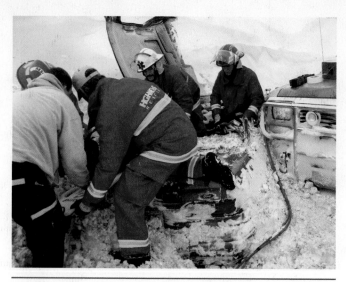

● **Figure 4-29** Rescue operations can involve multiple risks including environmental hazards, road hazards, and entrapment, as seen here. (© *Pat Songer*)

- Termination of CPR
- Treatment of crush injuries and compartment syndromes. (For a review of these trauma injuries, see Volume 5.)

A number of environmental issues can affect your assessment during a rescue situation (Figure 4-29 ●). Some of the most important issues include the following:

- *Weather/temperature extremes.* Extreme weather or temperature conditions increase the risk of patient hypo/hyperthermia. These conditions also make it difficult or impossible to expose the patient completely for full assessment and treatment. As a result, your physical examination may be compromised. Use of tarps, blankets, or plastic sheeting may help in some cases, but your assessment will usually be limited at best.

- *Limited patient access.* Parts of the patient may not be accessible for examination because they are pinned beneath debris or stuck in a confined space. Cramped space and low lighting conditions also make assessment difficult. For this reason, it is important that you carry a headlamp with extended battery packs.

- *Difficulty transporting street equipment.* Hazardous terrain often makes it difficult to transport typical street equipment to the patient. Tackle boxes and heavy equipment may be inappropriate to take into a confined space or the backwoods, or down a hasty rappel. As a result, equipment usually must be downsized. Often you will use a backpack to keep your hands free for carrying. Essential equipment for the initial assessment and management include:

  ○ *Airway*—oral and nasal airways, manual suction, intubation equipment

  ○ *Breathing*—thoracic decompression equipment, small oxygen tank/regulator, masks/cannulas, pocket mask/BVM

  ○ *Circulation*—bandages/dressings, triangular bandages, occlusive dressings, IV administration equipment, and BP cuff and stethoscope

  ○ *Disability*—extrication collars

  ○ *Expose*—scissors

  ○ *Miscellaneous*—headlamp/flashlight, space blanket, padded aluminum splint (SAM® splint), PPE (leather gloves, latex gloves, eye shields)

- *Cumbersome PPE.* Necessary, but cumbersome, PPE can restrict rescuer mobility. In certain instances, some of the PPE might be removed to perform care steps. For example, the heavy outer gloves worn in extremely cold conditions might be taken off during administration of an IV. However, all PPE should be reapplied as soon as possible.

- *Patient exposure.* Patients should be quickly covered to ensure thermal protection. During the extrication, place hard protection, such as a spine board, and take steps to prevent patient contact with sharp objects or debris. For example, use an aluminized blanket to prevent glass shards from contacting the patient.

- *Use of ALS skills.* Good basic life support skills are mandatory in hazardous terrains, but limit ALS skills to those that are really essential. More wires and tubing complicate the extrication process. Continuous oxygenation and definitive airway control and volume may be essential. However, rescuers cannot carry lots of oxygen tanks into rugged terrains. As a result, you may have to use your tank at a slower flow rate so it will last a longer period of time.

- *Patient monitoring.* Hazardous terrain can alter your use of monitoring equipment. In high-noise areas, for example, you may have to take BP by palpation or use a compact pulse oximetry unit. An ECG monitor can be cumbersome during extrication and will be more difficult to use than in a street situation.

- *Improvisation.* Improvisation is common in rescue situations. To minimize the amount of equipment carried over hazardous terrain, you may want to consider such techniques as tying upper extremity fractures to the torso or tying lower extremity fractures to the uninjured leg. Lightweight SAM splints can be very useful in the backwoods and should be part of your downsized medical gear. Whatever you do, continue talking to the patient and explain exactly what is happening. Answer any questions, particularly if you are improvising. The patient is already frightened by the entrapment. Do not worsen the situation by making the patient feel even more out of control.

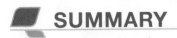 SUMMARY

All rescue operations can be divided into seven functional stages: arrival and size-up, hazard control, patient access, medical treatment, disentanglement, patient packaging, and removal/transport. Whenever you function in any one of these phases, you must be properly outfitted with protective equipment. You must also have training specific to the assigned rescue.

In any rescue, you must access the scene quickly so assessment and management can begin. Situational threats to the rescuer and/or patient should be identified and remedied as thoroughly as conditions permit. Patients should be reassessed throughout the rescue and repackaged as extrication and removal progress.

During the operational phases of the rescue, you must provide direct patient care and work with technical teams to ensure optimal patient management. Any paramedic assigned to rescue duties should have training in the care of patients who may require prolonged management. Such training results from the increased time to locate, access, remove, and/or transport a rescue patient.

Either you or a paramedic on your crew must accompany the patient throughout the transportation phase. This person should constantly monitor any changes in condition, while coordinating patient transport to an appropriate medical facility. If a specialized rescue team includes a trained paramedic, this person may fulfill these functions.

YOU MAKE THE CALL

You and your partner are working on Medic Ambulance 642 covering the north portion of town. You receive a call for a motor vehicle collision on Interstate I-94. Upon arrival, you quickly determine that the collision involves more than the average complications. Apparently, the vehicle swerved off the road and rolled down an embankment. Traffic is already backed up for about half a mile. Several motorists have gotten out of their cars.

When you look over the embankment, you discover that two bystanders have climbed down the hill and are standing near the overturned automobile. They yell up: "There's just one guy inside. He's breathing, so we know he's alive. But we can't get any response out of him. Do you want us to do something?" While you are directing the bystanders to stand clear of the car, "rubbernecking" in the other lane causes a low-speed collision right on the highway.

1. What are your immediate considerations as you size up the scene?

2. Why would you consider this a rescue operation?

3. What additional resources would you request?

See Suggested Responses at the back of this book.

REVIEW QUESTIONS

1. The best helmets have a _____ suspension system.
a. two-point, elastic
b. two-point, nonelastic
c. four-point, elastic
d. four-point, nonelastic

2. Although specific procedures in rescue operations vary from area to area and from rescue to rescue, most calls will go through _____ general phases.
a. ten
b. four
c. five
d. seven

3. _____ triggers the technical beginning of the rescue.
a. Access
b. Arrival
c. Size-up
d. Hazard control

4. This phase may be the most technical and time-consuming portion of a rescue operation.
a. hazard control
b. patient access
c. disentanglement
d. patient packaging

5. Decisions regarding patient transport should be coordinated based on advice from _____.
   a. the safety officer
   b. medical direction
   c. the liaison officer
   d. the communications officer

6. Examples of confined spaces include all of the following *except*_____.
   a. flat water
   b. drainage culverts
   c. wells and cisterns
   d. grain bins and silos

7. The types of confined-space emergencies most commonly encountered in the workplace are _____.
   a. falls
   b. explosions
   c. entrapment
   d. all of the above

8. A _____ is usually the easiest means of access to a motor vehicle.
   a. door
   b. window
   c. trunk
   d. windshield

9. As a rule, the primary role of EMS personnel in vehicle stabilization and removal is that of _____.
   a. extrication
   b. scene control
   c. patient care provider
   d. communications officer

10. A technique for securing rescuers to a vertical face is called a(n) _____.
    a. aid   c. anchor
    b. belay   d. rappel

See Answers to Review Questions at the back of this book.

REFERENCES

1. Ducharme, M. S. and D. S. Lounsbury. "Self-Rescue Swimming in Cold Water: The Latest Advice." *Appl Physiol Butr Metab* 32 (2007): 799–807.
2. Giesbrecht, G. G. "Prehospital Treatment of Hypothermia." *Wilderness Environ Med* 12 (2001): 24–31.
3. Driscoll, T. R., J. A. Harrison, and M. Steenkamp. "Review of the Role of Alcohol in Drowning Associated with Recreational Aquatic Activity." *Inj Prev* 10 (2004): 107–113.
4. Watson, R. S., P. Cummings, L. Quan, S. Bratton, and N. S. Weiss. "Cervical Spine Injuries among Submersion Victims." *J Trauma* 51 (2001): 658–662.

FURTHER READING

Auerbach, P. S. *Wilderness Medicine.* 5th ed. St. Louis, MO: Mosby–Year Book, 2012.

Martinette, Jr., C. V. *Trench Rescue.* 2nd ed. Sudbury, MA: Jones and Bartlett Publishers, 2007.

Tilton, B. and F. Hubbell. *Medicine for the Backcountry.* 3rd ed. Guilford, CT: Globe Pequot, 2000.

Vines, T. *High-Angle Rescue Techniques.* 3rd ed. St. Louis: Mosby, 2004.

Wilkerson, J. A. *Medicine for Mountaineering & Other Wilderness Activities.* 5th ed. Seattle: The Mountaineers, 2002.

5

Hazardous Materials

Bryan Bledsoe, DO, FACEP, FAAEM, EMT-P

STANDARD
EMS Operations (Hazardous Materials)

COMPETENCY
Applies knowledge of operational roles and responsibilities to ensure patient, public, and personnel safety.

OBJECTIVES

Terminal Performance Objective
After reading this chapter, you should be able to effectively perform the expected functions of EMS personnel in a hazardous materials incident.

Enabling Objectives
To accomplish the terminal performance objective, you should be able to:

1. Define key terms introduced in this chapter.

2. Describe the distribution of hazardous materials throughout the country.

3. Relate your training in response to toxicologic emergencies, multiple-casualty incidents, and terrorism to the response to hazardous materials.

4. Describe the need for specialized training at various levels to effectively manage hazardous materials incidents.

5. Describe the paramedic's role at hazardous materials incidents.

6. Recognize situations that may involve a hazardous material release.

7. Given a variety of scenarios involving hazardous material release, identify the substance and use resources to determine information about the substance and actions to take.

8. Describe the various control zones established at a hazardous materials incident.

9. Take actions to protect yourself and other responders from exposure at the scene of a hazardous materials incident.

10. Describe the levels of hazardous materials protective equipment available.

11. Describe approaches to decontaminating patients exposed to a variety of hazardous materials.

12. Given a variety of hazardous materials scenarios, demonstrate safe and effective patient care.

13. Describe the role of EMS personnel in monitoring and rehabilitating those responding to a hazardous materials incident.

KEY TERMS

acetylcholinesterase
  (AChE), p. 104
acute effects, p. 103
air-purifying respirator
  (APR), p. 109
biotransformation, p. 104
CAMEO®, p. 99
CHEMTEL, p. 99
CHEMTREC, p. 99
cold zone, p. 101
cytochrome oxidase, p. 105

delayed effects, p. 103
hazardous materials
  (hazmat), p. 93
hot zone, p. 101
local effects, p. 104
material safety data sheet
  (MSDS), p. 99
primary contamination, p. 103
secondary
  contamination, p. 103

semi-decontaminated
  patient, p. 107
shipping papers, p. 98
synergism, p. 104
systemic effects, p. 104
UN number, p. 96
warm zone, p. 101
warning placard, p. 95
weapons of mass destruction
  (WMD), p. 96

CASE STUDY

The radio dispatches your unit to a chemical burn incident at the Acme Chicken Processing Plant. You jump aboard the ambulance and travel to the address given by the dispatcher. On arrival, you observe about 50 workers standing in the parking lot. A security guard approaches the ambulance and points toward the loading dock. He tells you, "A couple of people were sprayed with refrigerant when the hose broke open. Some of them got burned."

You proceed to the loading dock and find six patients. All of them are experiencing shortness of breath. Several have burns, including one patient with obvious facial injuries. Bystanders have already begun flushing his eyes with water. The plant supervisor tells you the refrigerant was anhydrous ammonia. You relay the initial scene size-up to the dispatch center. Then you request additional ambulances, a supervisor, the fire department, and a local hazmat team.

As the first on-scene unit, you initiate the incident management system. You assume the role of incident commander while your partner acts as triage officer. She quickly tags three patients red and three patients yellow. She reports one patient with some facial burns and possible eye injuries. Two other patients have chemical burns on their backs and extremities and are suffering respiratory distress. The remaining three patients have no burns but are having difficulty breathing.

You instruct the patients to immediately remove all their clothing for decontamination. By this time, additional units have already begun to arrive. The fire chief requests a quick report and then initiates gross decontamination measures with large amounts of water. Meanwhile, you relocate all personnel to avoid contact with the runoff dilution.

You assign the patient with facial burns and eye injuries to a crew from one of the ALS ambulances. They complete decontamination and begin treatment. Other crews decontaminate and treat the remaining patients in the order established by triage. All patients receive oxygen. Paramedics establish intravenous lines and administer albuterol by small-volume nebulizer to the patients who are wheezing. Crews also apply dressings to the burn patients as necessary.

By now the supervisor has arrived, and you complete a face-to-face transfer of command. The supervisor oversees hazmat operations and notifies hospitals of incoming patients. The hazmat team dons the necessary equipment and provides paper garments for the patients. Because decontamination is not very demanding, transport begins quickly. Your ambulance remains on scene as a dedicated unit for the hazmat team.

You assess two hazmat crew members before they enter the plant. In analyzing the damage, the hazmat team determines that the anhydrous ammonia must be cleaned up by a contractor. However, if nobody enters the building, the chemical poses no immediate hazard to the workers, the public, or the environment.

You now perform a post-entry evaluation of the hazmat team. You find that they have not suffered significant heat stress during their entry. The supervisor then terminates the incident and orders the plant closed until the contractor completes the cleanup operation.

INTRODUCTION

Hazardous materials (hazmat) are all around us. Companies in the United States manufacture more than 50 billion tons of hazardous materials a year. Some 4 billion tons of hazardous materials are shipped throughout the United States by truck, pipeline, railroad, and tankers (Figure 5-1 ●).[1] They can exist as solids, liquids, or gases. They can irritate, burn, poison, corrode, or asphyxiate.

You learned about some hazardous materials in the chapters on toxicologic and environmental emergencies in Volume 4. This chapter deals with the hazardous materials spilled or released as a result of an accident, equipment failure, human error, or an intentional violation of the laws and regulations that govern their manufacture, use, and disposal.

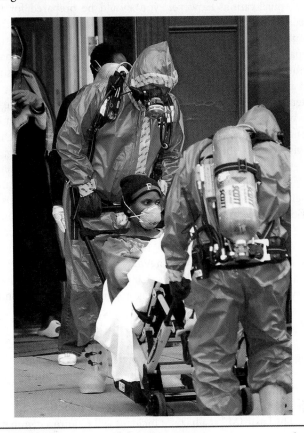

● **Figure 5-1**   A hazardous materials emergency can involve countless substances and occur in many situations. Warning placards on a truck should immediately alert you to the possible need of a hazmat team. (© *AP Images/Herald-Mail, Erick Gibson*)

For purposes of this chapter, keep in mind the definition of a hazardous material offered by the U.S. Department of Transportation (DOT). A hazardous material can be regarded as "any substance which may pose an unreasonable risk to health and safety of operating or emergency personnel, the public, and/or the environment if not properly controlled during handling, storage, manufacture, processing, packaging, use, disposal, or transportation."

ROLE OF THE PARAMEDIC

Hazardous materials incidents, or hazmat incidents, present some of the most challenging situations that you will face as a paramedic. As mentioned, a hazmat event can involve all kinds of substances: corrosive chemicals, pulmonary irritants, pesticides, chemical asphyxiants, hydrocarbon solvents, and radioactive wastes. The exposure to hazardous materials may be limited to just a few victims, or it may cause widespread destruction and loss of many lives. However, as the opening case study shows, even a small-scale incident is almost always a multijurisdictional event. For this reason, EMS agencies should train all their personnel how to respond to hazmat incidents and how to

CONTENT REVIEW

► Role of EMS Hazmat First Responders

- Size up incident
- Assess toxicologic risk
- Activate the IMS
- Establish command

interact with other agencies that might be summoned to the scene.[2]

Traditionally, paramedics do not perform defensive (containment) and offensive (control) functions at a hazardous materials response. Even so, paramedics are still an integral part of a community's hazmat response system. As you will learn in this chapter, EMS personnel fulfill a variety of tasks at a hazmat incident. As first responders, they may size up the incident, assess the toxicologic risk, and activate the incident management system (IMS) needed to handle the event. They will also be called on to evaluate decontamination methods, to treat and transport exposed patients, and to perform medical monitoring of hazmat teams that enter the area.[3]

Requirements and Standards

Two federal agencies, the Occupational Safety and Health Administration (OSHA) and the Environmental Protection Agency (EPA), have set forth a number of regulations and standards for dealing with hazmat emergencies. The most important of these are found in OSHA publication CFR 1910.120, *Hazardous Waste Operations and Emergency Response Standard* (2004). This standard provides specific response procedures, including use of an incident management system, use of personal protective equipment (PPE), use of a safety officer, and special training requirements. The EPA has published a mirror regulation, 40 CFR 311, that applies to those agencies that fall outside OSHA's jurisdiction.

In addition, the National Fire Protection Association (NFPA) has published NFPA 473, *Standard Competencies for EMS Personnel Responding to Hazardous Materials Incidents*. This standard, along with two other NFPA standards for hazmat response, deals with the training standards for EMS personnel assigned to hazmat incidents.

Levels of Training

The documents just mentioned set forth three levels of training appropriate to EMS response at hazmat incidents: Awareness Level, EMS Level 1, and EMS Level 2. The Awareness Level applies to responders who may arrive first at a scene and discover a toxic substance. Training focuses on recognition of hazmat incidents, basic hazmat identification techniques, and individual protection from involvement in the incident. All EMS personnel, as well as police officers and firefighters, need to be trained to the Awareness Level.

EMS Level 1 training, or the "operations level," is required for those who may perform patient care in the cold zone on patients who do *not* present a significant risk of secondary contamination. This training focuses on hazard assessment, patient assessment, and patient care for previously decontaminated patients.

EMS Level 2 training, or the "technician level," is required for those who may perform patient care in the warm zone on patients who still present a significant risk of secondary contamination.

This training focuses on personal protection, decontamination procedures, and treatment for patients who are beginning or undergoing decontamination.

The level of training required for each individual depends on that person's role in the hazmat response system. All systems require some individuals to be trained in both the EMS Level 1 and Level 2 standards. In this way, patient care can begin during decontamination and continue after the patient has been cleaned of contaminants.

INCIDENT SIZE-UP

Sizing up a hazardous materials incident is a very difficult task. You often receive inaccurate or incomplete information; in addition, events tend to develop very quickly during each phase of the incident. As already indicated, you can also expect a number of agencies to be involved in the response. As a result, you should be skilled in the use of the IMS discussed in Chapter 3 and practice it regularly with the other agencies that typically respond to a hazmat call.

IMS and Hazmat Emergencies

Priorities for a hazmat incident are the same as those for any other major incident: life safety, incident stabilization, and property conservation. However, you should be prepared for the special circumstances surrounding most hazmat emergencies. Some incidents, for example, will require immediate evacuation of patients from a contaminated area. Other incidents will have ambulatory contaminated patients who seek out EMS personnel as soon as you arrive on scene. In performing early hazmat interventions, you face the challenge of avoiding exposure to the hazardous material yourself. As a result, never compromise scene safety during the early phase of a hazmat operation. Otherwise, you risk becoming a contaminated patient. (The subject of "self-rescued" patients will be discussed later in the chapter.)

In setting priorities, you must also quickly determine whether the hazmat emergency is an open incident or a closed incident. That is, does the event have the potential for generating more patients? As you learned in Chapter 3, the answer to this question will determine the resources that you request, how you stage them, and the way in which you deploy personnel. In reaching your decision, remember that some chemicals have delayed effects. Triage must be ongoing, because patient conditions can change rapidly.

Finally, in employing the IMS at a hazmat incident, you must take into account certain special conditions when choreographing the scene. The most preferable site for deploying resources will be uphill and upwind. This will help prevent contamination from ground-based liquids, high-vapor-density gases, runoff water, and vapor clouds.

The basic IMS at a hazmat incident will require a command post, a staging area, and a decontamination corridor. Depending on the event, the incident commander may also establish separate areas, such as treatment areas and personnel staging areas, to prevent unnecessary exposure to contamination. A backup plan for areas of operations must be determined early in the event. For example, what would you do if the wind direction suddenly shifted and a cloud of chlorine gas headed toward your staging area?

Incident Awareness

One of the most critical aspects of any hazmat response is the simple awareness that a dangerous substance may be present. Virtually every emergency site—residential, business, or highway—possesses the potential for hazardous materials. For example,

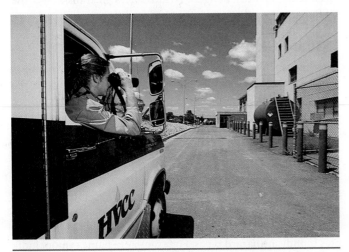

● **Figure 5-2** Don't take any chances. Use binoculars to make a visual inspection of a potentially hazardous situation—such as a suspicious storage tank—from a safe distance.

most households keep ammonia and liquid bleach in the kitchen or laundry room. When combined, these substances can produce a toxic gas. Homes with kerosene heaters or blocked flues can be filled with carbon monoxide. Do not take any chances. Always keep the possibility of dangerous substances in mind whenever you approach the scene of an emergency. If you suspect the presence of hazardous materials, use binoculars to inspect the scene from a distance (Figure 5-2 ●).

Transportation

Any transportation accident—automobile, truck, or railroad—should raise a suspicion of the presence of hazardous materials (Figure 5-3 ●). Maintain a high degree of hazmat awareness whenever you are summoned to collisions involving commercial vehicles, pest control vehicles, tanker trucks, tractor-trailers, or cars powered by alternative fuels. Do not rule out the presence of hazardous materials just because you do not see a **warning placard**. Hospitals and laboratories, for example, routinely and legally transport medical radioactive isotopes in unmarked passenger cars. You could look into the back seat of a crashed automobile and see a container with a label indicating radioactive contents.

Railroad accidents merit special attention for two reasons. First, railroad cars can carry large quantities of hazardous

CONTENT REVIEW

▶ Hazmat Requirements/ Standards

- OSHA publication CFR 1910.120
- EPA regulation 40 CFR 311
- NFPA standard 473

Establishing the Danger Zone

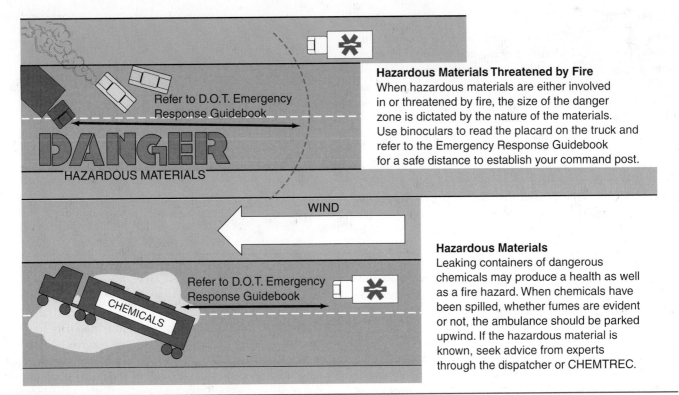

Hazardous Materials Threatened by Fire
When hazardous materials are either involved in or threatened by fire, the size of the danger zone is dictated by the nature of the materials. Use binoculars to read the placard on the truck and refer to the Emergency Response Guidebook for a safe distance to establish your command post.

Hazardous Materials
Leaking containers of dangerous chemicals may produce a health as well as a fire hazard. When chemicals have been spilled, whether fumes are evident or not, the ambulance should be parked upwind. If the hazardous material is known, seek advice from experts through the dispatcher or CHEMTREC.

● **Figure 5-3** Transportation incidents involving hazardous materials.

CONTENT REVIEW

► Potential Terrorist Targets

• Public buildings
• Multinational headquarters
• Shopping centers
• Workplaces
• Sites of assembly

materials. The largest tanker truck, for example, has about a 14,000-gallon capacity, whereas a railroad tank car can carry up to 34,000 gallons. Second, several tank cars may be hitched together on a freight train. Obviously, there is a greater chance for a major incident if one or more of these tanks are ruptured in an accident. Fortunately, railroads run along fixed lines, which means you can preplan your response in case a railroad accident occurs within your jurisdiction.

Fixed Facilities

Hazmat incidents can also take place at fixed facilities where dangerous substances are produced or stored. Chemical plants and all manufacturing operations have tanks, storage vessels, and pipelines used to transport products and/or wastes. Additional fixed sites with possible hazardous materials include warehouses, hardware or agricultural stores, water treatment centers, and loading docks. If you work in a rural area, keep in mind the number of places where you can find hazardous materials on a farm or ranch: silos, barns, greenhouses, and more. (For information on rural hazmat emergencies, see Chapter 7.)

Finally, remember that many communities have some kind of fixed pipelines, especially in urban settings. These pipelines can be damaged by acts of nature (earthquakes), by construction crews, or, if aboveground, by vehicle crashes. A rupture or leak in a gas or oil pipeline can spell disaster, especially if ignited.

Terrorism

Unfortunately, a new type of hazmat incident has emerged in the form of terrorism. Terrorists may use any variety of chemical, biological, or nuclear devices to strike at government or high-profile targets. These **weapons of mass destruction (WMD)** can be manufactured from materials as simple as those found on most farms, as was the case in the bombing of the Alfred P. Murrah Federal Building in Oklahoma City (see Chapter 8). The perpetrators can come from within the United States or from abroad.

The most frightening aspect of terrorism is the lack of predictability about when or where an attack might take place. Lacking a clear verbal or written threat, it can happen almost anywhere. However, terrorists usually select their targets by activity, particularly government or industrial, and by the number of people present. Potential targets include public buildings, multinational headquarters, shopping centers, workplaces, and sites of assembly such as arenas, stadiums, transportation centers, or places of worship. All of these locations should be identified in any mass casualty or disaster plan for your community.

In responding to a suspected terrorist incident, look for potential clues. Patients in a closed environment, such as a subway or an office building, will exhibit similar symptoms if they have been exposed to a chemical or biological weapon of mass destruction. In the case of an explosion, remember that a secondary device may exist. Take every precaution not to fall victim to a terrorist attack yourself. Make full use of the IMS and all specialized agencies able to respond to the scene of suspected terrorism.

For more on responding to terrorist acts, see Chapter 8.

Recognition of Hazards

To aid in the visual recognition of hazardous materials, two simple systems have been developed. The DOT has implemented placards to identify dangerous substances in transit, and the NFPA has devised a system for fixed facilities.

Placard Classifications

Although many vehicles are required by law to carry placards (Figure 5-4 ●), the absence of a placard does not mean the absence of a hazmat threat. Regulations depend on the type of substance and/or the amount of substance in transit.

Placards are easily spotted because of their diamond shape (Figure 5-5 ●). Each placard indicates hazmat classifications through use of a color code and hazard class number. Some placards also carry a **UN number**—a four-digit number specific to the actual chemical. For quick reference, keep in mind the general classifications listed in Table 5–1.

In addition to numbers and colors, placards also use symbols to indicate hazard types. For example, a flame symbol indicates a flammable substance, a ball-on-fire symbol indicates an oxidizer, a propeller symbol indicates a radioactive substance, and a skull-and-crossbones symbol indicates a poisonous substance. When combined with numbers and colors, these symbols help you to recognize the specific nature of the hazardous material. For instance, a red placard with the number 2 and a

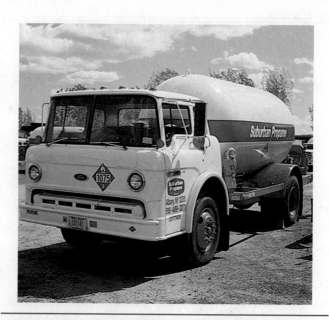

● **Figure 5-4** Vehicles carrying hazardous materials are required to display placards indicating the nature of their contents. Even if you have studied these placards earlier in your EMS career, you should regularly review the symbols, color codes, and hazard class numbers so that you can identify dangerous materials.

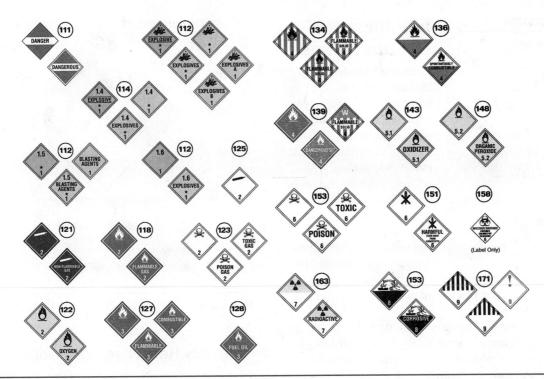

● **Figure 5-5** Sample labels and warning placards required by the DOT for all packages, storage containers, and vehicles containing hazardous materials. (*U.S. Department of Transportation*)

TABLE 5–1 | Hazard Classes and Placard Colors

Hazard Class	Hazard Type	Color Code
1	Explosives	Orange
2	Gases	Red or green
3	Liquids	Red
4	Solids	Red and white
5	Oxidizers and organic peroxides	Yellow
6	Poisonous and etiologic agents	White
7	Radioactive materials	Yellow and white
8	Corrosives	Black and white
9	Miscellaneous	Black and white

flame symbol means that the vehicle is carrying a flammable gas. Over time, you will become more familiar with these and other important symbols such as a "W" with a line through it, which means "reacts with water."

In using the placard system, keep in mind several short-comings. Although some substances are required to show a placard in any quantity, others need to be placarded only if they are transported in large quantities. This means that a truck may be carrying hazardous materials, but because the amount falls below the quantity required for placarding, no placard is shown. Also, the "Dangerous" placard means that there are two or more substances onboard between 1,000 and 5,000 pounds total weight. However, the generic placard tells you nothing about the hazardous nature of the materials. Finally, people can remove placards or fail to apply them in the first place. In this case, you have no immediate indication at all of a dangerous hazmat situation.

NFPA 704 System

The NFPA 704 System identifies hazardous materials at fixed facilities. Like the DOT placards, the system uses diamond-shaped figures, which are placed on tanks and storage vessels. The diamond is divided into four sections and color coded (Figures 5-6a ● and 5-6b ●). The top segment is red and indicates the flammability of the substance. The left segment is blue and indicates the health hazard. The right segment is yellow and indicates the product's instability. The bottom segment is white and indicates special information. The hazards listed may include water reactivity, oxidizing properties, or simple asphyxiant.

Flammability, health hazard, and reactivity are measured on a scale of 0 to 4. A designation of 0 indicates no hazard, whereas a designation of 4 indicates extreme hazard. The degrees of hazard are summarized in the figures. The NFPA 704 standard should be referred to for specific criteria used to rate the materials.

► Hazmat References

- *Emergency Response Guidebook* (ERG)
- Shipping papers
- Material safety data sheets
- Monitors/chemical tests
- Databases (CAMEO)
- Hazmat telephone hotlines (CHEMTREC; CHEMTEL)
- Poison control centers
- Toxicologists
- Reference books

Identification of Substances

Once you have determined that an incident involves hazardous materials, you must next try to identify the particular substance. This is the crux, or most difficult aspect, of dealing with a hazmat incident. You will often lack adequate on-scene information to make a positive identification, or you will get conflicting preliminary information. For this reason, you must be familiar with the resources that can assist you in identification of a hazardous material and become skilled at using each of them.

To prevent dangerous interpretations, try to locate two or more concurring reference sources. Do not take action until you find this information—otherwise you risk making mistakes and providing incorrect patient treatment.

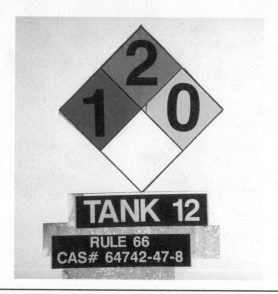

● **Figure 5-6b** NFPA 704 labeling on a tank.

Emergency Response Guidebook

You have already read about UN numbers, the four-digit numbers specific to actual chemicals. Some placards will include the UN number as well as the hazard class information. For example, you may see a tanker truck with a red (3) placard with the number 1203 in the middle. Based on what you already know, you can determine that the incident involves a flammable liquid. To identify the specific flammable liquid, you will need the *Emergency Response Guidebook* (ERG) (Figure 5-7 ●).

The ERG, published by the U.S. Department of Transportation, Transport Canada, and the Secretary of Communications and Transportation of Mexico, should be carried on every emergency vehicle. It lists more than a thousand hazardous materials, along with placards, UN numbers, and chemical names. It also cross-references each identification number to specific emergency procedures related to the chemical. The ERG includes, for example, a list of evacuation distances for the most hazardous substances. It is revised frequently, and the most up-to-date version should be readily available to all crew members. Newest updates are available on the Internet from the DOT.

When using the ERG, keep in mind two shortcomings. First, the reference provides only basic generic information on medical treatment. One recommendation, for instance, involves calling EMS. Obviously, this is not very helpful for EMS personnel. Second, more than one chemical often have the same UN number. For example, UN 1203 may be diesel fuel, gasohol, gasoline, motor fuels, or motor spirits. The difference between a gasoline leak and a diesel fuel leak, for instance, is dramatic, highlighting the need to use other methods of positive identification.

Shipping Papers

The most accurate information about a transported substance can be found in the **shipping papers**, or bill of lading. Trucks, boats, airplanes, and trains routinely carry these documents. Ideally, they should list the specific substances and quantities

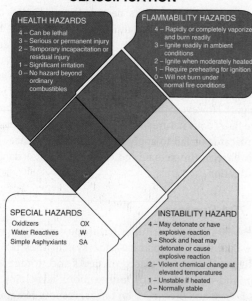

HAZARDOUS MATERIALS CLASSIFICATION

HEALTH HAZARDS
4 – Can be lethal
3 – Serious or permanent injury
2 – Temporary incapacitation or residual injury
1 – Significant irritation
0 – No hazard beyond ordinary combustibles

FLAMMABILITY HAZARDS
4 – Rapidly or completely vaporize and burn readily
3 – Ignite readily in ambient conditions
2 – Ignite when moderately heated
1 – Require preheating for ignition
0 – Will not burn under normal fire conditions

SPECIAL HAZARDS
Oxidizers   OX
Water Reactives   W̶
Simple Asphyxiants SA

INSTABILITY HAZARD
4 – May detonate or have explosive reaction
3 – Shock and heat may detonate or cause explosive reaction
2 – Violent chemical change at elevated temperatures
1 – Unstable if heated
0 – Normally stable

● **Figure 5-6a** NFPA 704 hazardous materials classification. *(Reprinted with permission from NFPA 704-2012, System for the Identification of the Hazards of Materials for Emergency Response, Copyright © 2011, National Fire Protection Association. This reprinted material is not the complete and official position of the NFPA on the referenced subject, which is represented solely by the standard in its entirety. The classification of any particular material within this system is the sole responsibility of the user and not the NFPA. The NFPA bears no responsibility for any determinations of any values for any particular material classified or represented using this system.)*

Monitors and Testing

If you are unable to secure positive identification using the preceding sources, you may have to rely on monitors and other means of testing. If you do not have the training and equipment to do the reconnaissance, leave testing to the hazmat team. Monitoring devices or materials typically include:

- *Air and gas monitors*—typically determine the percentage of oxygen in the air and measure the presence of explosive gases, carbon monoxide, and toxic gases such as hydrogen sulfide
- *Litmus paper*—measures the approximate pH of a liquid, indicating whether it is an acid or a base
- *Colorimetric tubes*—suction the air and search for specific chemicals

Other Sources of Information

Once you have identified the hazardous substance, you will need to determine its specific chemical or physical properties. You can consult textbooks, handbooks, or technical specialists. You might also make use of a computerized database such as CAMEO®—Computer-Aided Management of Emergency Operations. Developed by the EPA and the National Oceanic and Atmospheric Administration (NOAA), this website provides answers to technical questions, opportunities for skills practice, copies of software, links for networking, and more. Yet another source of information includes your local or regional poison control center. (For more on the use of poison control centers, see Volume 4, Chapter 8.)

Two other sources of information are CHEMTREC—the Chemical Transportation Emergency Center—and CHEMTEL. Established by the American Chemistry Council (formerly the Manufacturing Chemists Association), CHEMTREC maintains a 24-hour, toll-free hotline. It provides information on the chemical properties of a substance and explains how the material should be handled. If necessary, CHEMTREC will even contact shippers and manufacturers to find out more detailed information about the incident and provide field assistance. In the United States and Canada, the toll-free number for CHEMTREC is 800-424-9300. For collect calls and calls from other points of origin, contact 703-527-3887. CHEMTREC can also refer you to the proper agencies for emergencies involving radioactive materials.

CHEMTEL, Inc. maintains another 24-hour, toll-free emergency response communications center for the United States and Canada. In addition to providing support for chemical emergencies, CHEMTEL also supplies the names of state and federal authorities that deal with radioactive incidents. For toll-free calls, dial 800-255-3024. For collect calls and calls from other points of origin, contact 813-979-0626.[4]

The contact numbers given here are printed on the back cover of the ERG.

Hazardous Materials Zones

As already mentioned, your main priority at a hazmat incident is safety. First, you protect your own safety and the safety of your crew. Then you attend to the safety of the patient(s) and

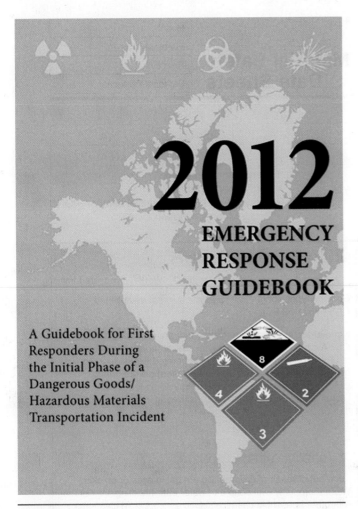

● **Figure 5-7** Carry a copy of the *Emergency Response Guidebook* in your vehicle at all times.

carried. However, drivers, pilots, or engineers may not take these papers when they exit the vehicle or craft, and you may find the scene too unstable to retrieve the documents yourself. In some cases, the papers may be incomplete or inadequate, requiring you to consult additional sources of identification.

Material Safety Data Sheets

In the case of fixed facilities, employers are required by law to post **material safety data sheets (MSDSs)**. These sheets contain detailed information about all potentially hazardous substances found on site. The sheets typically list the names and characteristics of the materials; what types of health, fire, and reactivity dangers the materials pose; any specific equipment or techniques required for safe handling of the materials; and suggested emergency first aid treatment.

Even simple chemicals, such as window cleaners, should have MSDSs posted in an easily accessible location. Figure 5-8 ● shows the MSDS posted for a familiar chemical—chlorine bleach. Among other information, it indicates possible adverse reactions in cases of accidental exposure, spills, leaks, and so on. Note, too, the range of substances that can produce toxic fumes if mixed with the bleach.

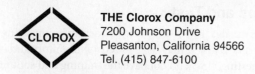

THE Clorox Company
7200 Johnson Drive
Pleasanton, California 94566
Tel. (415) 847-6100

Material Safety Data Sheets

Health	2+
Flammability	0
Reactivity	1
Personal Protection	B

I – CHEMICAL IDENTIFICATION

Name	regular Clorox Bleach	CAS No.	N/A
Description	clear, light yellow liquid with chlorine odor	RTECs No.	N/A

Other Designations
EPA Reg. No. 5813-1
Sodium hypochlorite solution
Liquid chlorine bleach
Clorox Liquid Bleach

Manufacturer
The Clorox Company
1221 Broadway
Oakland, CA 94612

Emergency Procedure
• Notify your supervisor
• Call your local poison control center   OR
• Rocky Mountain Poison Center
(303)573-1014

II – HEALTH HAZARD DATA

• Causes severe but temporary eye injury. May irritate skin. May cause nausea and vomiting if ingested. Exposure to vapor or mist may irritate nose, throat and lungs. The following medical conditions may be aggravated by exposure to high concentrations of vapor or mist: heart conditions or chronic respiratory problems such as asthma, chronic bronchitis or obstructive lung disease. Under normal consumer use conditions the likelihood of any adverse health effects are low.
FIRST AID: EYE CONTACT: Immediately flush eyes with plenty of water. If irritation persists, see a doctor. SKIN CONTACT: Remove contaminated clothing. Wash area with water.
INGESTION: Drink a glassful of water and call a physician.
INHALATION: If breathing problems develop remove to fresh air.

III – HAZARDOUS INGREDIENTS

Ingredients	Concentration	Worker Exposure Limit
Sodium hypochlorite CAS# 7681-52-9	5.25%	not established

None of the ingredients in this product are on the IARC, NTP or OSHA carcinogen list. Occasional clinical reports suggest a low potential for sensitization upon exaggerated exposure to sodium hypochlorite if skin damage (e.g., irritation) occurs during exposure. Routine clinical tests conducted on intact skin with Clorox Liquid Bleach found no sensitization in the test subjects.

IV – SPECIAL PROTECTION INFORMATION

Hygienic Practices: Wear safety glasses. With repeated or prolonged use, wear gloves.

Engineering Controls: Use general ventilation to minimize exposure to vapor or mist.

Work Practices: Avoid eye and skin contact and inhalation of vapor or mist.

V – SPECIAL PRECAUTIONS

Keep out of reach of children. Do not get in eyes or on skin. Wash thoroughly with soap and water after handling. Do not mix with other household chemicals such as toilet bowl cleaners, rust removers, vinegar, acid or ammonia containing products. Store in a cool, dry place. Do not reuse empty container; rinse container and put in trash container.

VI – SPILL OR LEAK PROCEDURES

Small quantities of less than 5 gallons may be flushed down drain. For larger quantities wipe up with an absorbent material or mop and dispose of in accordance with local, state and federal regulations. Dilute with water to minimize oxidizing effect on spilled surface.

VII – REACTIVITY DATA

Stable under normal use and storage conditions. Strong oxidizing agent. Reacts with other household chemicals such as toilet bowl cleaners, rust removers, vinegar, acids or ammonia containing products to produce hazardous gases, such as chlorine and other chlorinated species. Prolonged contact with metal may cause pitting or discoloration.

VIII – FIRE AND EXPLOSION DATA

Not flammable or explosive. In a fire, cool containers to prevent rupture and release of sodium chlorate.

IX – PHYSICAL DATA

Boiling point..................................212°F/100°C (decomposes)
Specific Gravity (H_2O = 1).............1.085
Solubility in Water........................complete
pH...11.4

● **Figure 5-8**   An example of a material safety data sheet (MSDS).

the public. To ensure that expert help arrives, request it right away—just as you would under the IMS. Establish command and hold it until relieved by somebody higher in the chain of command.

While waiting for additional support, keep a bad situation from becoming worse by evacuating people from the area around the incident. Do not risk anyone's safety by allowing "heroic" rescues. The result can be only an increased number of contaminated patients. Prepare for the arrival of additional resources by setting up the control zones shown in Figure 5-9 ●. They are:

- *Hot (red) zone:* The hot zone, also known as the exclusionary zone, is the site of contamination. Prevent anyone from entering this area unless they have the appropriate high-level PPE. Hold any patients that escape from this zone in the next zone, where decontamination and/or treatment will be performed.

- *Warm (yellow) zone:* The warm zone, also called the *contamination reduction zone,* lies immediately adjacent to the hot zone. It forms a "buffer zone" in which a decontamination corridor is established for patients and

EMS personnel leaving the hot zone. The corridor has both a "hot" and a "cold" end.

- *Cold (green) zone:* The cold zone, or "safe zone," is the area where the incident operation takes place. It includes the command post, medical monitoring and rehabilitation, treatment areas, and apparatus staging. The cold zone must be free of any contamination. No people or equipment from the hot zone should enter until they have undergone the necessary decontamination. You and your crew should remain inside this zone unless you have the necessary training, equipment, and support to enter other areas.

SPECIALIZED TERMINOLOGY

To prevent conflicts between the personnel or departments working at a hazmat incident, everyone should use the same terminology. This helps to eliminate dangerous misunderstandings during operations and treatment.

Terms for Medical Hazmat Operations

The following are the general terms that you can expect to encounter during a medical hazmat operation. They apply to situations involving chemical and/or radioactive materials.

- *Boiling point*—temperature at which a liquid becomes a gas.
- *Flammable/explosive limits*—range (upper and lower) of vapor concentration in the air at which an ignition will initiate combustion. The lower explosive limit (LEL) is the lowest concentration of chemical that will burn in the air. Below the LEL, there is not enough chemical to support combustion. The upper explosive limit (UEL) is the highest concentration of chemical that will burn in the air. Above the UEL, there is too much chemical and not enough oxygen to support combustion.
- *Flash point*—lowest temperature at which a liquid will give off enough vapors to ignite.
- *Ignition temperature*—lowest temperature at which a liquid will give off enough vapors to support combustion; slightly higher than the flash point.
- *Specific gravity*—the weight of a volume of liquid compared with an equal volume of water. Chemicals with a specific gravity greater than 1 will sink in water, whereas chemicals with a specific gravity less than 1 will float on water.
- *Vapor density*—the weight of a vapor or gas compared with the weight of an equal volume of air. Chemicals with a vapor density greater than 1 will fall to the lowest point possible, whereas chemicals with a vapor density less than 1 will rise.
- *Vapor pressure*—pressure of a vapor against the inside walls of a container. As temperatures increase, so do vapor pressures.
- *Water solubility*—ability of a chemical to dissolve into solution in water.

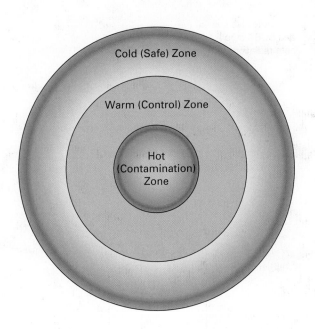

Hot (Contamination) Zone
- Contamination is actually present.
- Personnel must wear appropriate protective gear.
- Number of rescuers limited to those absolutely necessary.
- Bystanders never allowed.

Warm (Control) Zone
- Area surrounding the contamination zone.
- Vital to preventing spread of contamination.
- Personnel must wear appropriate protective gear.
- Lifesaving emergency care is performed.

Cold (Safe) Zone
- Normal triage, stabilization, and treatment are performed.
- Rescuers must shed contaminated gear before entering the cold zone.

● **Figure 5-9** The three zones typically established at a hazmat incident.

- *Alpha radiation*—neutrons and protons released by the nucleus of a radioactive substance (Figure 5-10 ●). This is a very weak particle and will only travel a few inches in the air. Alpha particles are stopped by paper, clothing, or intact skin. They are hazardous if inhaled or ingested.

- *Beta radiation*—electrons released with great energy by a radioactive substance. Beta particles have more energy than alpha particles and will travel 6 to 10 feet in the air. Beta particles will penetrate a few millimeters of skin.

- *Gamma radiation*—high-energy photons, such as X-rays. Gamma rays have the ability to penetrate most substances and to damage any cells within the body. Heavy shielding is needed for protection against gamma rays. Because gamma rays are electromagnetic (instead of particles), no decontamination is required. (For more information on the hazards and protection strategies of the three types of radiation, see Volume 5, Chapter 12, and Volume 4, Chapter 8.)

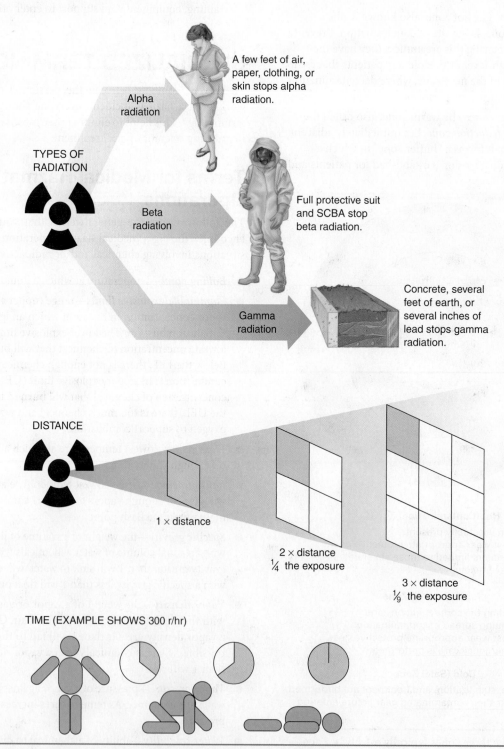

● **Figure 5-10** Alpha, beta, and gamma rays have different powers of penetration.

Toxicologic Terms

It is equally important to learn the terminology related to the toxic effects of hazardous materials. Here are the most important toxicologic terms used in the field:

- *Threshold limit value/time weighted average (TLV/TWA)*—maximum concentration of a substance in the air that a person can be exposed to for 8 hours each day, 40 hours per week, without suffering any adverse health effects. The lower the TLV/TWA, the more toxic the substance. The *permissible exposure limit (PEL)* is a similar measure of toxicity.

- *Threshold limit value/short-term exposure limit (TLV/STEL)*—maximum concentration of a substance that a person can be exposed to for 15 minutes (time weighted); not to be exceeded or repeated more than four times daily with 60-minute rests between each of the four exposures.

- *Threshold limit value/ceiling level (TLV-CL)*—maximum concentration of a substance that should never be exceeded, even for a moment.

- *Lethal concentration/lethal doses (LCt/LD)*—concentration (in air) or dose (if ingested, injected, or absorbed) that results in the death of 50 percent of the test subjects. Also referred to as the LCt50 or LD50.

- *Parts per million/parts per billion (ppm/ppb)*—representation of the concentration of a substance in the air or a solution, with parts of the substance expressed per million or billion parts of the air or solution.

- *Immediately dangerous to life and health (IDLH)*—level of concentration of a substance that causes an immediate threat to life. It may also cause delayed or irreversible effects or interfere with a person's ability to remove himself from the contaminated area.

CONTAMINATION AND TOXICOLOGY REVIEW

You have already covered some of the following material in Volume 4, Chapter 8. These points serve as a review, highlighting topics of particular relevance to hazmat situations. Keep this material in mind whenever you come onto any scene in which you suspect the presence of dangerous substances.

Types of Contamination

Whenever people or equipment come into contact with a potentially toxic substance, they are considered to be contaminated. The contamination may be either primary or secondary.

Primary contamination occurs when someone or something is directly exposed to a hazardous substance. At this point, the contamination is limited, that is, the exposure has not yet harmed others.

Secondary contamination takes place when a contaminated person or object comes in contact with an uncontaminated person or object—that is, the contamination is transferred. If you touch a contaminated patient, for example, you can become a contaminated care provider. Although gas exposure rarely results in secondary contamination, liquid and particulate matter are much more likely to be transferred.

To understand the difference between primary and secondary contamination, consider this example. A chemical pipeline ruptures and sprays several people with a hazardous substance. This is primary contamination. One of these patients walks out of the area and calls an ambulance. On arrival, this same patient climbs into the back of the ambulance, exposing the paramedics and the ambulance to the contaminant. This is secondary contamination. As a member of the EMS crew, you must make every effort not to become part of the incident through such secondary contamination.[5]

Routes of Exposure

As you know from Volume 4, Chapter 8 on toxicology, a person can be exposed to a hazardous substance in four ways. The most common method is respiratory inhalation. Gases, liquids, and particulate solids can all be inhaled through the nose or mouth. Once substances enter the bronchial tree, they can be quickly absorbed, especially in oxygen-deficient atmospheres. The substance then enters the central circulation system and is distributed throughout the body. As a result, inhaled substances often trigger a rapid onset of symptoms.

Toxic substances may also be introduced into the body through the skin, either by topical absorption or parenteral injection. Any toxic substance placed topically on intact skin and transferred into the person's circulation is considered a medical threat. In the case of injections, poisons directly enter the body via a laceration, a burn, or a puncture.

In hazmat situations, the least common route of exposure is through gastrointestinal ingestion, but it does happen. In occupations involving hazardous materials, people can be exposed to poisons by eating, drinking, or smoking around deadly substances. Foodstuffs can be exposed to a chemical and then eaten. People can forget to wash their hands and introduce the substance into their mouths.

Cycles and Actions of Poisons

Absorption—the rate at which a substance is delivered into the bloodstream—varies with the type and dosage of the poison. In general, the higher the dose, the greater the effect the substance will have on the body. Because of the wide variety of toxic substances, you will need to rely on the resources mentioned earlier to determine a given substance's actions, distribution to target organs, likely areas of deposit, and so on.

Basically, a poison's actions may be acute or delayed. **Acute effects** include those signs and symptoms that manifest themselves immediately or shortly after exposure. **Delayed effects** may not become apparent for hours, days, weeks, months, or even years. If a person is exposed to chlorine gas, for example, he

CONTENT REVIEW

▶ Common Routes of Hazmat Exposure

- Respiratory inhalation
- Topical absorption
- Parenteral injection
- Gastrointestinal ingestion

CONTENT REVIEW

▶ Hazmat Chemical
Classifications

• Corrosives—acids and
bases
• Pulmonary irritants—fumes
from chlorine and ammonia
• Pesticides—carbamates
and organophosphates
• Chemical asphyxiants—
carbon monoxide and
cyanides
• Hydrocarbon solvents—
xylene and methylene
chloride

immediately develops shortness of breath—an acute effect. If a person is exposed to a carcinogen, on the other hand, it may take many years before a malignancy develops—a delayed effect. Some substances, such as mustard gas (a military blister agent), cause immediate damage, but victims do not develop symptoms for many hours.

Once a substance is introduced into the body, it is distributed to target organs. Effects from a chemical may be local or systemic. **Local effects** involve areas around the immediate site and should be evaluated based on standard criteria such as the rule of nines, which was described in Volume 5, Chapter 6. You can usually expect some skin irritation (topical) or perhaps acute bronchospasm (respiratory). An acid sprayed on the skin, for example, creates immediate skin damage at the point of contact.

Systemic effects occur throughout the body. They can affect the cardiovascular, neurologic, hepatic, and/or renal systems. For example, although hydrofluoric acid may cause local skin burns on contact, it can also trigger hypocalcemia and arrhythmias. As a result, exposure to this substance can be potentially fatal.

The organs most commonly associated with toxic substances are the liver and the kidneys. The liver metabolizes most substances by chemically altering them through a process known as **biotransformation**. The kidneys can usually excrete the substances through the urine. However, both the liver and kidneys may be adversely affected by chemicals as are other organ systems. In such situations, the body may not be able to eliminate the toxic substances, creating a life-threatening situation.

When treating patients exposed to toxic substances, keep in mind that two substances or drugs may work together to produce an effect that neither of them can produce on their own. This effect, known as **synergism**, is part of the standard pharmacological approach to medicine. Before administering any medication, be sure to consult with medical direction or the poison control center on possible synergistic effects or treatments.

Treatment of Common Exposures

As noted several times, patients can be exposed to an incredibly large number of chemicals. Their treatment ranges from supportive care to specific antidotes. After ensuring your own safety, you should see that all patients receive the necessary supportive measures: airway support and suctioning, respiratory support, supplemental oxygen, circulatory support, and intravenous access. Before administering specific pharmacological treatment, at least two sources should agree on the medication. In addition, you should confer with medical direction, as previously mentioned.

The following subsections cover several of the most common classifications of chemicals to which patients may be exposed.

A brief overview of effects and treatment procedures is provided for each circumstance. Keep in mind that this is a generic discussion and is not intended to replace the specific identification resources already described.

Corrosives

Corrosives—acids and alkalis (bases)—can be found in many everyday materials. Most drain cleaners, for example, contain the alkali sodium hydroxide. Depending on the concentration, these substances can damage skin and other tissues. Corrosives can be inhaled, ingested, absorbed, or injected. Primary effects include severe skin burns, respiratory burns, and/or edema. Some corrosives may also have systemic effects.

When decontaminating a patient exposed to solid corrosives, brush off dry particles. In the case of liquid corrosives, flush the exposed area with large quantities of water. Tincture of green soap may help in decontamination. Irrigate eye injuries with water, possibly using a topical ophthalmic anesthetic such as tetracaine to reduce eye discomfort. In patients with pulmonary edema, consider the administration of furosemide (Lasix) or albuterol. If the patient has ingested a corrosive, *DO NOT* induce vomiting. If the patient can swallow and is not drooling, you may direct the person to drink 5 mL/kg water up to 200 mL. As with other injuries, maintain and support the ABCs: airway, breathing, and circulation.

Pulmonary Irritants

Many different substances can be pulmonary irritants, including the fumes from chlorine and ammonia. When inhaled, chlorine mixes with respiratory secretions to produce hydrochloric acid. Ammonia mixes with respiratory secretions to produce ammonium hydroxide, an alkali. In addition to tissue damage, these chemicals can cause pulmonary edema. The substances can also injure intact skin. Liquid ammonia, for example, will cause cold burns.

Primary respiratory exposure cannot be decontaminated. However, you should remove the patient's clothing to prevent any trapped gas from being contained near the body. You should also flush any exposed skin with large quantities of water. Irrigate eye injuries with water, possibly using tetracaine to reduce eye discomfort. Treat pulmonary edema with furosemide, if indicated. Again, treatment includes maintaining and supporting the ABCs.

Pesticides

Toxic pesticides or insecticides include primarily carbamates and organophosphates. Patients may come in contact with these chemicals through any of the four routes of exposure: inhalation, absorption, ingestion, or injection. The substances can act to block **acetylcholinesterase (AChE)**, an enzyme that stops the action of acetylcholine, a neurotransmitter. The result is overstimulation of the muscarinic receptors and the SLUDGE syndrome: **S**alivation, **L**acrimation, **U**rination, **D**iarrhea, **G**astrointestinal distress, and **E**mesis. Stimulation of the nicotinic receptor may also trigger involuntary contraction of the muscles and pinpoint pupils.

These chemicals will continue to be absorbed as long as they remain on the skin. As a result, decontamination with large amounts of water and tincture of green soap is essential. Remove all clothing and jewelry to prevent the chemical from being trapped against the skin. Maintain and support the ABCs. Secretions in the airway may need to be suctioned.

The primary treatment for significant exposure to pesticides is atropinization. The dose should be increased until the SLUDGE symptoms start to resolve. For carbamates, pralidoxime is *NOT* recommended. If an adult patient presents with seizures, administer 5 to 10 mg of diazepam. Do *NOT* induce vomiting if the patient has ingested the chemical.

Chemical Asphyxiants

The most common chemical asphyxiants include carbon monoxide (CO) and cyanides such as bitter almond oil, hydrocyanic acid, potassium cyanide, wild cherry syrup, prussic acid, and nitroprusside. Keep in mind that both CO and cyanides are by-products of combustion, so patients who present with smoke inhalation may need to be assessed for these substances as well. Most patients are exposed to CO and cyanides through inhalation. However, keep in mind that cyanides can also be ingested, absorbed, or injected.

These two chemicals have different actions once inhaled. Carbon monoxide has a very high affinity for hemoglobin—approximately 200 times greater than oxygen. As a result, it displaces oxygen in the red blood cells. Cyanides, however, inhibit the action of **cytochrome oxidase**. This enzyme complex, found in cellular mitochondria, enables oxygen to create the adenosine triphosphate (ATP) required for all muscle energy. Primary effects of CO exposure include changes in mental status and other signs of hypoxia such as chest pain, loss of consciousness, or seizures. Primary effects of cyanides include rapid onset of unconsciousness, seizures, and cardiopulmonary arrest.

Decontamination of patients exposed to CO and cyanide asphyxiants is usually unnecessary. However, these patients must be removed from the toxic environment without exposing rescuers to inhalation. Take off the patient's clothing to prevent entrapment of any toxic gases, while maintaining airway, breathing, and circulatory support. Definitive treatment for CO inhalation is oxygenation. In some cases, it may be provided through hyperbaric therapy, which increases the displacement of carbon monoxide from hemoglobin molecules by oxygen.

Definitive treatment for cyanide exposure can be provided by one of two cyanide antidotes. The older system, generally referred to as a cyanide antidote kit (also called a Pasadena, Lilly, or Taylor kit) contains three medications: amyl nitrite, sodium nitrite, and sodium thiosulfate. If this kit is used, first administer amyl nitrite. This short-acting vasodilator has the ability to convert hemoglobin to methemoglobin, which forms a nontoxic complex with cyanide ions. Wrap an ampule in gauze or cloth and crush it between your fingers. Then place it in front of a spontaneously breathing patient for 15 seconds. Repeat at 1-minute intervals until an infusion of sodium nitrite is ready. Keep in mind that amyl nitrite is volatile and highly flammable when mixed with air or oxygen. Next, administer the sodium nitrite, 300 mg IV push over 5 minutes. (Sodium nitrite also produces methemoglobin.) Quickly follow the sodium nitrite with an infusion of sodium thiosulfate, 12.5 g IV push over 5 minutes. The sodium thiosulfate converts the cyanide/methemoglobin complexes into thiocyanate, which can be excreted by the kidneys. If the signs and symptoms reappear, the process should be repeated at half the original doses.

A safer and less toxic antidote is now available (Figure 5-11 ●). This antidote, called hydroxocobalamin, is commercially available and packaged as Cyano-Kit™. Hydroxocobalamin is a precursor to cyanocobalamin (vitamin B_{12}). When hydroxocobalamin is administered, it binds cyanide from cytochrome oxidase and forms cyanocobalamin. Excess cyanocobalamin is excreted from the body via the kidneys.[6]

CONTENT REVIEW

► Use of Cyanide Kit

- Administer ampule of amyl nitrite for 15 seconds.
- Repeat at 1-minute intervals until sodium nitrite is ready.
- Administer infusion of sodium nitrite, 300 mg IV push over 5 minutes.
- Follow with infusion of sodium thiosulfate, 12.5 g IV push over 5 minutes.
- Repeat at half original doses, if necessary.

Hydrocarbon Solvents

Many different chemicals can act as solvents, including xylene and methylene chloride. Usually found in liquid form, they give off easily inhaled vapors. Primary effects include arrhythmias, pulmonary edema, and respiratory failure. Delayed effects include damage to the central nervous system and the renal system. Exposure to these chemicals may be intentional, such as among drug abusers seeking the central nervous system effects (euphoria) produced by the fumes. If the patient ingests the chemical and vomits, aspiration may lead to pulmonary edema.

Treatment varies with the route of exposure. In cases of topical contact, decontaminate the exposed area with large quantities of warm water and tincture of green soap. If the patient has ingested the solvent, *DO NOT* induce vomiting. If the adult patient presents with seizures, administer 5 to 10 mg of diazepam. In the case of inhalation, maintain and support the ABCs.

APPROACHES TO DECONTAMINATION

Decontamination, as you have read, attempts to reduce or remove hazardous substances from people and/or equipment to prevent adverse health effects. Decontamination can be accomplished by physical or chemical means. Physical decontamination involves the removal of chemicals by separating them from the person or equipment, whereas chemical

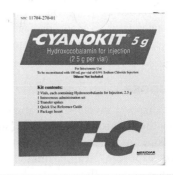

● **Figure 5-11**   The Cyano-Kit. (*© Dr. Bryan E. Bledsoe*)

CONTENT REVIEW

► Methods of
Decontamination

- Dilution
- Absorption (blotting)
- Neutralization
- Isolation/disposal

decontamination focuses on changing the hazardous substance into something less harmful.

Decontamination (decon) procedures serve several purposes. First, decon reduces the dosage of the material to which patients are exposed. Second, it reduces the risk of secondary contamination of rescuers, on-scene personnel, bystanders, hospital personnel, the families of rescuers, and the general public.

Methods of Decontamination

The four methods of decontamination are dilution, absorption, neutralization, and isolation/disposal. The method used depends on the type of hazardous substance and the route of exposure. In many instances, rescuers will use two or more of these methods during the decontamination process.

Dilution

Dilution involves the application of large quantities of water to the contaminated person or item. Water is considered the universal decon solution, especially for reducing topical absorption. It may be aided by use of a soap, such as tincture of green soap. Mixing hazardous substances with water significantly reduces their concentration, hopefully to a level at which they are no longer dangerous. Be aware that a small number of chemicals should never be mixed with water.

Absorption

Absorption entails the use of pads or towels to "blot" up the hazardous material. The process is usually applied after washing with water—that is, as a means of drying the patient. Absorption further reduces the contamination levels but is not usually a primary method of decon. Absorption is more commonly used during environmental cleanup.

Neutralization

Neutralization occurs when one substance reduces or eliminates the toxicity of another substance, such as adding an acid to a base. Although this is a third method of patient decontamination, it is almost never used by EMS personnel. In a field setting, it is difficult to identify the exact hazardous substance and the proper neutralizing agent. In addition, neutralization often produces an exothermic reaction, or release of large quantities of heat. The heat can be just as damaging as, or even more damaging than, the original chemical. Lavage usually dilutes and removes the chemical faster and is more practical given the typical on-scene equipment.

Isolation/Disposal

Isolation and/or disposal involves separating the patient or equipment from the hazardous substance. Isolation begins by establishing zones at the incident to prevent any further contamination or exposure. Next, hazmat teams remove patients from the hot zone to the warm zone. Last, any items that might contain or trap a hazardous substance should be removed, including a patient's clothing and jewelry. All contaminated items should be properly disposed of or stored.

Decontamination Decision Making

In performing decontamination, always recall the priorities of incident management: life safety, incident stabilization, and property conservation. These priorities should guide your decision making throughout the incident. For example, you should try to prevent any water runoff used for decontamination from damaging the environment. However, environmental considerations form a major concern only in cases in which there are no life threats—that is, when patients are stable and not expected to deteriorate during the decon process. If life threats exist, the patients come first; environmental considerations come last.

Modes of Operation

In general, EMS personnel engage in one of two modes of operation at hazmat incidents that generate patients: "fast-break" decision making or long-term decision making. Fast-break decision making occurs at incidents that call for immediate action to prevent rescuer contamination and/or to handle obvious life threats. Long-term decision making takes place at extended events in which hazmat teams retrieve patients, identify the hazardous substance, and determine methods of decontamination and treatment.

Fast-Break Decision Making   At hazmat incidents where patients are conscious, contaminated victims will often self-rescue. They will walk from the primary incident site to the EMS units. In such cases, you must make fast-break decisions to prevent rescuer contamination. Keep in mind that it may take time for a hazmat team to arrive and set up operations. In the interim, the conscious, contaminated patients may try to leave the scene entirely. As a result, all EMS units must be prepared for gross decontamination. Basic personal protective equipment should be onboard and all personnel should be familiar with the two-step decontamination procedures covered later in this chapter.

Implement this mode of decision making at all incidents with critical patients and unknown or life-threatening materials. Fire apparatus often respond very quickly and carry large quantities of water that can be used for decon. Remove patient clothing, treat life-threatening problems, and wash with water. Although it is preferable to use warm water to prevent hypothermia, this option is not always available. Please remember the first rule of EMS: *Do not become a patient!* At no time should you or other crew members expose yourselves to contaminants—even to rescue a critically injured patient. Instead, contain and isolate the patient as best you can until the proper support arrives.

When treating critically injured hazmat patients, it is important to perform a rapid risk-to-benefit assessment. Ask yourself these questions: How much risk of exposure will I incur by intubating a patient during decon? Does the patient really need an intravenous line established right now? Few ALS procedures will truly make a difference if performed rapidly, but one mistake can cause any rescuer to become a patient. Take a few moments, and think before you act.

At incidents where patients are noncritical, rescuers can take a more contemplative approach, especially if they can identify the substance. Decontamination and treatment proceed simultaneously, following the general steps already mentioned. However, depending on whether the substance has been identified, you may be able to give special attention to other matters. For example, you might contain water runoff. You might better protect patient privacy by grossly decontaminating ambulatory patients in a more controlled setting. You might also spend time on patient monitoring, reclothing patients, isolating or containing patients, and so on.

Long-Term Decision Making   At more extended events, you will engage in long-term decision making. This mode of operation most often occurs when patients remain in the hot zone and have not self-rescued. Traditionally, EMS personnel have not been trained or equipped to enter the hot zone to retrieve these patients. Instead, a hazmat team is summoned promptly, and the EMS crew awaits the team's arrival. The team will not make their entry until you or members of your crew perform the necessary medical monitoring and establish a decontamination corridor. It often takes 60 minutes or more for actual team deployment.

This mode of operation provides a number of advantages: a better opportunity for thorough decontamination, better PPE, less chance of secondary decontamination, greater consideration of the environment, and more detailed research of the actual hazardous substance. Obviously, long-term decision making presents less opportunity for error and is preferable to fast-break decision making. Unfortunately, self-rescued patients often force a decision about the mode of operation the minute you arrive on the scene. Be prepared for fast-break operations whenever you suspect a potential hazmat incident.

Field Decontamination

As mentioned, the decontamination method and type of PPE depend on the substance involved. If in doubt, assume the worst-case scenario. When dealing with unknowns, do not attempt to neutralize. Brush dry particles off the patient before the application of water to prevent possible chemical reactions. Next, wash with great quantities of water—the universal decon agent—using tincture of green soap if possible. Isopropyl alcohol is an effective agent for some isocyanates, and vegetable oil can be used to decon water-reactive substances.

Two-Step Process

Use the two-step decon process for gross decontamination of patients who cannot wait for a more comprehensive decon process, usually patients at a fast-break incident.

● *Step 1:* Rescuers remove or instruct patients to remove all clothing, including shoes, socks, and jewelry. (Remember to have some method of accounting for personal effects *before* hazmat incidents occur.)

● *Step 2:* Rescuers wash and rinse the patients with soap and water, making sure that they do not stay in contact with the runoff. Repeat the process, allowing the fluid to drain away each time. It is important to pay special attention to

difficult contamination areas such as the scalp and hair, ears, nostrils, axillae, fingernails, navel, genitals, groin, buttocks, behind the knees, between the toes, and toenails.

Eight-Step Process

The eight-step process takes place in a complete decontamination corridor and is much more thorough. To leave the hot zone, the hazmat rescuers follow these steps:

● *Step 1:* Rescuers enter the decon area at the hot end of the corridor and mechanically remove contaminants from the victims.

● *Step 2:* Rescuers drop equipment in a tool-drop area and remove outer gloves.

● *Step 3:* Decon personnel shower and scrub all victims and rescuers, using gross decontamination. As surface decontamination is removed, the dilution is conducted into a contained area. Victims may be moved ahead to Step 6 or Step 7.

● *Step 4:* Rescuers remove and isolate their self-contained breathing apparatus (SCBA). If reentry is necessary, the team dons new SCBA from a noncontaminated side.

● *Step 5:* Rescuers remove all protective clothing. Articles are isolated, labeled for disposal, and placed on the contaminated side.

● *Step 6:* Rescuers remove all personal clothing. Victims who have not had their clothing removed have it taken off here. All items are isolated in plastic bags and labeled for later disposal or storage.

● *Step 7:* Rescuers and victims receive a full-body washing, using soft scrub brushes or sponges, water, and mild soap or detergent. Cleaning tools are bagged for later disposal.

● *Step 8:* Patients receive rapid assessment and stabilization before being transported to hospitals for further care. EMS crews medically monitor rescuers, complete exposure records, and transport rescuers to hospitals as needed.

These procedures are not set in stone. Small variations may exist from system to system. You should become familiar with the specific procedures in the jurisdiction where you practice.

Transportation Considerations

Remember that no patient who undergoes field decontamination is truly decontaminated. Field-decontaminated patients, sometimes called **semi-decontaminated patients**, may still need to undergo a more invasive decon process at a medical facility. Depending on the type of exposure, wounds may need debridement, hair or nails may need to be trimmed or removed, and so on. However, it is always better to deliver a grossly decontaminated living patient to the hospital than a perfectly decontaminated corpse. Just make sure that field-decontaminated patients are transported to facilities capable of performing more thorough decon procedures.

When transporting field-decontaminated patients, always recall that they may still have some contamination in or on them. For example, a patient may have ingested a chemical, which can be expelled if the patient coughs or vomits. As a result, use as much disposable equipment as possible. Keep in mind that any airborne hazard not only can incapacitate the crew in the back of the ambulance but can affect the driver as well. Although it is not practical to line the ambulance in plastic, you can isolate the patient using a stretcher decon pool. The pool can help contain any potentially contaminated body fluids. Plastic can also be used to cover the pool, adding yet another protective barrier.

HAZMAT PROTECTION EQUIPMENT

As you know, the personal protective equipment used at a hazmat incident is specifically designed to prevent or limit rescuer injuries (Figures 5-12a ● through 5-12d ●). Hard hats, for example, protect rescuers against impacts to the head. There are

basically four levels of hazmat protective equipment, ranging from Level A (the highest level) to Level D (the minimum level).

● *Level A*—provides the highest level of respiratory and splash protection. This hazmat suit offers a high degree of protection against chemical breakthrough and fully encapsulates the rescuer, even covering the SCBA. The sealed, impermeable suits are typically used by hazmat teams entering hot zones with an unknown substance and a significant potential for both respiratory and dermal hazards.

● *Level B*—offers full respiratory protection when there is a lower probability of dermal hazard. The Level B suit is nonencapsulating, but chemically resistant. Seams for zippers, gloves, boots, and mask interface are usually sealed with duct tape. The SCBA is worn outside the suit, allowing increased maneuverability and greater ease in changing SCBA bottles. The decon team typically wears Level B protective equipment.

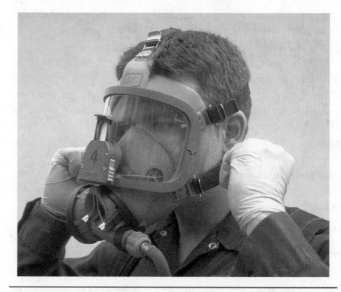

● **Figure 5-12b**   Putting on a mask.

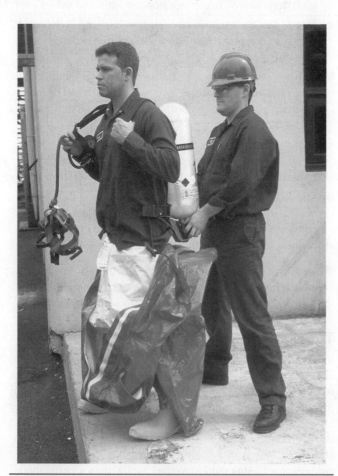

● **Figure 5-12a**   Assisting with an air tank.

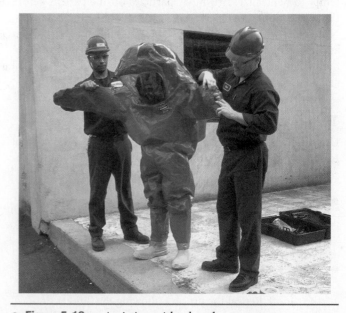

● **Figure 5-12c**   Assisting with a hood.

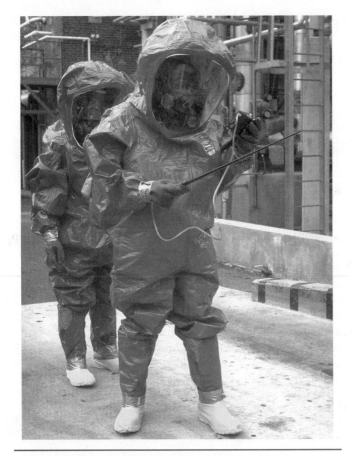

● **Figure 5-12d** Hazmat team fully suited.

- *Level C*—includes a nonpermeable suit, boots, and gear for protecting eyes and hands. Instead of SCBA, Level C protective equipment uses an **air-purifying respirator (APR)**. The APR relies on filters to protect against a known contaminant in a normal environment. As a result, the canisters in the APR must be specifically selected and are not usually implemented in a hazmat emergency response. Level C clothing is usually worn during transport of patients with the potential for secondary contamination.
- *Level D*—consists of structural firefighter, or turnout, gear. Level D gear is usually not suitable for hazmat incidents.

The level of hazmat protective gear worn depends on the chemical or substance involved. Ideally, the chemical should be identified so a permeability chart can be consulted to determine the breakthrough time. No single material is suitable to all hazmat situations. Some materials are resistant to certain chemicals and nonresistant to others.

EMS personnel should not become involved in any hazmat situation without the proper PPE. All ambulances carry some level of PPE, even if not ideal. If the situation is emergent and the chemical unknown, use as much barrier protection as possible. Full turnout gear (Level D) or a Tyvek suit is better than no gear at all. High-efficiency particulate air (HEPA) filter masks and double or triple gloves offer good protection against some hazards. Keep in mind that latex gloves are not chemically resistant. Instead, use nitrile gloves, which have a high resistance to most chemicals.

Also remember that leather boots will absorb chemicals permanently, so be sure to don rubber boots.

MEDICAL MONITORING AND REHABILITATION

As noted, one of the primary roles of EMS personnel at a hazmat incident is the medical monitoring of entry personnel. All hazmat team members should undergo regular annual physical examinations, with baseline vital signs placed on file.

Entry Readiness

Prior to entry, you or other EMS crew members will assess rescuers and document the following information on an incident flow sheet: blood pressure, pulse, respiratory rate, temperature, body weight, ECG, and mental/neurologic status. If you observe anything abnormal, do not allow the hazmat team member to attempt a rescue.

Hazmat team members will enter the hot zone only in groups of two, with two more members in PPE remaining outside the hot zone as a backup team. The PPE used at hazmat incidents can cause significant stress and dehydration. As a result, entry team personnel should prehydrate themselves with 8 to 16 ounces of water or sports drinks. Because sports drinks are more effective at half strength, dilute them with 50 percent water when possible.

Post-Exit Rehab

After the hazmat entry team exits the hot zone and completes decontamination, they should report back to EMS for post-entry monitoring (Figure 5-13 ●). Measure and document the

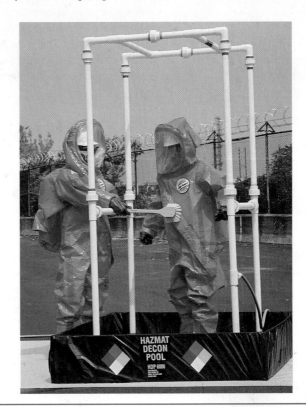

● **Figure 5-13** Rescuers involved in the decontamination process.

CONTENT REVIEW

► Pre-Entry/Post-Exit
Documentation

- Blood pressure
- Pulse
- Respiratory rate
- Temperature
- Body weight
- ECG
- Mental/neurologic status

same parameters on the flow sheet. Rehydrate the team with more water or diluted sports drinks. You can use weight changes to estimate any fluid losses. Check with medical direction or protocols to determine fluid replacement by means of PO or IV. Entry team members should not be allowed to reenter the hot zone until they are alert, nontachycardic, normotensive, and within a reasonable percentage of their normal body weight.

Heat Stress Factors

In evaluating heat stress, you will need to take many factors into account. Primary considerations include temperature and humidity. Prehydration, duration and degree of activity, and the team member's overall physical fitness will also have a bearing on your evaluation. Keep in mind that Level A suits protect a rescuer, but prevent cooling. A rescuer essentially works inside an encapsulated sauna. The same suit that seals out hazards also prevents heat loss by evaporation, conduction, convection, and radiation. Therefore, place heat stress at the top of your list of tasks for post-exit medical monitoring.

IMPORTANCE OF PRACTICE

As a paramedic, you will play an important role at any hazmat incident. You may establish command, make the first incident decisions, and help protect all on-scene personnel, including the hazmat team. As a result, you should practice skills that you can expect to use in most EMS systems.

Here are some things you should routinely do. Put on and take off Level B hazmat protective equipment. Set up a rapid two-step decontamination process and an eight-step decontamination process, preferably with the help of the local hazmat team. With a crew member, identify a simulated chemical, determine the correct PPE, and establish the proper decontamination methods. Practice pre-entry and post-exit medical monitoring and documentation. Prepare a patient and ambulance for transport. Because these skills may be rarely used except in the busiest EMS systems, you should work closely with your local hazmat team to practice these skills on a regular basis.

 SUMMARY

Every member of an EMS team should be prepared to face the challenges of a hazmat incident. At all times, keep in mind the high potential for rescuer involvement in a hazmat incident, especially during the early phases. As with any EMS operation, the primary consideration is your own safety. No patient's life is worth your own. This is especially true at a fast-break incident in which you must resist heroic efforts that will place you in contact with ambulatory, self-rescued patients. You become useless at a hazmat incident if you become contaminated yourself.

 YOU MAKE THE CALL

You are dispatched to a motor vehicle collision on an interstate highway. You arrive on scene and find that a car has rear-ended a tractor-trailer. Two people exit the cab of the truck and begin to walk toward the ambulance. Both have obvious respiratory distress. You note that the driver of the car appears to be unresponsive behind the steering wheel.

You do a quick windshield size-up for hazards and see a black-and-white placard on the rear of the truck. The placard bears a skull and crossbones and two numbers, 6 and 2783. You notice some liquid dripping from the rear door of the truck onto the hood of the car.

The occupants of the truck walk up to the side of the ambulance. You observe that they are drooling, tearing, and sweating profusely. One of them knocks on your window and says, "Please help us. We can't breathe."

1. What do you suspect has happened based on your quick scene size-up?

2. What are your initial priorities?

3. How will you identify the substance involved in the accident?

4. What additional resources would you request?

5. Is this a fast-break or a long-term incident? Explain.

6. What are your first actions?

See Suggested Responses at the back of this book.

REVIEW QUESTIONS

1. This standard, along with two other NFPA standards for hazmat response, deals with the training standards for EMS personnel assigned to hazmat incidents.
   a. CRF 1910.120
   c. NFPA 473
   b. 40 CFR 311
   d. ASTM 1147

2. Which of the following does *not* represent one of the three levels of training appropriate to EMS response at hazmat incidents?
   a. Awareness Level
   c. EMS Level 1
   b. Paramedic Level 4
   d. EMS Level 2

3. The basic IMS at a hazmat incident will require a _____.
   a. command post
   b. staging area
   c. decontamination corridor
   d. all of the above

4. The _____ has implemented placards to identify dangerous substances in transit.
   a. UN
   c. NFPA
   b. DOT
   d. NIOSH

5. Which source of information maintains a 24-hour, toll-free hotline; provides information on the chemical properties of a substance; and explains how the material should be handled?
   a. EPA
   c. CHEMTREC
   b. NOAA
   d. CAMEO

6. The control zone, where the incident operation takes place, including the command post, medical monitoring and rehabilitation, treatment areas, and apparatus staging, is the _____.
   a. hot (red) zone
   b. warm (yellow) zone
   c. exclusionary zone
   d. cold (green) zone

7. The most common method by which a person can be exposed to a hazardous substance is _____.
   a. respiratory inhalation
   b. topical absorption
   c. parenteral injection
   d. gastrointestinal ingestion

8. _____ is considered the universal decon solution, especially for reducing topical absorption.
   a. Water
   b. Oxygen
   c. Atropine
   d. Sodium nitrite

See Answers to Review Questions at the back of this book.

REFERENCES

1. United States Department of Transportation, Pipeline and Hazardous Materials Safety Administration. [Available at http://www.phmsa.dot.gov/public/definitions]

2. Keim, M. M. "The Public Health Impact of Industrial Disasters." *Am J Disaster Med* 6 (2011): 265–272.

3. Decker, R. J. "Acceptance and Utilization of the Incident Command System in the First Response and Allied Disciplines: An Ohio Study." *J Bus Contin Emer Plan* 5 (2011): 224–230.

4. Oberg, M., N. Palmen, and G. Johanson. "Discrepancy among Acute Guidelines for Emergency Response." *J Hazard Mater* 184 (2010): 439–447.

5. Scanlon, J. "Chemically Contaminated Casualties: Different Problems and Possible Solutions." *Am J Disaster Med* 5 (2010): 95–105.

6. Hall, A. H, J. Saiers, and F. Baud. "Which Cyanide Antidote?" *Crit Rev Toxicol* 39 (2009): 514–552.

FURTHER READING

De Lorenzo, R. A., and R. S. Porter. *Weapons of Mass Destruction: Emergency Care.* Upper Saddle River, NJ: Pearson/Prentice Hall, 2000.

Emergency Response Guidebook: A Guidebook for First Responders During the Initial Phase of a Dangerous Goods/Hazardous Materials Transportation. Washington, DC: U.S. Department of Transportation, 2008.

Leonard, J. E., and G. D. Robinson. *Managing Hazardous Materials.* Rockville, MD: Institute of Hazardous Materials Management, 2002.

Meyer, E. *Chemistry of Hazardous Materials.* 4th ed. Upper Saddle River, NJ: Pearson/Prentice Hall, 2005.

NFPA 473. *Standard Competencies for EMS Personnel Responding to Hazardous Materials Incidents.* 2008 ed. Quincy, MA: National Fire Protection Agency.

NFPA 704. *Standard for Identification of the Fire Hazards of Materials.* 2012 ed. Quincy, MA: National Fire Protection Agency.

Noll, G. G., M. S. Hildebrand, and J. G. Yvorra. *Hazardous Materials: Managing the Incident.* 3rd ed. Chester, MD: Red Hat Publishing, 2005.

Stutz, D. R., and S. Ulin. *Haztox: EMS Response to Hazardous Materials Incidents.* Miramar, FL: GDS Communications, 1994.

6

Crime Scene Awareness

Bryan Bledsoe, DO, FACEP, FAAEM, EMT-P
Daniel Limmer, AS, EMT-P

STANDARD
Assessment (Scene Size-Up)

COMPETENCY
Integrates scene and patient assessment findings with knowledge of epidemiology and pathophysiology to form a field impression. This includes developing a list of differential diagnoses through clinical reasoning to modify the assessment and formulate a treatment plan.

OBJECTIVES

Terminal Performance Objective
After reading this chapter, you should be able to integrate the special considerations involved in response to crime scenes and increased risk of violence into the overall approach to scene management and patient care.

Enabling Objectives
To accomplish the terminal performance objective, you should be able to:

1. Define key terms introduced in this chapter.
2. Describe the demographics of violence.
3. Recognize indications that you may encounter violence on a call.
4. Describe the actions you should take to protect your safety when you are advised of danger before you reach the scene, to observe danger on arriving at the scene, and when danger arises during a call.
5. Take steps to avoid the types of dangers you may encounter when responding to calls on the roadside or highway.
6. Take steps to avoid the types of dangers you may encounter when responding to violent street events.
7. Describe particular safety concerns related to responding to clandestine drug laboratories.
8. Implement the tactical options of retreat, concealment, cover, distraction, evasion, contact and cover, warning signals, and communication when situations call for their use.
9. Describe the advantages and limitations of using body armor.
10. Describe the role of tactical EMS.
11. Given a crime scene scenario, interact cooperatively with law enforcement to provide patient care while maintaining awareness of crime scene and evidence considerations.

KEY TERMS
blood spatter evidence, p. 123
body armor, p. 121
concealment, p. 120
CONTOMS, p. 122

cover, p. 120
EMT-Tacticals (EMT-Ts), p. 122
hate crimes, p. 117
particulate evidence, p. 124

special weapons and tactics
  (SWAT) team, p. 121
tactical emergency medical
  service (TEMS), p. 114

At 10:30 P.M. your paramedic unit receives a call for an unknown problem at 4926 Magnolia Boulevard. The residence lies in a well-kept part of the city. As you turn onto Magnolia, you shut off the vehicle's emergency lights. Before arriving on scene, you request further information from dispatch. The dispatcher tells you that an older male requested an ambulance because "someone is sick and needs help, now!" He then quickly hung up without providing any further details, which makes you suspicious. Computer-aided dispatch shows no prior calls at the residence and no history of violence at the location.

Your partner stops the ambulance two houses away from the scene. You both observe the quiet single-family residence. Because you see no signs of danger, your partner moves the rig closer. Both you and your partner exit the vehicle and approach the residence with only the necessary equipment. The two of you take separate, unpredictable paths to the residence, keeping each other in sight. This provides a better view of the dwelling.

Your partner looks in the front window and observes an older man standing over a woman about the same age. She seems to be very ill. There are no signs of fighting, intoxication, or other unusual behavior.

You and your partner decide that it is safe to approach the door. You knock, and the man urges you to enter quickly. "My wife is so sick," he exclaims. "I don't know what to do. Please follow me."

You introduce yourself and immediately notice that the man has difficulty hearing you. He is older than you had suspected and is obviously distraught. The combination of factors explains why he may have failed to provide adequate information to dispatch.

You learn that the patient is experiencing chest discomfort and has been vomiting. You treat her according to ALS protocols and then transport both the patient and her husband to the hospital.

No violence on this call! Yet neither you nor your partner has any doubt about your cautious approach to the call. You have learned from experience that quiet calls can be just as worrisome as those made with loud voices. At least with loud voices, you have some reason to suspect trouble. Although you discovered a reasonable explanation for this suspicious call, you know all too well that your personal safety depends on your ability to detect potentially violent situations before you even step outside your ambulance.

INTRODUCTION

Violence can occur anywhere. Regardless of where you work as a paramedic—the inner city, the suburbs, or rural America—you can be affected by violence. The violence can take all forms, from interpersonal abuse in the home to gang activities in the street. The violence can also involve any number of weapons, ranging from fists to guns to explosives.

Although people of all ages and backgrounds commit acts of violence, the past two decades have seen a dramatic increase in violence among youth. According to the Division of Violence Prevention at the National Center for Injury Prevention and Control, arrest rates for homicide, rape, robbery, and aggravated assault are consistently higher for people ages 15 to 34 than for all other age groups. Even more alarming, an average of 16 youth (ages 10–24) homicides occur in the United States every day. Among 10- to 24-year-olds, homicide is the leading cause of death for African Americans and the second leading cause of death for Hispanics.[1]

Approximately one of six victims of violent crimes requires medical attention, often by the emergency medical services. Several studies suggest that a substantial number of these victims fail to report the violence to the police. As a result, the emergency medical services may be a victim's only contact with professionals who can intervene to prevent further harm.

A more recent phenomenon is bullying. Bullying is a form of youth violence and can result in physical injury, social and emotional distress, and even death. Victimized youth are at increased risk for mental health problems such as depression and anxiety, psychosomatic complaints such as headaches, and poor school adjustment. Youths who bully others are at increased risk for substance use, academic problems, and violence later in adolescence and adulthood.

Despite the increased presence of violence, EMS providers find it almost impossible to predict exactly when and where a violent incident will occur. Nearly all calls that you or any other paramedic handle on a given day will progress without any threat of danger. In fact, you have a higher risk of being injured by oncoming traffic than by a violent act. Even so, you cannot let down your "crime scene awareness." Otherwise, you risk becoming a victim or hostage of a violent situation.

As this chapter shows, your most important safety tactic is an ability to identify potentially violent situations as soon as possible. Although you cannot predict violence hours in advance, you can remain alert to signs of danger. You can also become aware of local issues that hold a potential for violence, such as the presence of street gangs or a known area of drug activity.

Equally as important, you should familiarize yourself with standard operating procedures (SOPs) for handling violent situations and/or the specialized resources that you can call on for backup. Find out, for example, whether your unit has access to a **tactical emergency medical service (TEMS)**, which is a unit that provides on-site medical support to law enforcement.[2, 3] If so, know how and when to access it. Above all else, remain alert to the signs of danger from the start of a call to the time you return your ambulance to service.

APPROACH TO THE SCENE

Your safety strategy begins as soon as you are dispatched on a call. Even the most basic information can provide important tactical clues. Emergency medical dispatchers try to keep callers on the line to obtain as much information as possible. They remain alert to background noises such as fighting or intoxicated persons, so they can warn incoming units of these dangers. Modern computer-aided dispatch programs provide instant information on previous calls at a particular location and display "caution indicators" to notify dispatchers when a location has a history of violence.

Even in the age of computers, however, some of your best information can still come from your own experience and that of other crews. Your memory of previous calls can serve as an important indicator of trouble. For example, if a bar or club has a reputation for fights and you are summoned there, you will already have a high suspicion of danger before you arrive.

Possible Scenarios

There are three possible scenarios in which you might observe violence during an EMS call. The dispatcher may advise you of a potentially violent scene en route to the call. Obviously, you will be alert to danger from the start. In other cases, you may not spot danger until you arrive on the scene and begin your size-up and approach. In yet a third scenario, you may not face danger until the start of patient care or transport.

Advised of Danger En Route

When the dispatcher reports possible danger, do not approach the scene until it has been secured by law enforcement personnel. Remember that lights and sirens can draw a crowd and/or alert the perpetrator of a crime, so use them cautiously or not at all.

Never follow police units to the scene. To do so might place you at the center of violence. If you arrive first, keep the ambulance out of sight so the rig does not attract the attention of bystanders or any of the parties involved in the incident. While you wait for police to secure the scene, set up a staging area.

Management of the incident depends on interagency cooperation. Communicate with the police—you are in this together. Be sure you understand any differences in dispatch terminology. For example, a code 1 emergency for police units is a code 3 emergency for EMS units. Work with police to determine if and when you should approach the scene.

Keep in mind that violence can occur or resume even with the police present. Furthermore, depending on your uniform colors and the use of badges, people might mistake you for the police, especially if you exit from a vehicle with flashing lights and siren. They might expect you to intervene in a violent situation, or they might direct aggression toward you as an authority figure. If the scene cannot be made safe, retreat immediately (Figure 6-1 ●).

Observing Danger on Arrival

Even if dispatch has not alerted you to danger, you must still keep this possibility in mind once you arrive on scene. One of the main purposes of the scene size-up is to search for any possible hazards. This includes nonviolent dangers such as downed power lines, dangerous pets, unstable vehicles, or hazmat. As you look for these dangers, observe for other signs of trouble such as crowds gathering on the street, an unusual silence, or a darkened residence. Obviously, you will adopt a different approach for a confirmed medical emergency than for an "unknown problem, caller hang-up." Even so, do not exit the vehicle until you have ruled out all immediate hazards.

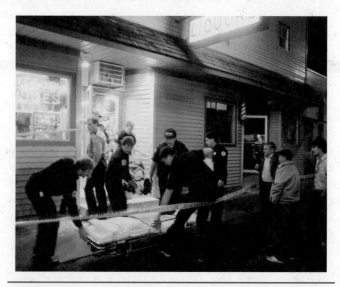

● **Figure 6-1** Never approach the scene until you have been advised that the scene is secure. Remember, even if a scene has been declared secure, violence may still erupt. (*© Craig Jackson/In the Dark Photography*)

If you have any doubts about a call, park away from the scene. If you must park in view of the location, take an unconventional approach to the door (Figure 6-2 ●). People will expect you to use the sidewalk. Therefore, approach from the side, on the lawn, or flush against the house. Avoid getting between a residence and the lighted ambulance so you do not "backlight" yourself. In addition, hold your flashlight to the side rather than in front of you (Figure 6-3 ●). Armed assailants often fire at the light.

Before announcing your presence, listen and observe for signs of danger. If you can, look in windows for evidence of fighting, the presence of weapons, or the use of alcohol or drugs. Gradually make your way to the doorknob side of the door, or the side of the door opposite the hinges (Figure 6-4 ●). Listen for any signs of danger such as loud noises, items breaking, incoherent speech, or the lack of any sounds at all.

If you spot danger at any time during your approach, immediately stop and reevaluate the situation. Decide whether it is in the interest of your own safety to continue or to retreat until law enforcement officials can be summoned. Rather than risk becoming injured or killed, err on the side of safety.

Eruption of Danger During Care or Transport

Remain alert throughout a call, especially in areas with a history of violence. You may enter the scene and spot weapons or drugs. Additional combative people may arrive on scene. The patient or bystanders may become agitated or threatening. Even if

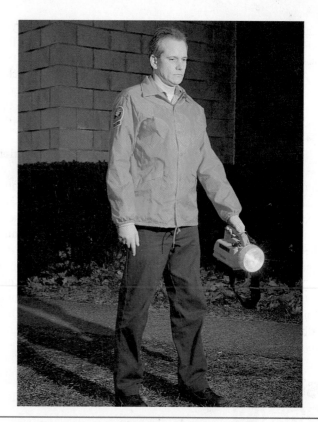

● **Figure 6-3** Hold a flashlight to the side of your body, not in front of it. Armed assailants usually aim at the light.

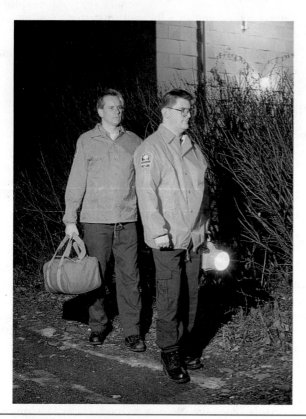

● **Figure 6-2** Approach potentially unstable scenes single file along an unconventional path.

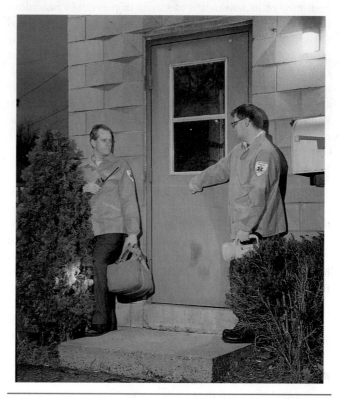

● **Figure 6-4** Stand to the side of the door when knocking. Do not stand directly in front of a door or window, making yourself an unwitting target.

CONTENT REVIEW

▶ Potentially Dangerous
Scenes

• Highway encounters
• Violent street incidents
• Drug-related crimes
• Clandestine drug labs
• Domestic violence

treatment has begun, you must place your own safety first. You now have two tactical options: (1) quickly package the patient and leave the scene with the patient or (2) retreat without the patient.

Your choice of action depends on the level of danger. Abandonment is always a concern. However, in most cases, you can legally leave a patient behind when there is a *documented* danger. As discussed later in the chapter, keep accurate records of incidents involving violence. If you must defend yourself, use the minimum amount of force necessary. Immediately summon police and retreat as needed.

Regardless of the situation, always have a way out. Your failure to plan will undoubtedly lead to an emergency at some point in time. Make sure that SOPs include an escape plan. Then adhere to this plan so you do not become a victim of violence yourself.

SPECIFIC DANGEROUS SCENES

Most prehospital services were developed to meet the needs of individual patients in controlled situations. However, in recent years, EMS personnel trained for this limited role have been pressed increasingly into service in potentially hazardous situations. The result has been the employment of specialized resources with the tactical judgment and skills not normally taught in EMS programs. Your ability to survive a violent street encounter depends on recognition of threats and an understanding of some of the things that can be done to provide for rescuer and patient safety. The following sections describe some of the known dangers that you may face while "on the street." (A discussion of tactical safety strategies appears later in the chapter.)

Highway Encounters

The preceding examples of known dangers have focused largely on residences. However, EMS units frequently report to roadside calls involving motor vehicle collisions, disabled vehicles, or sick and/or unresponsive people inside a car—for example, "man slumped over wheel" calls. Chapters 1 and 4 have already indicated the dangers of highway operations and the steps that you should take to protect yourself. However, highway operations also hold the risk of violence from occupants who may be intoxicated or drugged, fleeing from the police, or in possession of weapons. Some potential warning signs of danger include:

● Violent or abusive behavior

● An altered mental state

● Grabbing or hiding items inside the vehicle

● Arguing or fighting among passengers

● Lack of activity where activity is expected

● Physical signs of alcohol or drug abuse (e.g., liquor bottles, beer cans, or syringes)

● Open or unlatched trunks (a potential hiding spot for people or weapons)

● Differences among stories told by occupants

To make a safe approach to a vehicle at a roadside emergency, follow these steps:

● Park the ambulance in a position that provides safety from traffic.

● Notify dispatch of the situation, location, the vehicle make and model, and the state and number of the license plate.

● Use a one-person approach. The driver should remain in the ambulance, which is elevated and provides greater visibility.

● The driver should remain prepared to radio for immediate help and to back or drive away rapidly once the other medic returns.

● At night, use the ambulance lights to illuminate the vehicle. However, do not walk between the ambulance and the other vehicle. You will be backlighted, forming an easy target.

● Because police approach vehicles from the driver's side, you should approach from the passenger's side—an unexpected route.

● Use the A, B, and C door posts for cover.

● Observe the rear seat. Do not move forward of the C post unless you are sure there are no threats in the rear seat or foot wells.

● Retreat to the ambulance (or another strategic position of cover) at the first sign of danger.

● Make sure you have mapped out your intended retreat and escape with the ambulance driver.

Violent Street Incidents

You can encounter many different types of violence while working on the streets. You see examples on the news all the time. Incidents can range from random acts of violence against individual citizens to organized efforts at domestic or international terrorism. Some of the dangerous street situations that you may face at some point in your EMS career are discussed next.

Murder, Assault, and Robbery

Although the overall crime rate has dropped in recent years, millions of violent acts still occur annually. They take place at residences, at schools, and at commercial establishments. However, according to the U.S. Department of Justice, the most common location for violent crimes is on the streets—often within 5 miles of the victim's home. In order of occurrence, the most frequent crimes include simple assaults, aggravated assaults, rapes and sexual assaults, robberies, and homicides.

In one-quarter of the incidents of violent crime, offenders used or threatened the use of a weapon. Homicides are most commonly committed with handguns, but knives, blunt objects, and other types of guns or weapons may also be used. About one in five violent victimizations involves the use of alcohol.

Although motives vary, the late 1990s and early 2000s saw a rise in **hate crimes**—crimes committed against a person solely on the basis of the individual's actual or perceived race, color, national origin, ethnicity, gender, disability, or sexual orientation. A number of states or communities have passed legislation on the management of hate crimes, including the steps to be taken on scene. Determine whether these laws exist in your area, and establish protocols that your agency should follow. Crew assignments, for example, should be well thought out in advance of the response to a hate crime. You should also know the specific type of information that must be documented for later use by the courts.

In responding to the scene of any violent crime, keep these precautions in mind:

- Dangerous weapons may have been used in the crime.
- Perpetrators may still be on scene or could return to the scene.
- Patients may sometimes exhibit violence toward EMS, particularly if they risk criminal penalties as a result of the original incident.

Dangerous Crowds and Bystanders

As mentioned earlier, you must remain aware of crowd dynamics whenever you respond to a street incident. Crowds can quickly become large and volatile, especially in the case of a hate crime. Violence can be directed against anyone or anything in the path of an angry crowd. Your status as an EMS provider does not give you immunity against an out-of-control mob.

Whenever a crowd is present, look for these warning signs of impending danger:

- Shouts or increasingly loud voices
- Pushing or shoving
- Hostilities toward anyone on scene, including the perpetrator of a crime, the victim, and police
- Rapid increase in the crowd size
- Inability of law enforcement officials to control bystanders

To protect yourself, constantly monitor the crowd and retreat, if necessary. If possible, take the patient with you so you do not have to return later. Rapid transport may require limited or tactical assessment at the scene with more in-depth assessment done inside the safety of the ambulance. Be sure to document reasons for the quick assessment and transport.

Street Gangs

Gangs include groups of people who band together for a variety of reasons: fraternization, self-protection, creation of a surrogate family, or, most frequently, the pursuit of criminal enterprises. Street gangs can be found in big cities, suburban towns, and lately in rural America. No EMS unit is totally immune from gang activity. In fact, some organized gangs have purposely branched out into smaller towns in an effort to escape surveillance and expand their illicit businesses.

Youth gangs account for a disproportionate amount of youth violence across the nation. Gang activity is associated with high levels of delinquency, illegal drug use, physical violence, and possession of weapons. Young people from all demographic backgrounds report some knowledge of gangs or gang activity.

Some of the largest and best-known gangs include the Crips, Bloods, Almighty Latin King Nation (Latin Kings), Hell's Angels, Outlaws, Pagans, and Banditos. Local variations of these and other gangs can be found throughout the country. In some places, gangs have used firebombs, Molotov cocktails, and, on a limited basis, military explosives (hand grenades) as weapons of revenge and intimidation. Links have been drawn between street gangs and the sale of drugs, which in turn finance gang activities.

Commonly observed gang characteristics include the following:

- *Appearance*—Gang members frequently wear unique clothing specific to the group. Because the clothing is often a particular color or hue, it is referred to as the gang's "colors." Wearing a color, even a bandana, can signify gang membership. Within the gang itself, members sometimes wear different articles to signify rank.
- *Graffiti*—Gangs have definite territories, or "turfs." Members often mark their turf with graffiti broadcasting the gang's logo, warning away intruders, bragging about crimes, insulting rival gangs, or taunting police.
- *Tattoos*—Many gang members wear tattoos or other body markings to identify their gang affiliation. Some gangs even require these tattoos. The tattoos will be in the gang's colors and often contain the gang's motto or logo.
- *Hand signals/language*—Gangs commonly create their own methods of communication. They give gang-related meanings to everyday words or create codes. Hand signs provide quick identification among gang members, warn of approaching law enforcement, or show disrespect to other gangs. Gang members often perform signals so quickly that an uninformed outsider may not spot them, much less understand them.

EMS units venturing into gang territory must be extremely cautious because of the potential for violence. Danger is increased if your uniform looks similar to the uniform worn by police. Gangs with a history of arrest may in fact make every effort to prevent you from transporting one of their members to a hospital or any other place beyond the reach of the gang. Do not force the issue if your safety is at stake.

Drug-Related Crimes

The sale of drugs goes hand in hand with violence (Figure 6-5 ●). Hundreds of people die each year in drug deals gone bad. In addition, drug dealers protect their drug stashes and "shooting galleries" with booby traps, weapons, and abused dogs that are likely to attack. The combination of high cash flow, addiction, and automatic weapons threatens anyone who unwittingly walks onto the scene of a drug deal or threatens to uncover an illicit drug operation.

A number of signs can alert you to the involvement of drugs at an EMS call:

- Prior history of drugs in the neighborhood of the call
- Clinical evidence that the patient has used drugs of some kind
- Drug-related comments by bystanders

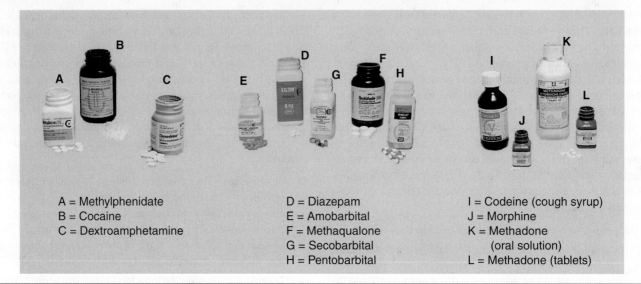

A = Methylphenidate
B = Cocaine
C = Dextroamphetamine

D = Diazepam
E = Amobarbital
F = Methaqualone
G = Secobarbital
H = Pentobarbital

I = Codeine (cough syrup)
J = Morphine
K = Methadone
    (oral solution)
L = Methadone (tablets)

● **Figure 6-5** Substances abused and sold come in all forms. Some of the most commonly prescribed substances sold or used on the streets are shown here. Persons who abuse or deal in drugs may exhibit violent behavior.

- Drug paraphernalia visible at the scene such as the following:
  ○ Tiny zip-top bags or vials
  ○ Sandwich bags with the corners torn off (indicating drug packaging) or untied corners of sandwich bags (indicating drug use)
  ○ Syringes or needles
  ○ Glass tubes, pipes, or homemade devices for smoking drugs
  ○ Chemical odors or residues

Whenever you observe any of the preceding items, assume the use or presence of drugs at the scene. Even if the patient is not involved, others at the scene may still pose a danger. Keep in mind that not all patients who use drugs will be seeking to harm you. Some may, in fact, be looking for help. Evaluate each situation carefully. Above all else, remember to retreat and/or request police backup at the earliest sign of danger.

Clandestine Drug Laboratories

Drug dealers often set up "laboratories" to manufacture controlled substances or to otherwise refine or convert a controlled substance to another more profitable or usable form, such as tablets. One of the most common types of substances manufactured in drug laboratories is methamphetamine, also known by street names such as "crank," "speed," or "crystal." Other drugs include LSD and "crack."

Clandestine drug laboratories, or "clan labs," have three requirements: privacy, utilities, and equipment such as glassware, chemical containers, and heating mantles or burners (Figure 6-6 ●). Most clan labs are uncovered by neighbors who report suspicious odors, deliveries, or activities.

Drug raids on clan labs have a way of turning into hazmat operations. All too often, the labs contain toxic fumes and volatile chemicals. The people on scene complicate matters by fighting or shooting at the rescuers who come to extricate them from the toxic

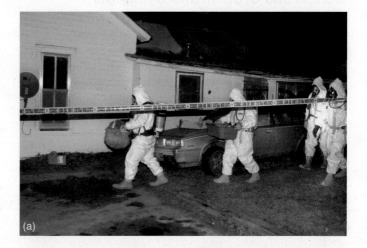

(a)

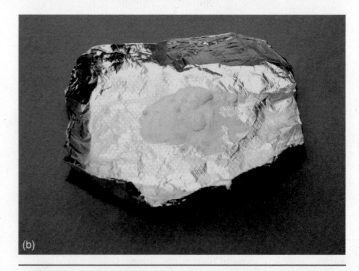

(b)

● **Figure 6-6** (a) Clandestine labs, particular methamphetamine ("meth") labs, pose a risk for rescuers. Many of the solvents and reagents are toxic and highly explosive. (© *Mikael Karlsson/Arresting Images.com*) (b) Powdered meth. (*Photo courtesy of US Drug Enforcement Administration*) environment. As they retreat, drug dealers may also trigger booby traps or wait for police or EMS personnel to trigger them. If you ever come upon a clan lab, take these actions:

- Leave the area immediately.
- Do not touch anything.
- Never stop any chemical reactions already in progress.
- Do not smoke or bring any source of flame near the lab.
- Notify the police.
- Initiate IMS and hazmat procedures.
- Consider evacuation of the area.

Remember that laboratories can be found anywhere—on farms, in trailers, in city apartments, and elsewhere. They may be mobile, roaming from place to place in a camper or truck. Or they may be disassembled and stored in almost any variety of locations. The job of raiding clan labs belongs to specialized personnel—not EMS crews.

Domestic Violence

Domestic violence involves people who live together in an intimate relationship. The violence may be physical, emotional, sexual, verbal, or economic. It may be directed against a spouse or partner, or it may involve children and/or older relatives who live at the residence.

When called to the scene of domestic violence, the abuser may turn on you or other members of the crew. You have two main concerns: your own personal safety and protection of the patient from further harm. For more on the indications of domestic violence and the appropriate actions of EMS crews, see Volume 6, Chapter 6.

TACTICAL CONSIDERATIONS

As mentioned on several occasions, your best tactical response to violence is observation. Know the warning signs and stay out of danger in the first place. If the dispatcher alerts you to hazards, resort to staging until the appropriate authorities can resolve the situation.

Nevertheless, you still may find yourself in situations with a potential for danger—a suspicious call that you must check out, the eruption of violence during treatment, and so on. In such instances, you must have a "game plan" in place. This section presents some of the actions you can take to protect your own safety while attempting to provide tactical patient care.

Safety Tactics

Dangerous situations mean extreme stress. As a result, your response to danger will be most effective if you practice tactical options frequently. Even on routine calls, think about safety, contact and cover, escape routes, and other strategies that can help you make a better decision when you are faced with actual danger. To borrow a phrase from professional sports, "You will play the game the way you practice." If you have rehearsed the responses to danger before you actually need them, you will be more likely to use them successfully. The following sections describe some proven methods for EMS safety in dangerous situations.

Retreat

The prudent strategy is to retreat whenever you spot indicators of violence or potential physical confrontations, particularly with fleeing criminals or people with emotional disturbances (Figure 6-7 ●). Retreat in a calm, but decisive, manner. Be aware that the danger is now at your back and integrate cover into your retreat.

CONTENT REVIEW

▶ Safety Tactics
- Retreat
- Cover and concealment
- Distraction and evasion
- Contact and cover
- Warning signals and communication

Ideally you will retreat to the ambulance so that you can summon help. However, if a dangerous obstacle, such as a crowd, blocks access to your rig, retreat by foot or by whatever means possible. Nothing in the ambulance is worth your life.

In deciding how far to retreat, your primary goal is to protect yourself from any potential danger. You must be out of the immediate line of sight. You must also seek cover from gunfire. Finally, you must allow enough distance to react if a person or crowd attempts to move toward you again. You need time and space to respond to changing situations.

As soon as possible, notify other responding units and agencies of the danger. Activate appropriate codes, SOPs, and/or interagency agreements, particularly with law enforcement departments. Be sure to document your observations of danger and your specific responses. Include information such as the following:

- Actions taken while on scene
- Reasons you retreated
- Time at which you left and/or returned to the scene
- Personnel or agencies contacted

Also keep in mind that retreat does not mean the end of a call. As already mentioned, you should seek to stage at a safe area until police secure the scene and you can respond once again. Staging, along with thorough documentation, will reduce liability and provide evidence to refute charges of abandonment.

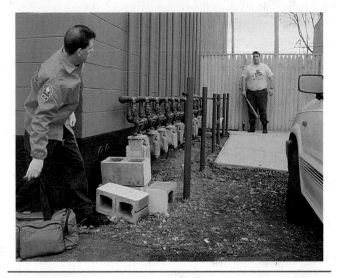

● **Figure 6-7** A patient's stance and position can indicate a potential for violence. If you suspect such a situation, put your own personal safety first. Retreat and request police backup.

Cover and Concealment

When faced with danger, two of your most immediate and practical strategies are cover and concealment (Figures 6-8a ● and 6-8b ●). **Concealment** hides your body, such as when you crouch behind bushes, wallboards, or vehicle doors. However, most common objects do not stop bullets. During armed encounters, seek **cover** by hiding your body behind solid and impenetrable objects such as brick walls, rocks, large trees or telephone poles, and the engine block of vehicles.

For cover and concealment to work, they must be used properly. In applying these safety tactics, keep in mind the following general rules.

● As you approach any scene, remain aware of the surroundings and any potential sources of protection in case you must retreat or are "pinned down."

● Choose your cover carefully. You may have only one chance to pick your protection. Select the item that hides your body adequately, while shielding you against ballistics.

● Once you have made your choice of cover, conceal as much of your body as possible. Be conscious of any reflective

clothing that you may be wearing. Armed assailants can use it as a target, especially at night.

● Constantly look to improve your protection and location.

Distraction and Evasion

Distraction and evasion can be integrated into any retreat. Some specific techniques to avoid physical violence include:

● Throwing equipment to trip, slow, or distract an aggressor

● Wedging a stretcher in a doorway to block an attacker

● Using an unconventional path while retreating

● Anticipating the moves of the aggressor and taking countermoves

● Overturning objects in the path of the attacker

● Using preplanned tactics with your partner to confuse or "throw off" an aggressor

The key to the success of these safety tactics is your own physical well-being. Regular exercise and good health ensure that you will have the strength to outrun or, if necessary, defend yourself against an attacker. Some units provide basic training in self-defense or have protocols on its use. Make sure you take advantage of this training and/or know the protocols related to the application of force.

Contact and Cover

The concept of contact and cover comes from a police procedure developed in San Diego, California, where several officers were injured or killed while interviewing suspects. Studies of the incidents revealed that the officers focused directly on the suspect, reducing their ability to observe the "big picture." This left them exposed to threats of physical violence and/or encounters with edged weapons or firearms.

To solve this problem, the San Diego Police Department adopted an interview approach in which one officer "contacts" the suspect while another officer stands 90 degrees to the side. By standing at a different angle, the second officer can provide "cover" to the officer dealing with the suspect.

When adapted to EMS practice, the procedure assigns the roles shown in Table 6–1. As with any tactic adopted from another discipline, contact and cover has obvious correlations and drawbacks. The tactic is ideal for street encounters with intoxicated

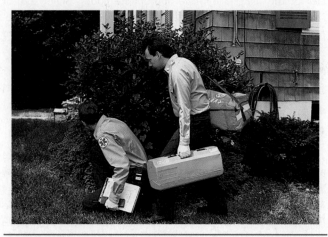

● **Figure 6-8a** Concealing yourself is placing your body behind an object that can hide you from view.

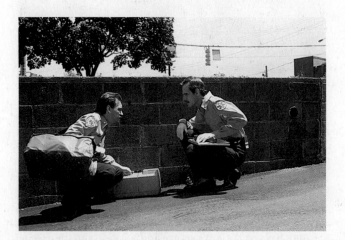

● **Figure 6-8b** Taking cover is finding a position that both hides you and protects your body from projectiles.

TABLE 6–1	Contact and Cover	
Contact Provider	**Cover Provider**
Initiates and provides direct patient care.	Observes the scene for danger while the contact provider cares for the patient.
Performs patient assessment.	Generally avoids patient care duties that would prevent observation of the scene.
Handles most interpersonal scene contact.	In small crews, may perform limited functions such as handling equipment.

persons or subjects acting in a suspicious manner. An obvious drawback is that two medics working on a cardiac arrest will not be able to designate one person to act solely as a "cover" medic.

Perhaps the best application of this police procedure to EMS is its emphasis on the importance of observation and teamwork. A crew that works well together will assign roles—formally or informally—to guarantee safety and patient care. In its most basic form, contact and cover means that you will watch your partner's back while he watches yours.

Warning Signals and Communication

Communication forms a vital part of EMS regardless of the situation. In the case of "street survival," it is an invaluable safety tool. Every team or crew should develop methods of alerting other providers to danger without alerting the aggressor. Devise prearranged verbal and nonverbal clues and then practice them.

Be sure to involve dispatch in the process. Choose signals that will indicate a variety of circumstances while sounding harmless to an attacker. This can be a lifesaving technique in situations where you find yourself, the crew, and/or the patient held hostage. Your so-called "routine" radio reports can spell out the nature of the trouble and summon help from a **special weapons and tactics (SWAT) team,** a trained police unit equipped to handle hostage holders or other difficult law enforcement situations.

Tactical Patient Care

The increased involvement of care providers in violent situations has raised discussion and debate over the tactical training and protection offered to the EMS community. Interagency planning is essential, especially for clarifying the duties and roles of EMS and law enforcement agencies at crime scenes, riots, or terrorist events. Other aspects of tactical patient care include the use of body armor by EMS providers and the training of special tactical EMS personnel.

Body Armor

Several years ago, few EMS providers would have considered wearing **body armor,** or bulletproof vests, while on duty. However, today more and more providers are taking "tactical patient care" seriously. To protect EMS personnel against danger, an increasing number of EMS agencies have chosen to supply body armor or to provide a sum of cash toward its purchase. Body armor manufacturers have responded by designing and marketing vests specifically for the EMS community.

Unlike conventional armor, body armor is soft. A series of fibers such as Kevlar™ are woven tightly together to form the vest. The tight weave and strength of the material offer protection from many handgun bullets, most knives, and blunt trauma. The number of layers of fiber determine the rating or "stopping power" of a vest. Most body armor is rated from level 1 (least protective) to level 3 (most protective). Specialty vests with steel inserts and other materials are available for use by the military or by SWAT teams.

Some critics of body armor claim that wearers may feel a false sense of security. They point out that body armor offers reduced protection when wet. They also note that it provides little or no protection against high-velocity bullets, such as those fired by a rifle, or from thin or dual-edged weapons. An ice pick, for example, can penetrate between the fibers of most vests.

Supporters of body armor feel that it should be viewed just like any other PPE offered to rescuers. They point to the new threats faced by emergency responders, such as paramilitary groups, international terrorists, drug-related violence, and the widespread possession of handguns.

Whether you purchase or wear body armor is a personal decision (Figure 6-9 ●). However, for it to be effective, you must follow several guidelines:

● Keep in mind the limitations of body armor. Never do anything you would not do without it.

● Remember that body armor does not cover the whole body. You can still get seriously injured or killed.

● Even though body armor can prevent many types of penetration, you can still experience severe cavitation.

● For body armor to work, it must be worn. The temptation not to wear it, especially in hot temperatures, can render even the best body armor useless.

Tactical EMS

As already mentioned, the provision of care in violent or tactically "hot" zones, such as sniper situations, often necessitates risks far beyond those found on most EMS calls. Medical personnel assigned to such incidents require special training and

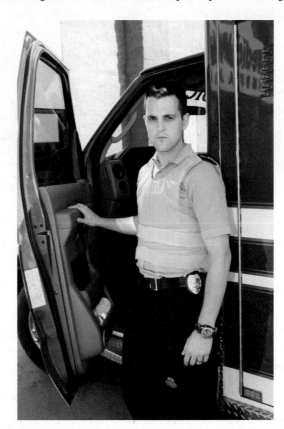

● **Figure 6-9** Body armor has been shown to save lives in the military and police setting. As a result, an increasing number of EMS providers have started wearing body armor (bulletproof vests) while on duty. (© Dr. Bryan E. Bledsoe)

authorization. Like hazmat teams, they must don special equipment, function with compact gear, and, in most cases, work as medical adjuncts to the police or military.

The patient care offered by TEMS differs from routine EMS care in several ways:

- A major priority is extraction of the patient from the hot zone.
- Care may be modified to meet tactical considerations.
- Trauma patients are more frequently encountered than medical patients.
- Treatment and transport interventions must almost always be coordinated with an incident commander.
- Patients must be moved to tactically cold zones for complete assessment, care, and transport.
- Metal clipboards, chemical agents, and other tools may be used as defensive weapons.

Local protocols, standing orders, and issues of medical direction must be resolved before the employment of a TEMS unit. The units may be composed of EMTs, paramedics, and/or physicians who operate as part of a tactical law enforcement team. Certification of SWAT-Medics and **EMT-Tacticals (EMT-Ts)** is offered by several organizations including the **CONTOMS** (Counter-Narcotics Tactical Operations) program and the National Tactical Officers Association (NTOA).

The training required of EMT-Ts or SWAT-Medics involves strenuous physical activity, under a variety of conditions. In a CONTOMS program, medics may be exposed to scenarios or skills such as the following:

- Raids on clandestine drug laboratories
- Emergency medical care in barricade situations
- Wounding effects of weapons and booby traps
- Special medical gear for tactical operations
- Use of CS, CN (mace), capsaicin (pepper spray), CR, or other riot-control agents
- Blank-firing weapons
- Helicopter operations
- Pyrotechnics (smoke and distraction devices)
- Operation under extreme conditions, darkness, and psychological stress
- Firefighting and hazmat operations

In summoning or working with a TEMS unit, follow the same general approaches and procedures as with other units and teams. If you have not had exposure to such a unit, find out more about EMT-Ts or SWAT-Medics from local law enforcement officials or from sites sponsored by CONTOMS or NTOA on the Internet.

EMS AT CRIME SCENES

A crime scene can be defined as a location where any part of a criminal act has occurred and where evidence relating to a crime may be found. The goal of performing EMS at a crime scene is to provide high-quality patient care while preserving

evidence. *Never* jeopardize patient care for the sake of evidence. However, do not perform patient care with disregard of the criminal investigation that will follow.

EMS and Police Operations

Often emergencies arise in which police and EMS personnel respond to the same crisis. Both are there for specific purposes. The EMS crew has arrived on scene to treat patients and save lives. Law enforcement officers have come to protect the public and to solve a crime. These two primary goals sometimes create tension between the two teams. For example, police and paramedics often work under different time constraints. As a paramedic, you have a limited time at the scene. The police, on the other hand, spend much more time at the location of a crime. In some major cases, police can remain at the scene for days or weeks as they methodically look for evidence (Figure 6-10 ●).

The key to cooperation between EMS and law enforcement personnel is communication. You should become aware of the nature and significance of physical evidence at a crime scene and, if possible, keep that evidence intact. Police, on the other hand, should be aware that the first and foremost responsibility of a paramedic is to save the life of the victim. However, police and paramedics can usually reach a common ground. By preserving evidence, you can help the police to lock up a criminal before the person hurts, injures, or kills someone else. Remember: EMS personnel and law enforcement are really on the same side. Talk to each other.

Preserving Evidence

To prevent future violent injuries, be aware that anything on and around the patient may be evidence. You never know when a seemingly unimportant item may, in fact, be crucial evidence that could help solve a crime. Whenever in doubt, save or treat an object as evidence.

If you are the first person at the scene of a crime, be aware that anything you touch, walk on, pick up, cut, wipe off, or move could be evidence. Developing an awareness of evidence will

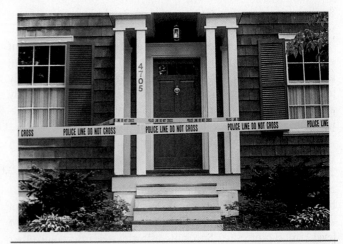

● **Figure 6-10** Police can remain at the scene of a crime for days, methodically searching for evidence. An EMS crew has a limited time at the scene. During that time, they must protect themselves, treat the patient, *and* preserve potential evidence, if at all possible.

Preserving Evidence at a Crime Scene

Modern science has made solving crimes easier. The advent of forensic science and DNA technology has greatly increased the ability of authorities to link a person to a crime scene.

EMS personnel are often the first to arrive at the scene of a crime—sometimes ahead of law enforcement personnel. Although the paramedic's primary responsibilities are scene safety and care of the patient, it is important to be cognizant of crime scene evidence and make every effort to avoid contaminating or disturbing it. For example, when cutting away the clothing of a gunshot or stabbing victim, take care not to cut through the gunshot or stab entrance wound. Furthermore, never handle any weapons found at the scene. If you arrive at a scene and find your victim dead, your responsibility should turn to protecting the scene and any evidence until law enforcement personnel arrive and release you from the scene.

It is important for EMS and law enforcement personnel to work together. Although our jobs are different, we share a common dedication to justice, and protection of crime scene evidence is just one way to accomplish this.

even affect the way you treat patients. You will need to observe the patient carefully and to disturb as little direct evidence as possible. For example, if clothing must be removed, never cut through a gunshot or knife wound. Instead, try to cut as far away from the wound as possible. Instead of placing the cut cloth or garment in a plastic bag, put it in a brown paper bag so condensation does not build up and destroy body fluid evidence.

In addition, when examining a patient, remember that you may be at risk. The victim may have a concealed weapon, such as a knife or gun. Or the person who committed the crime may be intent on finishing it and reappear to attack the patient. As a result, your first responsibility is to protect yourself. If you have any suspicions at all about the patient or the safety of the scene, wait for the police to frisk the patient and/or secure the scene.

Types of Evidence

Gathering evidence is a specialized and time-consuming job. Although it is unrealistic to train EMS personnel in the details of police work, it is not unrealistic to ask them to develop an awareness of the general types of evidence that they may expect to encounter at a crime scene. Some of the main categories of evidence are prints, blood and body fluids, particulate evidence, and your own observations at the scene.

Prints Prints include fingerprints, footprints, and tire prints. Of the three, fingerprints can be the most valuable source of evidence. No two people have identical fingerprints—the distinctive patterns left on a surface by the natural oils and moisture that form on a person's fingertips. The patterns can be compared with the millions of fingerprints already on file or compared to the fingerprints of a suspect charged with the crime.

As a paramedic, you have two concerns when it comes to fingerprints. First, try not to disturb any fingerprint evidence that

may be present. Second, do not leave behind your own fingerprints at a crime scene.

The only way to preserve fingerprints is simply not to touch anything. Of course, this is impossible when treating a patient. However, you can and should minimize what you touch. If you must touch or move an item, remember to tell the police that you did so.

Because of Standard Precautions, you will be wearing disposable gloves as a part of infection control. These gloves prevent you from leaving your own fingerprints—but they will not prevent you from smudging existing prints. Again, touch as little as possible. In addition, bring in only the necessary equipment. The more equipment you have, the more evidence you can potentially disturb, including fingerprints.

Scan the approach to the scene and the scene itself for footprints or tire prints. These prints have value because they give the police an idea of what a perpetrator was wearing (e.g., sneakers vs. work boots) or the type of tread on a vehicle's tires. These patterns may be later matched to the footwear or vehicle used by an alleged perpetrator.

Blood and Body Fluids Blood and body fluids also give police a lot of information about a crime. For example, if the victim scratched or injured the perpetrator, blood samples might be found under the fingernails, on clothing, on hands, or elsewhere. By ABO blood typing these samples, the field of suspects can be narrowed down.

Identification of DNA (deoxyribonucleic acid) has been called "genetic fingerprinting." Matching the DNA found in blood samples or other body fluids to the DNA of a suspect is nearly 100 percent accurate. There is only one chance in several million that the DNA could be from someone else. The high cost of DNA testing prevents its widespread use. However, when performed, medical technologists need only a small sample to ascertain the genetic code of the person from which it came.

The way in which blood is splattered or dropped at the scene provides yet other clues for police. This so-called **blood spatter evidence** can indicate the type of weapon used, the position of the attacker in relation to the victim, and the direction or force used in the attack.

Preserving blood evidence can be performed in the following ways:

- Avoid mixing samples of blood whenever possible. Cross-contamination of blood will render blood evidence useless.

- Avoid tracking blood on your shoes. You will leave your own footprints, plus you risk contaminating other blood evidence.

- If you must cut bloody clothing from a victim, place each piece in a separate brown paper bag. If the garment is wet, gently roll it in the paper bag to layer it. Place the entire contents in a second paper bag and then in a plastic bag for body fluid protection.

CONTENT REVIEW

► Types of Evidence

- Prints—fingerprints, footprints, tire prints
- Blood and blood spatter
- Body fluids
- Particulate evidence
- On-scene EMS observations

- Do not throw clothes stained with blood or other body fluids in a single pile or in a puddle of blood.

- Do not clean up or smudge blood spatter left at a scene.

- If you leave behind blood from a venipuncture, notify police.

- Because blood can be a biohazard, ask police whether the scene should be secured for evidence collection.

Particulate Evidence   Particulate evidence, also known as *microscopic* or *trace evidence*, refers to evidence that cannot be readily seen by the human eye, such as hairs or carpet and clothing fibers. Particulate evidence can help identify the actual crime scene, such as in cases where a body has been moved, or the DNA of the perpetrator. Minimal handling of a victim's clothes by EMS personnel may help to preserve this evidence.

On-Scene Observations   Everything that you and other members of the EMS crew see and hear can serve as evidence. Your observations of the scene will become part of the police record—and ultimately part of the court record. Be sure to look for and record the following information:

- Conditions at the scene (e.g., absence or presence of lights, locked or unlocked doors, open or closed curtains)

- Position of the patient/victim

- Injuries suffered by the patient/victim

- Statements of persons at the scene

- Statements by the patient/victim

- Dying declarations

- Suspicious persons at, or fleeing from, the scene
- Presence and/or location of any weapons

If the victim is deceased by the time you arrive, any staff not immediately needed on the scene should leave to minimize the risk of disturbing evidence. If a gun is seen or found on the deceased victim, do not touch or move it unless it must be secured for the safety of others. Pick it up only as a last resort, and touch it only by the side grips or handles. The grips are coarse and will not generally leave good fingerprints. *Never* put anything into the barrel of the gun to lift or move it. The barrel of a gun can house the majority of the evidence used by the police: traces of gunpowder, rifling patterns, and even flesh or blood from the victim.

Documenting Evidence

Record only the facts at the scene of a crime, and record them accurately. Otherwise, they might be thrown out of court as evidence. Use quotation marks to indicate the words of bystanders and any remarks made by the patient. Avoid opinions not relevant to patient care. If the patient has died, do not offer any judgments that might contradict later findings by the medical examiner. For example, a knife wound is not a knife wound until it is proven that a knife caused the laceration. Instead, describe the shape and anatomic location of the puncture or cut.

Also keep in mind the protocols, local laws, and ethical considerations in reporting certain crimes such as child abuse, rape, geriatric abuse, and domestic violence. (For more on reporting abuse and assault, see Volume 6, Chapter 6.) Finally, follow local policies and regulations regarding confidentiality surrounding any criminal case. Any offhand remarks that you make might later become testimony in a courtroom along with other documents that you prepare at the scene.

 SUMMARY

Your first priority at any crime scene is your own safety. To protect your life and the lives of others, you need to develop a "crime scene awareness." Whenever you survey the scene of any call, keep in mind some of the telltale signs of potential violence such as a suspiciously darkened house, or a lack of activity. Do not needlessly expose yourself to dangers better left to professional emergency medical personnel such as SWAT-Medics or EMT-Ts. When you do treat the victim(s) at a crime scene, keep in mind that police and EMS personnel must work together to preserve the evidence that may lead to conviction of the perpetrator. Touch only those items or objects that pertain directly to patient care.

 YOU MAKE THE CALL

Your ambulance receives a call about a 65-year-old man with chest pain. You arrive at the scene and scan for dangers. Detecting no visible hazards, you enter the patient's home and begin assessment. The patient describes the pain as crushing and points to the center of his chest. You observe labored breathing and begin care. You direct your partner to administer oxygen, while you look for a peripheral IV site.

While treatment progresses, the patient's son bursts through the door. He appears intoxicated and is obviously agitated at the presence of an ambulance. The patient whispers, "My son isn't quite right when he's drinking. You better be careful."

While you introduce yourself to the son, your partner slips away to radio the police. The dispatcher advises her that it could be a few minutes before the police can arrive on scene. Meanwhile, you tell the son why it is important that you start an IV. The son yells, "You're no doctor. Get away from my father. He needs to get to a hospital, not stay here in the living room. Get out of here before I throw you out."

1. What is your evaluation of this situation from a safety perspective?

2. What are your options?

See Suggested Responses at the back of this book.

REVIEW QUESTIONS

1. The most common place where violent crime takes place is in _____.
   a. a bar
   c. the street
   b. the home
   d. a school

2. Crimes committed against a person solely on the basis of the individual's actual or perceived race, color, national origin, ethnicity, gender, disability, or sexual orientation are termed _____ crimes.
   a. bias
   c. personal
   b. hate
   d. prejudice

3. Which of the following are warning signs of impending danger whenever a crowd is present?
   a. pushing or shoving
   b. rapid increase in crowd size
   c. inability of law enforcement officials to control bystanders
   d. all of the above

4. The contact-and-cover tactic is ideal to use to _____.
   a. escape from imminent danger
   b. interview a victim on the street
   c. signal incoming departments of potential danger
   d. retreat and then return to the scene at a later time

5. A trained police unit equipped to handle hostage holders or other difficult law enforcement situations describes a _____ team.
   a. TEMS
   c. SWAT
   b. EMT-T
   d. HAZMAT

6. How should you hold your flashlight when approaching a dark house at a potential crime scene?
   a. behind you
   c. to your side
   b. over your head
   d. in front of you

7. At a crime scene, you should preserve evidence containing body fluids by placing it in a(n) _____.
   a. sterile container
   b. sealed plastic bag
   c. brown paper bag
   d. airtight container

8. Which of the following is an appropriate way for the paramedic to avoid crime scene evidence contaminations?
   a. clean up blood spatter
   b. wear gloves while on scene
   c. place small articles of clothing in a plastic bag
   d. fold blood-stained clothes and place them in a single pile

See Answers to Review Questions at the back of this book.

REFERENCES

1. Centers for Disease Control and Prevention. Violence Prevention. [Available at http://www.cdc.gov/violenceprevention/]

2. Tang, N. and G. D. Kelen. "Role of Tactical EMS in Support of Public Safety and the Public Health Response to a Hostile Mass Casualty Event." *Disaster Med Public Health Prep* 1(1Suppl) (2007): S55–S56.

3. Rinnert, K. J. and W. L. Hall, 2nd. "Tactical Emergency Medical Support." *Emerg Med Clin North Am* 20 (2002): 929–952.

FURTHER READING

DeLorenzo, R. A. and R. S. Porter. *Weapons of Mass Destruction: Emergency Care.* Upper Saddle River, NJ: Pearson/Prentice Hall, 2000.

Eliopilos, L. N. *Death Investigator's Handbook: A Field Guide to Crime Scene Processing, Forensic Evaluation, and Investigation Techniques.* Expanded and updated edition. Boulder, CO: Paladin Press, 2003.

Schwartz, R. D., J. G. McManus, and R. E. Swienton. *Tactical Emergency Medicine.* Philadelphia: Lippincott Williams and Wilkins, 2007.

7

Rural EMS

Bryan Bledsoe, DO, FACEP, FAAEM, EMT-P
Deborah J. McCoy-Freeman, BS, RN, NREMT-P

STANDARDS

Assessment (Scene Size-Up); EMS Operations (Air Medical)

COMPETENCY

Integrates scene and patient assessment findings with knowledge of epidemiology and pathophysiology to form a field impression. This includes developing a list of differential diagnoses through clinical reasoning to modify the assessment and formulate a treatment plan.

Applies knowledge of operational roles and responsibilities to ensure patient, public, and personnel safety.

OBJECTIVES

Terminal Performance Objective

After reading this chapter, you should be able to effectively perform the expected functions of EMS personnel in a rural setting.

Enabling Objectives

To accomplish the terminal performance objective, you should be able to:

1. Define key terms introduced in this chapter.

2. Describe the demographics, health status, and health access issues of rural populations.

3. Describe the special problems faced by rural EMS systems.

4. Suggest solutions to solving special problems faced by rural EMS systems.

5. Given a variety of scenarios, integrate the special challenges and considerations of rural EMS into patient care decision making.

6. Recognize the particular hazards and considerations involved in agricultural emergencies.

7. Anticipate injuries associated with various recreational activities.

KEY TERMS

air bags, p. 133
compartment syndrome, p. 133
cribbing, p. 133
crush points, p. 136
lock-out/tag-out, p. 133
pinch points, p. 134
prompt care facilities, p. 131
rust out, p. 129
shear points, p. 134
silo gas, p. 133
wrap points, p. 134

It's a warm sunny afternoon in July when a call comes in to your paramedic unit for "a man down in a farmyard." The communications officer has dispatched the local volunteer basic life support (BLS) squad. However, because the call involves an unresponsive patient, the dispatcher has also requested backup from the nearest paramedic unit. Your unit, which is stationed more than 29 miles away, receives the call.

It takes the local volunteer squad 5 minutes to assemble and get an ambulance en route to the farm, which lies at the edge of the squad's district. Your unit—a full-time paid agency—is off the floor in less than 1 minute. Because both units must travel quite a distance, they race against the clock to reach the scene safely.

The BLS squad arrives at the farm just a few minutes ahead of your unit. Crew members meet the patient's wife at the door of the house. She says, "Please hurry. Follow me. I'll show you where my husband is." The squad leader informs the wife that crew members will proceed as soon as they ensure that the scene is safe. By this time, the man's wife is frantic. She yells, "You've got to help my husband right now!"

At this point, your unit arrives on the scene and you assist the squad leader in calmly obtaining information. As the woman gestures toward a silo, you notice a man lying at its base. About a foot away from the patient, you see a ladder propped up against the silo. A rope runs up the ladder to the top of the silo.

When the squad leader asks the woman what may have happened, she says, "My husband was going to clean the silo today. Everything seemed OK, until I heard him yelling. When I looked out the window, my husband was having trouble climbing down the ladder. As he got near the ground, he seemed to keel over and fall."

The squad leader then finds out whether the woman's husband was using any hazardous materials and whether she has had any ill effects from being near the silo. She responds "no" to both questions. You and the squad leader agree that the scene is probably safe and relay this information to the dispatch center.

As you move toward the base of the silo, you note no apparent trauma to the victim. You ask the woman, "How far do you think your husband fell?" The patient's wife now says that he did not actually fall to the ground, but slumped forward to his current face-down position. Her comment corroborates your initial observation.

Because the patient is unresponsive, you assume control of the situation. You and your partner carefully log-roll the patient to assess the airway. You note that the man is breathing, but his respirations are less than 8 per minute. He is diaphoretic, ashen, and unconscious. His pulse is slow and weak.

The downtime is now 40 minutes. Because the patient must be ventilated, your partner assists breathing with a bag-valve-mask (BVM) unit. Meanwhile, you place a monitor on the patient and note a bradycardia. You establish an IV, using aseptic techniques, while your partner obtains vitals. She reports blood pressure 60 by palpation and a pulse of 40 bpm.

The patient is now receiving ventilations at 14 bpm, using capnography as a guide. You order the airway secured with a number 8.0-mm ET tube. Using a landline, you report the situation to medical direction. The medical director orders 0.5 mg of atropine IV push (IVP). Because this is a rural setting, you realize that the ambulance may experience communication blackouts. As a result, you must anticipate any problems that may arise en route to the hospital. In case the atropine does not help, you request orders for transcutaneous pacing (TCP) and/or additional doses of atropine according to advanced cardiac life support (ACLS) protocols.

After receiving approval from medical direction, you administer the prescribed atropine and load the patient into the ambulance. The total time of treatment prior to transport is 11 minutes. En route, you apply the TCP and achieve mechanical capture at 60 milliamperes (ma) on the rate of 70 bpm. The patient responds well to the treatment and is taken to a local hospital 33 miles away. At the hospital, he receives a temporary pacemaker. The patient is then transferred to the regional cardiac center for an internal pacemaker. The actions of the BLS and paramedic crews in this rural emergency have made the difference between life and death.

INTRODUCTION

Recent census data indicate that more than 53 million people in the United States live in rural areas. In fact, some states have rural populations of nearly 50 percent or more. In the West, states with large rural populations include Alaska, Montana, North Dakota, and South Dakota. In the South, they include Arkansas, Kentucky, Mississippi, North Carolina, South Carolina, and West Virginia. In the Northeast, they include Maine, New Hampshire, and Vermont.

People choose to live in rural areas for a variety of reasons. Their families have always lived there. They work at occupations such as farming, ranching, or mining. They like the solitude, open space, or recreational activities found in rural areas. Regardless of the reason, most rural dwellers face a similar problem: lack of easy access to the health care facilities found in most urban and suburban areas.

In the rural setting, resources such as full-service hospitals, fire departments, and EMS units are often as thinly distributed as the population. Specialty teams may be nonexistent. One of the challenges for rural EMS providers is to ensure that their patients receive the same high-quality care as people living elsewhere in the nation.[1] The following sections outline some of the obstacles and decisions typically faced by rural EMS providers.

PRACTICING RURAL EMS

In general, the U.S. government defines rural areas in terms of their sparse populations and distances from cities, towns, or villages. In relation to health care, rural areas can also be characterized by their higher percentage of people over age 65 and their lower physician-to-patient ratios.[2] Whereas one in five people in the United States lives in rural settings, only about one in ten doctors chooses to practice in these locations.

It has been found that rural residents experience a disproportionate number of serious injuries and chronic health conditions. Because of the greater distances to health care facilities, rural residents suffer a higher level of mortality associated with trauma and medical emergencies. In many cases, an EMS unit may provide the definitive care. In meeting the challenge of practicing rural EMS, paramedics and other health care personnel need to be aware of the special problems facing them.

Special Problems

As already indicated in this text, the cost of medical care and the rise of health maintenance organizations have expanded the roles and responsibilities of EMS personnel in the 21st century. The need for nonemergent transports, especially in rural areas, has increased. The shortage of specialized doctors and well-equipped hospitals in rural areas has become an even more critical problem. In the years ahead, a growing number of patients may have to be transported to urban areas to receive the care unavailable to them in rural facilities.

PATHO PEARLS

Quality Considerations in Rural EMS

It has been said that the farther a person is from a hospital, the more sophisticated the prehospital care should be. This is an ideal situation in an ideal world—yet rarely true. Many rural EMS providers routinely make emergent patient transports of an hour or longer. In some parts of this great land, especially in the frontier regions, air medical transport is not even available, thus forcing paramedics to transport critically ill or injured patients for hours before they reach any level of health care facility. The paradox is this: Although the level of prehospital care in rural areas should be high, the less frequent call volumes prevent this from occurring. Furthermore, it is much more difficult to get the required education in a rural setting, and skills decay is a particular problem. However, through outreach programs and skills retention programs, these problems can be overcome.

Rural paramedics must have and develop skills that will allow them to care for patients for a prolonged period of time: These skills include definitive airway management, fluid replacement therapy (possibly with hemoglobin-based oxygen-carrying solutions), selected fracture and dislocation reduction, and other aspects of prolonged patient care. Nasogastric tube and Foley catheter placements are often helpful during prolonged patient transports. Likewise, the ability to provide adequate analgesia, second-line antidysrhythmic agents, and, in certain cases, fibrinolytic therapy can often mean the difference between life and death.

Rural EMS has been neglected for a long time. Now, through several initiatives, attention has once again turned to rural EMS and the plight of the rural EMT and paramedic and their patients.

In the case of natural disasters, such as tornadoes, floods, or hurricanes, the situation is equally serious. In such instances, EMS personnel may be the *only* available medical support until state or federal agencies can be transported into the area.

Regardless of the circumstances surrounding a call, rural EMS crews face a number of obstacles and challenges not found in most urban areas. If you currently work for a rural EMS unit, you may already be aware of some of these situations from first-hand experience. As a paramedic, you will assume an expanded leadership role in directing other EMS personnel on how best to handle or overcome the following special problems.

Distance and Time

Rural EMS often relies on volunteer services. In responding to calls, volunteers must first travel varying distances to a squad building. Once aboard the ambulance, they then travel the distance to the patient and later the distance to the hospital. As a result, every decision that a paramedic makes in a rural setting needs to be made with the thought of distance in mind. (The "distance factor," one of the most critical aspects of rural EMS, will be discussed in more detail later in this chapter.)

Communication Difficulties

In rural areas, poor or old communication equipment often hampers public access to EMS. A rural area, for example, may not have universal access to 911 (Figure 7-1 ●). Lack of 911 service will delay response time or, in many cases, lead people to turn telephone operators into dispatchers.

Rural EMS crews can also be hampered by inadequate communications. Antiquated "fire phones" or "crash bars" might notify them of an emergency call, but crew members may have no way of communicating with each other en route to the service vehicle. Crews may also lack information from dispatch until they arrive at the squad building or are onboard the ambulance.

While traveling on the ambulance, rural EMS providers may experience dead spots where they cannot transmit

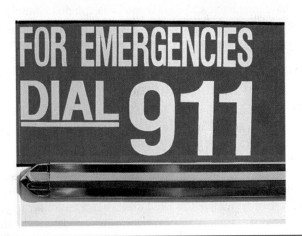

● **Figure 7-1** A universal access number, such as 911, is essential for rapid public access to the EMS system. However, many rural areas lack such a number, hampering communications and increasing response times.

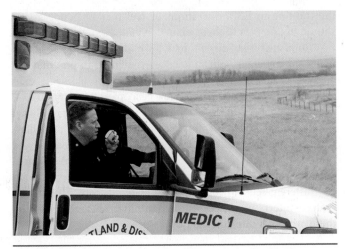

● **Figure 7-2** A rural paramedic must anticipate radio dead spots and request orders to treat any possible medical conditions that may arise during transport. (© *Kevin Link*)

(Figure 7-2 ●). Frequencies can also be overloaded with static from highway departments and school buses. This impairs a paramedic's ability to communicate with other ambulance crews or with medical direction. As a result, rural paramedics must often think ahead, asking for orders in anticipation of medical conditions that might develop while traveling within a dead spot.

Enrollment Shortages

Because many rural EMS providers work on a volunteer basis, units or squads can experience enrollment shortages. Volunteers must respond to calls from their jobs or homes. The greater distances and time involved in many rural EMS calls can take volunteers from their work or families for lengthy periods. This situation can affect their ability to earn a living or to raise their children. As a result, they often serve for only short stretches or resign entirely.[3]

Training and Practice

Access to training and continuing education is not readily available in many rural areas. In addition, the cost and amount of time required for certification as a paramedic has increased. For the volunteer, this means increased personal expense and time away from home. The net effect can be EMS providers with a less advanced level of training than their paid urban counterparts.

This situation can be further complicated by the low volume of EMS calls in some rural areas. EMS providers simply do not have the opportunity to practice their skills on a consistent basis. Members of rescue squads may experience what has become known as **rust out**, or an inability to keep abreast of new technologies and standards. The networking opportunities or volume of calls simply do not exist.[4]

Inadequate Medical Support

As might be expected, rural areas sometimes have difficulty obtaining EMS medical direction. Local physicians may lack the training in EMS operations or feel that EMS operations should not be part of their job.

Rural areas also may not have the budgets to buy new equipment and ambulances. In addition, air medical transport may not always be readily available because of many factors such as distance, lack of landing areas, cost, or too few helicopters for a large area.

Finally, hospitals and rural EMS agencies may not always implement protocols or standards for prehospital providers. Roles may not be clearly defined, or hospitals may have varying protocols. A rural paramedic faced with the decision to transport a patient to two different hospitals may have to deal with two different sets of protocols for prehospital care. That means that volunteers must seek out and familiarize themselves with these protocols often on their own.

Creative Problem Solving

To overcome the obstacles involved in the practice of rural EMS, agencies have turned to creative problem solving. The following sections outline some of the possible solutions available to rural EMS providers.

Improved Communications

In recent years, some rural counties have been fortunate enough to receive grants to modernize or supplement their communications equipment. In other areas, rural counties have joined together to share in the cost of implementing 911 systems. As 911 systems enter rural areas, dispatchers gain valuable education in medical priority dispatch and medical-assist dispatch. Dispatchers with specialized training can provide lifesaving instructions while rural crews are en route to emergencies.

Radio dead spots and crowded frequencies can be handled by requesting additional frequencies and/or by upgrading radio equipment. One possible solution is more powerful base station radios and towers. A group effort in the form of a 911 user advisory board or consortium of agencies can help reduce or eliminate the problem of radio traffic overcrowding. Such advisory boards or consortiums can also provide a forum for discussion of common communication concerns and other issues.

A technological innovation that promises to improve communications in rural areas is the cell phone. Through the use of cell phones, rural paramedics can communicate with emergency department physicians or their medical directors. Another innovation currently under consideration is the designation of cells for EMS use only.

Recruitment and Certification

One of the most important ways being used to improve rural EMS centers is the effort to increase the number of trained paramedics in rural areas. Recognizing the problem of distance, units with paramedics onboard can intercept basic life support (BLS) crews that require advanced life support measures for their patients. Paramedic units can thus help ensure the highest level of service in rural counties.

The issues of recruitment and certification of paramedics in rural areas can be addressed through flexible training sessions and ongoing education. Agencies can pool their resources with neighboring squads to offer education to all their members.

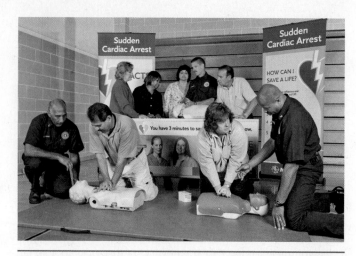

● **Figure 7-3** Public education is a critical part of fulfilling enrollment shortages in rural areas. As a paramedic, you should involve yourself in the training of techniques used by first responders such as CPR.

To increase interest in volunteer EMS, rural agencies can utilize "explorer" and "ride-along" programs, when appropriate. Paramedics can serve as "recruiters" by taking the lead in training rural residents as CPR drivers or first responders (Figure 7-3 ●). The goal is to involve them in ambulance service or quick response units as soon as possible. Once part of the EMS system, these volunteers can be encouraged to advance to the EMT and paramedic levels of training.

Some of the most important training advancements for rural areas have come through the use of computers and the Internet. Using the Internet, of course, means accessing valid sources of information. However, once these sources are identified, EMS personnel can use "distance learning" to develop an awareness of new standards and procedures. The Internet also provides rural squads with a cost-effective way to interface with other agencies. Networking over the Internet can be an excellent way to promote creative problem solving or to share new ideas.

Even without benefit of the Internet, agencies or units can purchase interactive CD-ROMs and EMS computer simulation programs. These programs allow crew members to maintain a high level of knowledge and skills. They also help EMT-Basics or EMT-Intermediates to train as paramedics (Figure 7-4 ●).[5]

Improved Medical Support

The National Association of EMS Physicians provides numerous educational opportunities for physicians interested in learning more about the supervision and oversight of EMS operations. Conferences held by this organization offer courses in EMS medical direction. Although many doctors choose to practice in urban areas, some highly trained physicians live in rural areas. If you live in a rural area, you or an officer in your agency might approach such physicians and determine their willingness to serve as an emergency medical director. If it is impossible to find a medical director among local physicians, you may need to search at the nearest urban hospital.

Regardless of where a paramedic lives, positive relationships with a hospital depend on good communications. A medic should spend time at the hospitals that serve his district and,

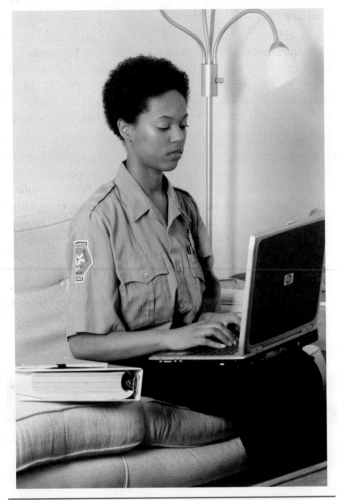

● **Figure 7-4** As a rural paramedic, your education should never end. You can overcome lack of access to classroom instruction through use of the Internet or computerized programs and simulations. You have a responsibility to provide patients with the same high-level care as your urban counterparts.

when possible, request to sit in on relevant in-service training sessions provided for the hospital staff.

Ingenuity and Increased Responsibilities

Rural EMS requires ingenuity. For most rural agencies, it is a constant struggle to retain members, supplement budgets, update equipment, provide quality education programs, and network with other health care facilities. As a rural paramedic, you will be involved in most, if not all, of these aspects of rural EMS.

As a rural paramedic, you can expect your role to grow as counties attempt to fill the "health care gap" between rural and urban areas. You may find yourself involved in hospital outreach programs such as **prompt care facilities**, or agencies that provide limited care and nonemergent medical treatment. In such cases, you may work under the direction of a physician or a physician's assistant (PA) and administer immunizations, handle wound care, and provide emergent transport as necessary.

Governments in some rural areas are also considering the involvement of paramedics in the public health system when not responding to emergency calls. Whatever the future may hold,

you will be challenged as a rural paramedic to raise the standard of prehospital care offered to the rural residents who make up nearly one-quarter of the nation's population.

TYPICAL RURAL EMS SITUATIONS AND DECISIONS

Rural paramedics must be highly skilled and highly practiced to compensate for the extended run times and more complicated logistics found in many rural settings. The following sections discuss some of the unique factors a rural paramedic must consider. The scenarios that appear at the end of each section challenge you to consider some of the complex decisions faced by paramedics working in rural areas. In reviewing this material keep in mind one key point: Increased time and distance mean an increased chance of shock.

The Distance Factor

In rural settings, it is often necessary to travel great distances. As a result, you may spend far more time with the patient on board the ambulance than at the scene itself. With this in mind, actions taken by a rural paramedic during transport can have a definitive impact on the patient's outcome. During transport, for example, you could treat a CHF patient with nitrates, CPAP, and an ACE inhibitor. By the time you reach the hospital, the patient may be completely out of crisis. For this reason, you must keep accurate and complete documentation during any lengthy transport.

Another factor to consider during transport is the availability of emergency staff at the local hospital. In most urban areas, hospitals stay active all night. They have full-time emergency departments with around-the-clock staffing able to handle complicated procedures 24 hours a day, 7 days a week. Some rural hospitals, however, may only have a part-time emergency department with only one or two doctors on staff. In such cases, you may have to call the hospital from the patient's home to arrange for the necessary personnel to be in the building when you arrive. You may also have to make a judgment call on whether or not to transport a critically injured patient to a more distant full-time trauma center. In the case of cardiac problems, the availability of fibrinolytic therapy or PCI might be the deciding factor.

In rural EMS, every decision depends on the situation. Because paramedics live in a world of advanced cardiac life support and trauma life support, you may have access to advanced equipment that is unavailable at your local hospital. A rural hospital under budget constraints, for example, may be unable to purchase equipment such as 12-lead ECG monitors and similar technology. In such instances, you might decide with approval of medical direction to use your equipment at the local hospital or to transport the patient to a definitive treatment center at a more distant location.

In treating seriously ill or injured patients, keep in mind that you may see all phases of a patient's death before reaching a distant medical facility. Consider a motor vehicle collision patient with a serious head trauma. At first, your patient may be alert, conscious, and oriented. The patient then becomes agitated and aggressive. He may begin to have memory lapses and become more confused. You notice dilated pupils. If the transport is long enough, the patient will go into a decorticate posture, then a decerebrate posture. You face this situation knowing that there is little or nothing you can do to change the patient outcome because of the unavoidable transport time.

Given scenarios such as the one just described, rural paramedics must know when and how to use air transport. (For more on air transport, see Chapter 2.)

To assess the effect of distance on the decisions made in many rural emergencies, consider Rural Scenario 1 and the questions that appear at the end of it.

Agricultural Emergencies

Agriculture provides one of the major sources of income in the rural setting. Emergencies related to farming or ranching can range from equipment-related injuries to pesticide poisoning to any number of medical problems exacerbated by agricultural labor.[6] When faced with an agricultural emergency, keep in mind the considerations discussed in the following sections.

Safety

As in any emergency situation, you must place crew safety first. Interpret the situation described by the dispatcher and think of all the scenarios that could be connected with this situation. In agricultural emergencies, many possibilities for injury exist. Potential dangers include livestock, chemicals, fuel tanks, fumes in storage bins and silos, and heavy or outdated farm equipment.

Farm Machinery   If you live in an agricultural area, you must familiarize yourself with the range of equipment used on farms or ranches (Figures 7-5a to 7-5c). Farm equipment can be very different from a car, in which a simple turn of the key shuts off the vehicle.

To prevent on-scene injuries, you need to make sure that farm equipment is both stable and locked down. Keep in mind that many types of farm equipment have fuel line shut-offs or power-kill switches. For this reason, it is important that you place personnel familiar with the equipment in charge of shutting off and locking down all machinery. Keep in mind this safety

RURAL SCENARIO 1

You are a rural volunteer paramedic. It's a foggy night, and you are en route to conduct training at an outlying quick response unit (QRU). On your radio, you hear dispatch sending this same QRU to a car-versus-train collision 10 miles ahead of you.

In approximately 10 minutes, you arrive at a very foggy scene with many flashing lights. You determine that the QRU and its fire department have already arrived. You also see a vehicle in the ditch near a railroad crossing. The first responder unit recognizes you as a paramedic and asks for your assistance. Crew members direct you to a 35-year-old man trapped behind the wheel of his vehicle.

On assessment, you find the patient alert and oriented but very anxious. Your physical exam shows blunt chest trauma, decreased breath sounds on the left, a rigid painful abdomen, and several lacerations and abrasions on the head and arms. You record the following vital signs: HR 160; RR 32 and shallow; BP 90/60.

Fire department personnel inform you that it will take approximately 20 minutes to extricate the patient. A volunteer BLS ambulance will be on scene in 15 minutes. The closest hospital is a 20-bed, Level IV trauma facility located 30 miles east. The nearest Level II trauma center, with an advanced life support (ALS) ambulance service, is 75 miles east and south of the scene.

1. On arrival on scene, you notice that the first responders with the QRU were not attempting to stabilize the cervical spine. They also were not using recommended Standard Precautions. How and when would you correct this situation?

   (After taking control of the scene, you correct any deficiencies that you might note right away. You would tell

the first responders to stabilize the head and neck using manual stabilization and don the necessary gear.)

2. To which of the two trauma facilities would you transport this patient? Why?

   (Because the patient is in decompensated shock with a possible pneumothorax and abdominal bleeding, the need for surgery is imminent. As a result, you should transport the patient to the Level II trauma center.)

3. What resources would you call on to help ensure that this patient receives the highest level of care?

   (Because of the mechanism of injury and distance to the appropriate hospital, you would request air transport as well as dispatch of the closest ALS unit. This will ensure that you receive the correct equipment on scene. Keep in mind that the foggy weather may make it impossible for the helicopter to land or necessitate intercept at a safer landing zone.)

4. Having no ALS equipment with you, are there any liability issues that might dictate your actions at the scene and during transport? Explain.

   (You have a duty to act in this situation. As a result, there will be no liability solely for the fact that you do not have gear. Remember you are always a paramedic and, in this case, your knowledge is as important as your equipment. This does not, however, cover any harm that you may cause to the patient in your treatment. Because you provided treatment on this patient, you must fully document all your actions.)

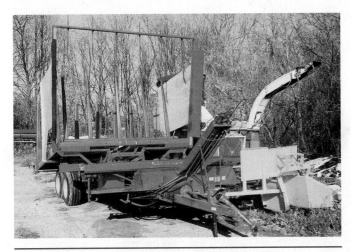

● **Figure 7-5a** Hay bale stacker. (© *Mark Foster*)

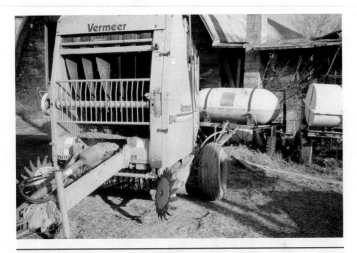

● **Figure 7-5b** Round hay baler. (© *Mark Foster*)

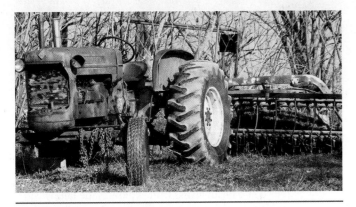

● **Figure 7-5c** Tractor and hay rake, typical of the old equipment found on many rural farms. (© *Mark Foster*)

principle: **lock-out/tag-out**. After you shut off the equipment, you lock off the switch and place a tag on the switch stating why it is shut off. This prevents accidental retripping of switches.

Remember, too, that the possibility for injury exists even after the equipment has been turned off. Engines fueled by gasoline, diesel, or propane hold the potential for explosion. Equipment that is not properly stabilized or chained can still roll or turn over. When lifting equipment, the center of gravity can shift, increasing the pressure on the patient or causing injury to crew members.

Hazardous Materials Hazardous materials can be found in many places on a farm or ranch (Figures 7-6 ● and 7-7 ●). They exist in greenhouses, bins used to store pesticides, the equipment used to spray or dust crops, and the manure storage pits on large livestock facilities. For this reason, a self-contained breathing apparatus (SCBA) should be standard equipment on every rural EMS unit.

Be especially wary of rescues involving grain tanks and silos. Over time, grain and silage will ferment if stored long enough. During fermentation, crops release high levels of CO_2, **silo gas** (oxides of nitrogen, or NO_2), and methane.[7] In rescues involving silos, you face the added risk of high angles, confined spaces, and the possibility of entombment under grain or silage. In such cases, determine whether any other agencies might be needed at the scene. Keep in mind the distance factor; don't arrive at the scene to find out you lack the correct apparatus or support for the call. (For more on management of hazardous materials, see Chapter 5.)

Potential for Trauma

Many farmers or ranchers work seven days a week, from sunrise to sunset. They endure extremes of heat, cold, and all kinds of weather conditions. They may spend a large part of the day in remote areas, far from telephones and help if injured.

The risk of serious agricultural accidents and injuries is increased by the equipment and machines routinely used by farmers. In some cases, farmers rely on old or outdated equipment because they cannot afford to replace it. They often wear little or no protective gear and may attempt to repair dangerous equipment themselves. All these situations expose farm workers to equipment-related trauma. Depending on the type of machinery, the mechanism of injury could be crushing, twisting, tearing, penetrating, or a combination of mechanisms.

Equipment-related trauma is complicated by a number of factors related to agriculture. First, a wound may become contaminated by pesticides or manure. Second, a patient may become easily trapped or entangled under heavy equipment, making extrication both difficult and time consuming. Standard extrication devices that are used efficiently for automobiles may be unable to handle the weight of heavy farm equipment. In some cases, extrication equipment may be unavailable and crews will need to improvise using other farm equipment.

Lengthy extrications can worsen the patient's condition. You might use **air bags** (inflatable high-pressure pillows that, when inflated, can lift up to 20 tons) or **cribbing** (wooden slats used to shore up equipment) to relieve some of the equipment's weight. However, if extrication goes on too long, a patient may suffer from **compartment syndrome** or similar problems (e.g., rhabdomyolysis, renal failure). This occurs when circulation to a portion of the body is cut off. Over a period of time (usually hours), toxins develop in the blood, and when circulation is restored the patient goes into shock. This is a serious complication that can be fatal unless proper treatment is given in a timely manner. (For more on the treatment of shock, see Volume 5, Chapters 4 and 13. For more about extrication and rescue, review Chapter 4 in this volume.)

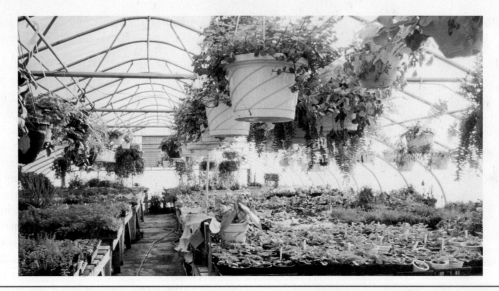

● **Figure 7-6** Greenhouses hold many hidden dangers such as pesticides, insecticides, and fertilizers. Remember that fertilizers contain nitrites. When mixed with diesel fuel, as in the Oklahoma federal building bombing, they can form powerful explosives. (© *Mark Foster*)

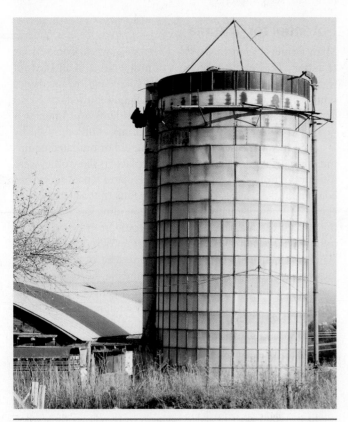

● **Figure 7-7** This old silo looks harmless, but it possesses the potential for entombment in a confined space and exposure to toxic silo gas. (© *Mark Foster*)

Mechanisms of Injury

Suspect many different mechanisms of injury in accidents involving agricultural equipment. For example, most farm machinery have spinning parts, such as fans, power takeoff (PTO) shafts, augers, pulleys, and wheels. These can cause sprains, strains, avulsions, fractures, and possible amputations. Common mechanisms of injury include:

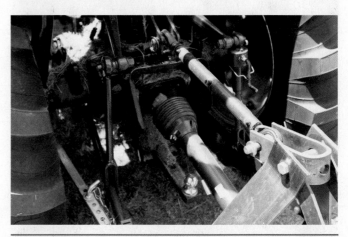

● **Figure 7-8** A tractor's PTO is a prime example of a possible mechanism for a wrap point injury. (© *Dr. Bryan E. Bledsoe*)

- *Wrap points:* **Wrap points** are points at which an appendage can get caught and significantly twisted (Figure 7-8 ●). As noted earlier, spinning parts such as fans, PTO shafts, augers, pulleys, and wheels can catch and twist arms, hands, legs, and feet.

- *Pinch points:* **Pinch points** occur when two objects come together and catch a portion of the patient's body between them. This could be anything from a plow blade falling on somebody's foot to catching a hand in a log splitter (Procedure 7–1 ●).

- *Shear points:* Like **pinch points**, shear points result when two objects come together. However, in this instance, the pinch points either meet or pass, causing amputation of a body part. An example of farm equipment able to cause a shear point is a sickle bar mower.

- *Crush points:* **Crush points** develop when two or more objects come together with enough weight or force to crush the affected appendage. A common crush point mechanism of injury is a tractor rollover.

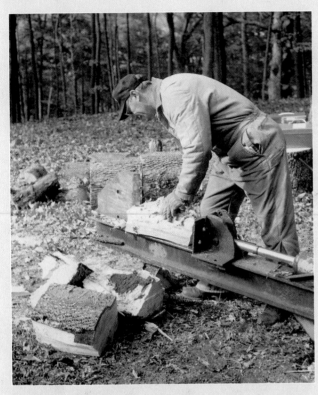

7-1a ● Log splitter—a typical mechanism for a pinch-point injury in a rural setting. Note the absence of protective gear on the farmer, except for lightweight work gloves. (© Mark Foster)

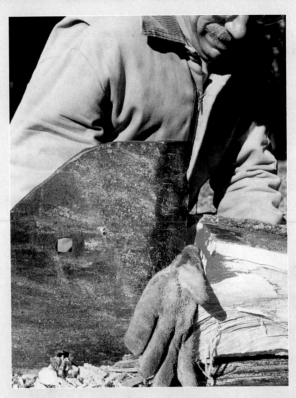

7-1b ● Hand caught in pinch-point mechanism of injury, with the possibility of compartment syndrome. (© Mark Foster)

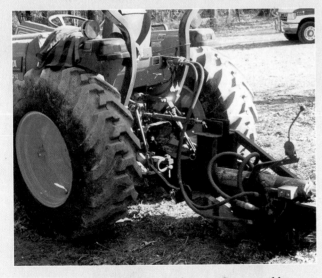

7-1c ● Determine whether machinery is operated by other equipment—in this case, a tractor. If so, use the machinery to extricate the patient. Then lock-out/tag-out the appropriate levers or switches. (© Mark Foster)

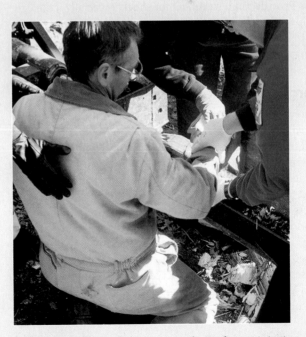

7-1d ● Stabilize both fractures and circulatory injuries during extrication. (© Mark Foster)

(Continued)

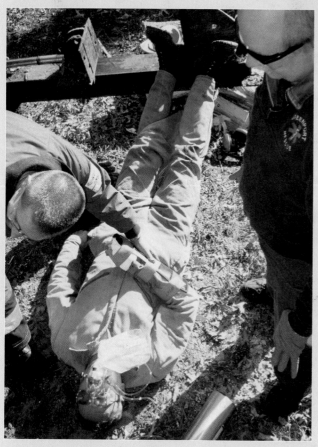

7-1e ● Provide rapid treatment for shock, especially if the call for help was delayed for a lengthy period. (© *Mark Foster*)

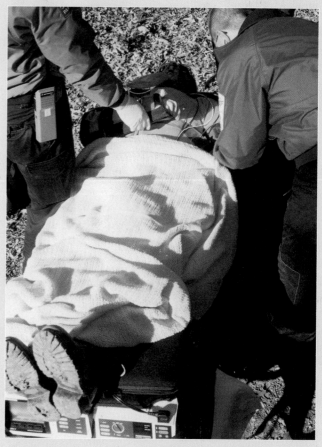

7-1f ● Package and transport to the nearest appropriate medical facility, using the most effective means of transport. (© *Mark Foster*)

Emergency Medical Care

In general, provide the same emergency medical care to patients involved in agricultural emergencies as you would to any other patient with similar injuries. However, at all times, keep in mind the effect of time and distance on the potential for shock. A farmer involved in a minor accident, for example, may lie injured for hours in harsh weather conditions before someone suspects any trouble. In cases involving long response and/or transport times, any serious bleeding injury can result in inadequate tissue perfusion if not treated promptly and effectively (Figure 7-9 ●). In addition, because of unsanitary work conditions, sepsis and poisoning are very real possibilities.

To assess the decisions in an agricultural emergency, consider Rural Scenario 2.

Recreational Emergencies

Recreational activities have always drawn people to rural settings. Depending on the season and the activity, the population in a rural community can swell dramatically as vacationers, sports enthusiasts, music fans, or "adventure seekers" arrive in an area. Small hill towns, for example, can grow to two or three times their normal size when a ski slope opens. Such a situation presents unique challenges to EMS units in the area (Figure 7-10 ●).

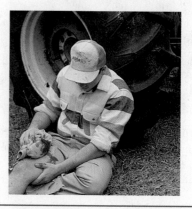

● **Figure 7-9** In rural settings, any serious bleeding injury can result in shock if distance delays treatment or transport.

It's late afternoon on a warm day in May. You are the on-duty paramedic at a rural rescue squad. The squad's staff consists of a 24-hour paid paramedic and a supplemental BLS ambulance crew. Having just completed a call, you are in the bay of the squad building restocking your ALS bag and checking your gear. Suddenly a car enters the squad's parking lot, and a very anxious man jumps out. The man rushes up to you. He declares, "My father is trapped under a tractor. He's hurt real bad, and I don't know what to do."

You load the four-wheel-drive quick response vehicle and tell the man that you will follow him to the scene of the accident. However, he speeds off before you can get precise directions to the farm.

En route to the emergency, you contact the county dispatcher and request that she tone out the BLS crew and the local fire rescue squad. Although you still cannot report an address, the dispatcher begins to assemble emergency personnel.

You follow the man into a field, using the four-wheel-drive vehicle to travel over the rough terrain. When you arrive at the site of the overturned tractor, you call county dispatch and provide your exact location before exiting the quick response vehicle. You also request that a helicopter be dispatched.

As you approach the scene, you see an elderly man trapped underneath a tractor from the waist down. Before beginning assessment, you ask the patient's son to make sure the tractor is shut down and the fuel shut-off switch is in place. You also look for fuel leaks, but find none.

On primary assessment, you observe that the patient has multiple contusions to his head and chest and an open humerus fracture on his right arm. Because of the position of the tractor, you are unable to access his lower extremities. The patient is unconscious, unresponsive, ashen, and diaphoretic. Vitals include pulse 132, respirations 32 and shallow, blood pressure 130/88.

Ten minutes later, the fire and BLS crews arrive on the scene. The helicopter is still 30 minutes out.

1. What would have made this call go smoother in the response phase?

   (The best scenario would be to have the son ride in your vehicle. A car chase is never a good idea, especially when you do not have a clue about where you are going. You should also specify the need for extrication, giving the crew time to assemble the necessary equipment.)

2. During the 10 minutes you are alone, what care would you provide to the patient?

   (You would protect the airway and use all appropriate ALS procedures such as IV and monitor to treat for shock. Just because you are alone does not mean you cannot provide treatment.)

3. As the on-scene paramedic, what directions would you provide to BLS and fire crews?

   (Directions: Treat for shock and accomplish rapid extrication.)

4. What steps might you take to reduce compartment syndrome?

   (The best treatment is rapid extrication. If you suspect compartment syndrome may have set in, be prepared to treat for septic shock.)

5. What details of this scenario are common to other calls you might make in a rural setting?

   (Details might include use of volunteers, lengthy distances, patients located in isolated areas, the use of many organizations to facilitate the treatment of your patient, and consideration of air transport.)

A ski slope, for instance, may have its own first aid station and ski patrol, but cannot usually provide advanced care or transport to a patient involved in a skiing accident.

As a rural paramedic, you need to be familiar with the recreational or wilderness pursuits in your area. If you live near a lake, local lifeguards can perform basic first aid and CPR, but they cannot abandon their beach patrol. Further treatment and transport falls to local EMS units. In such cases, a paramedic would need to be well versed in the procedures and skills related to water emergencies.

If you live in a wilderness or mountainous area, you might need to be aware of the accidents commonly encountered by hunters, backpackers, mountaineers, rock climbers, or mountain bikers. You might decide to take courses to receive certification in wilderness rescue. You might also practice rescues in extreme weather conditions, such as those found on New Hampshire's Mt. Washington, where harsh and unpredictable

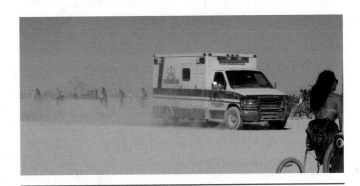

● **Figure 7-10** The recreational activities that draw people to rural settings for vacations, adventure, and sports activities also increase the chances for EMS involvement in environmental emergencies. The "Burning Man" event brings more than 50,000 people to the arid desert of northwestern Nevada. (© Dr. Bryan E. Bledsoe)

weather patterns can trap or injure even the most experienced climber. (For more information on treating environmental emergencies, see Volume 5, Chapter 12.)

In wilderness rescues, distance and extrication time play an important part in your decisions. For example, if a rock climber is injured in the Shawangunks in New Paltz, New York, several hospitals lie within a 30-minute range. However, if the patient is injured on the second pitch of a three-pitch climb, evacuation will delay transport, especially if the injury occurs on a class 5.10 or 5.11 route.

A helicopter might seem the obvious choice of transport for wilderness rescues. However, you must take into account weather conditions, availability of suitable landing zones, and the time it will take a helicopter to arrive. In some instances, ground transport may be more efficient, even if it means carrying a patient out in a basket stretcher. In other instances, a helicopter might be able to provide a higher level of care, depending on regional and state protocols. For example, if a rock climber has sustained a severe head injury and if ground transport lacks protocols for rapid sequence intubation, the patient's needs might be better served with helicopter transport.

Keep in mind that the helicopter is not a panacea. It has specific uses, tied to distance and level of care. Indiscriminate use of air transport can sometimes add dangerous minutes to patient treatment or even carry the risk of further patient injury. For example, high-altitude sickness can be worsened by an increase in altitude due to unpressurized flight. Decompression syndrome patients are definitely candidates for low-altitude transport. (For more on diving-related injuries, see Volume 5, Chapter 12.)

To assess the decisions in a recreational emergency, consider Rural Scenario 3.

➥ RURAL SCENARIO 3 ⇇

Shifting his weight from side to side, Jim compensates for the boat's wake as he glides across New York's Hudson River on water skis. His girlfriend Renee is piloting Jim's new boat, while two of Jim's friends enjoy the ride. As Jim shifts to tack in the opposite direction, he catches a wave and drops into the water. Renee sees Jim fall and turns the boat around to pick him up. She does her best to bring the boat gently to him, but piloting is new to her. She realizes too late that the boat is going hit Jim and puts the motor in reverse.

When the boat strikes Jim, the motor sucks his legs into the propeller. Both of his legs become twisted in and around the shaft. Fearing the worst, Jim's friends jump into the water to hold up his head so that he does not drown. They then yell to the nearest boat for help. The owner of that boat uses his cell phone to call 911.

The 911 dispatcher receives the call. Using prearrival dispatch instructions, the dispatcher initiates bystander treatment and gathers the necessary information. Meanwhile, the dispatcher's partner tones out the local rescue squad and the fire department extrication team. Because of the seriousness of the situation, the dispatcher also tones out the nearest ALS unit, where you serve as a paid 24-hour paramedic. Listening to other dispatches on the scanner, you had already begun to move closer to the scene. You now respond rapidly.

On arrival, you find that members of the rescue squad and fire department have entered the water to relieve the patient's exhausted friends. By this time, the patient is unconscious and unresponsive. He has a patent airway and does not have any trauma to his upper body. Postextrication assessment reveals the following vitals: a weak, rapid pulse of 130; respirations 24 and shallow; blood pressure 90/PALP. On physical examination, you note that both legs have multiple fractures. Deep lacerations run from the patient's groin to his ankles. Included in the lacerations are two arterial bleeders.

1. What would be the appropriate BLS and ALS treatment for this patient?

(BLS treatment includes high-concentration O_2, removal of wet clothing, passive warming for hypothermia, and direct pressure on the lesser bleeders. ALS treatment includes airway management, manual tamponading of arterial bleeders, IV therapy with moderate fluid challenges, monitoring, and rapid transport to a trauma center. Desired blood pressure should remain approximately 90/PALP.)

2. Would the PASG (pneumatic anti-shock garment) be appropriate in this situation? Explain.

(PASG would not be advised due to the fact that application will not tamponade arterial bleeding and will hide large blood loss inside the pants.)

3. What could be done to ensure better long-term management of this patient in the rural emergency setting?

(Because saline does not carry oxygen, better long-term management would include moderate fluid challenges instead of large fluid challenges. Also, tamponading of specific arterial bleeding, rather than tamponading of a large area, increases blood flow to the extremities. This makes the extremities more salvageable.)

4. Suppose air transport was unavailable. How would this change treatment provided by the paramedic?

(The paramedic could transport the patient to the nearest local hospital for stabilization and possible blood transfusions. This action, of course, would depend on equipment and services rendered by the local hospital.)

5. How did the availability of universal access to a 911 number affect the outcome of this patient?

(The 911 number provided rapid dispatch of all necessary equipment and personnel. It also allowed bystander actions to be guided by a highly trained dispatcher.)

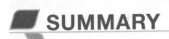

SUMMARY

Rural EMS presents the paramedic and other health care personnel with special challenges such as lengthy distances, radio dead spots, shortages of EMS providers and medical directors, lack of around-the-clock emergency departments, and fewer opportunities for skills practice. To meet these challenges, many rural EMS units have turned to creative problem solving. Counties have joined together to share in the cost of universal access to the 911 system. Squads have adopted flexible training sessions, making use of computerized instruction and networking through the Internet.

Paramedics play an important part in filling the "health care gap" between rural and urban areas. They take a leading role in training rural residents as CPR drivers and first responders. They intercept volunteer BLS units traveling over long distances and provide definitive care. They develop the specialized skills and training to handle the agricultural and/or recreational emergencies unique to their county or district. Because distance often increases the contact time between paramedics and their rural patients, decisions about treatment and use of air transport literally make the difference between life and death.

YOU MAKE THE CALL

The stone quarry in your district was abandoned after it flooded several years ago. Since then, the county has used it as a water source and placed it off limits to recreational users. However, the quarry's clear water and high cliffs serve as a magnet to teenagers who want to go swimming. To you, the quarry holds nothing but trouble for the teens. It is isolated and filled with old rusted equipment. Nothing, not even a well-traveled road, lies near the quarry.

One hot sunny afternoon in August, three teenagers—John, Todd, and Stacey—decide to hike into a remote part of the quarry for a swim. Once at the quarry, Todd rushes to the top of one of the 50-foot cliffs and jumps into the water. Misjudging the water's depth, he hits bottom. When Todd doesn't come up for air, Stacey realizes something is wrong. She and John dive into the water and pull Todd to shore.

The two teens now panic. Todd is breathing, but unconscious. Blood is pouring from a wound in his leg. Stacey tries to stop the bleeding by applying direct pressure. Meanwhile, John races to get help. It takes him nearly 30 minutes to reach a telephone. Lacking a universal access number, he calls the local fire department, which in turn places a call to your volunteer ALS unit. By the time you get into your ambulance, 45 minutes have passed since the accident took place. Although it will only take you about 10 minutes to reach the quarry, you will still need to gain access to the patient at the distant location where the teens chose to swim.

1. What apparatus or support are you going to need to perform this rescue?

2. Based on the mechanism of injury, what injuries should you suspect?

3. What will you do to stabilize this patient?

4. What factors made it impossible for you to meet response, treatment, and transport times in the rural setting when compared with the urban or suburban setting?

See Suggested Responses at the back of this book.

REVIEW QUESTIONS

1. Every decision that a paramedic makes in a rural setting needs to be made with the primary thought of _____ in mind.
- a. budget
- b. distance
- c. insurance
- d. rust out

2. A technological innovation that promises to improve communications in rural areas is the _____.
- a. CAD
- b. computer
- c. cell phone
- d. base station

3. Regardless of where a paramedic lives, positive relationships with a hospital depend on good _____.
   a. equipment
   b. pay schedules
   c. technology updates
   d. communications

4. Rural paramedics must be highly skilled and highly practiced to compensate for the _____.
   a. extended run times
   b. more complicated logistics
   c. inadequate number of volunteers
   d. all of the above

5. Hazardous materials can be found in many places on a farm or ranch. For this reason, a _____ should be standard equipment on every rural EMS unit.
   a. CAD   c. QRU
   b. SCBA   d. PTO

6. Common mechanisms of injury in accidents involving agricultural equipment include _____.
   a. wrap points   c. shear points
   b. pinch points   d. all of the above

See Answers to Review Questions at the back of this book.

REFERENCES

1. Key, C. B. "Operational Issues in EMS." *Emerg Med Clin North Am* 20 (2002): 913–927.

2. Shah, M. N., T. V. Caprio, P. Swanson, et al. "A Novel Emergency Medical Services-Based Program to Identify and Assist Older Adults in a Rural Community." *J Am Geriatr Soc* 58 (2010): 2205–2211.

3. Whyte, B. S. and R. Ansley. "Pay for Performance Improves Rural EMS Quality: Investment in Prehospital Care." *Prehosp Emerg Care* 12 (2008): 495–497.

4. Studnel, J. R., A. R. Fernandez, and G. S. Margolis. "Assessing Continued Cognitive Competence among Rural Emergency Medical Technicians." *Prehosp Emerg Care* 13 (2000): 357–363.

5. Warren, L., R. Sapien, and L. Fullerton-Gleason. "Is On-Line Pediatric Continuing Education Effective in a Rural State?" *Prehosp Emerg Care* 12 (2008): 498–502.

6. Gilpen, J. L., Jr, H. Carabin, J. L. Regens, and R. W. Burden Jr. "Agriculture Emergencies: A Primer for First Responders." *Bisecur Bioterror* 7 (2008): 187–198.

7. Shepherd, L. G. "Confined-Space Accidents on the Farm: The Manure Pit and Silo." *CJEM* 1 (1999): 108–111.

FURTHER READING

Farabee, C. R., Jr. *Death, Daring, and Disaster: Search and Rescue in the National Parks.* Boulder, CO: Roberts, Rinehart Publishers, 1999.

Tilton, Buck, and Frank Hubbel, *Medicine for the Backcountry.* 3rd ed. Guilford, CT: Globe Pequot, 2000.

Wilkerson, James A. *Medicine for Mountaineering & Other Wilderness Activities.* 5th ed. Seattle, WA: The Mountaineers, 2002.

chapter

8

Responding to Terrorist Acts

Bryan Bledsoe, DO, FACEP, FAAEM, EMT-P

STANDARD
EMS Operations (Terrorism and Disaster)

COMPETENCY
Applies knowledge of operational roles and responsibilities to ensure patient, public, and personnel safety.

OBJECTIVES

Terminal Performance Objective
After reading this chapter, you should be able to effectively perform the expected functions of EMS personnel when responding to terrorist acts.

Enabling Objectives
To accomplish the terminal performance objective, you should be able to:

1. Define key terms introduced in this chapter.
2. Identify likely targets of terrorist attacks.
3. Identify information and observations that can indicate a potential terrorist attack when responding to calls.
4. Describe the characteristics of explosive, incendiary, nuclear, chemical, and biological weapons used in terrorism.
5. Be aware of the likelihood of secondary explosions when responding to reports of an explosion.
6. Predict injury patterns and patient problems associated with explosions and the use of incendiary devices.
7. Describe the precautions in responding to a nuclear incident.
8. Anticipate the patient presentations and risks to responders associated with chemical agent exposures.
9. Describe the specific treatment for chemical agent exposures.
10. Describe the keys to recognizing a biological terrorist attack.
11. Describe the specific actions to be taken by responders to protect themselves when responding to a biological terrorist attack.

KEY TERMS
biological agents, p. 148
biotoxin, p. 147
chemical, biological, radiologic, nuclear, and explosive (CBRNE), p. 143

dirty bomb, p. 145
dosimeter, p. 145
erythema, p. 147
explosives, p. 143
fallout, p. 145

fasciculations, p. 146
Geiger counter, p. 145
incendiary agents, p. 144
Mark I kit, p. 146
miosis, p. 146

nerve agents, p. 146
nuclear detonation, p. 144
pulmonary agents, p. 147
rhinorrhea, p. 146

specific gravity,
 p. 146
terrorist act, p. 143
vesicants, p. 146

volatility, p. 146
weapons of mass destruction
 (WMDs), p. 143

CASE STUDY

Late Monday morning, during the first real cold spell of winter, Adam and Sean are called to transport a 54-year-old physician from a local OB/GYN clinic. He is found to have some "chest tightness" but no ECG abnormalities, and the rest of his assessment is unremarkable. Shortly after delivering him to the emergency department, the pagers go off again, and Adam and Sean are requested to respond to the same address, where several people are now complaining of fatigue, shortness of breath, and headache. Adam remembers that the clinic was the subject of a news report last week when anti-abortion demonstrators became violent during a protest. As Adam and Sean call in service and en route, Adam requests that the fire department respond for a possible hazardous environment. Sean uses the cell phone (and a secure line) to contact the dispatch center to make his concerns known and suggests that dispatch call the clinic and request evacuation of the facility. Sean also requests that the center activate the community's weapons of mass destruction plan.

Adam and Sean are on the first unit to arrive, so they establish incident command. They size up the scene and notice a dozen or so people in the parking lot but no signs of any smoke or gas clouds coming from the clinic. Adam notes the flag blowing gently from a northwesterly breeze. Sean parks the ambulance north and west of the building and, using the ambulance's public address system, requests the clinic employees to approach his location. He also contacts dispatch with an approximate number of people at the scene and suggests that the fire department approach the building from the northwest. Both paramedics don high-efficiency particulate air (HEPA) respirators and gloves. Sean speaks with some of the employees to ensure that all personnel are accounted for and out of the building.

When the fire department arrives, Captain James approaches, receives a situation update from Adam, and assumes incident command. He reports that a team with self-contained breathing apparatus (SCBA) gear is entering the building to investigate the problem. Adam and Sean establish a treatment sector and begin to assess the victims and administer high-concentration oxygen to the patients with the worst complaints. Their initial evaluation reveals that most patients are complaining of general fatigue, headache, some ringing in the ears, and mild dyspnea. Two other ambulances arrive and, at the direction of Adam, begin oxygen administration to the remaining patients. A pulse CO-oximeter reveals the presence of elevated carboxyhemoglobin levels in virtually all clinic employees and patrons. Captain James answers a radio call from the entry team and reports that carbon monoxide readings are very high in the building.

Adam and Sean remain at the scene but direct the other ambulances to begin transporting patients to the two local hospitals. Sean contacts medical direction and provides the number of patients, their signs and symptoms, and the likely cause of their problems. As Sean and Adam prepare the last of the patients for transport, Captain James reports that the furnace flue was intentionally redirected into the furnace room, generating the carbon monoxide. It is presumed to be a terrorist act, as many believe the clinic to be an abortion clinic. The police are informed and the area becomes a crime scene.

INTRODUCTION

The events of September 11, 2001, have had a great impact on our society and our sensitivity to the threat of terrorist acts. The extensive planning and coordination needed to bring down the World Trade Center, damage the Pentagon, and achieve such a great loss of life show just how intent some people are on causing public harm. This new awareness forces the EMS community to prepare itself to respond to acts of terrorism. These acts can come in many forms.

The weapon of choice used by terrorist groups worldwide is the conventional explosive. Conventional explosives have been used frequently in the Middle East and in the British Isles and were used by the Unabomber in the United States. We have also experienced major explosive events, such as the destruction of the Physics Annex at the University of Wisconsin in the mid-1960s, the first attempt to destroy the World Trade Center in 1993, and the bombing of the Oklahoma City federal building in 1995. All of these incidents involved the use of vehicles filled with high-nitrogen-content fertilizer soaked with diesel fuel and parked under or adjacent to the facility.

It is clear that the 21st century will bring new terrorism threats using more unconventional means, such as commercial aircraft to bring down structures (Figure 8-1 ●) and **weapons of mass destruction (WMDs)** including **chemical, biological, radiologic, nuclear, and explosive (CBRNE)** weapons.[1, 2] Harbingers of such acts include the attack on the Tokyo subway system with sarin gas in 1996 and letters laced with anthrax spores sent through the mail in North America in 2001. Both events underscore the real potential for massive and widespread injury and death caused by those intending to incite terror using WMDs. With the increasing likelihood of a **terrorist act**, EMS personnel become responsible for maintaining a higher index of suspicion for such an event. As a paramedic, you also must prepare to protect yourself and your crew, your patients, and the public from the effects of such an attack.

Terrorists may be of foreign or domestic origin. They are likely to target locations that are symbolic of the government (a federal building, such as the Pentagon) or that represent the influence of a country (such as an embassy). Domestic terrorists may further target corporations or their executives who represent a threat to their cause. They may also target their own employer or the public through their employer's products (as in tainted food or pharmaceuticals). The objective of both the domestic and the foreign terrorist is to incite terror in the public.

The likely mechanisms of mass destruction used by terrorists include explosive and incendiary agents, nuclear detonation or contamination, and the release of either chemical or biological agents.

EXPLOSIVE AGENTS

Explosives are the most likely method by which terrorists will strike. The bomb may range from a suicide bomber carrying a few sticks of dynamite to a large vehicle filled with highly explosive material. More recently, terrorists have attempted to detonate explosives on commercial airliners (e.g., the "shoe bomber" on American Airlines Flight 63 on December 22, 2001, and the "underwear bomber" on Northwest Airlines Flight 253 on December 25, 2009). In an instant, the device detonates and causes damage to the human body through several mechanisms (Figure 8-2 ●). The blast pressure wave causes compression/decompression injury as it passes through the lungs, the ears, and other hollow, air-filled organs. This damage may be enhanced when the explosion occurs in a confined space, such as the interior of a building or other structure. Debris thrown by the blast produces penetrating or blunt injuries, and similar additional injury occurs as the victim is thrown by the blast wind. Secondary combustion induces burn injury, and structural collapse causes blunt and crushing injuries. After the initial explosion, associated dangers include structural collapse, fire, electrical hazard, and combustible or toxic gas hazards. *Also be wary of*

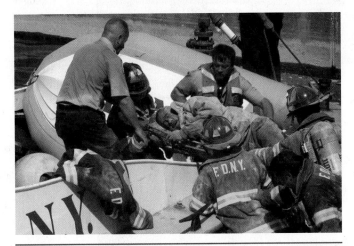

● **Figure 8-1** Providing treatment to a victim of the World Trade Center attack in New York City on September 11, 2001. (*© AP Images/Matt Moyer*)

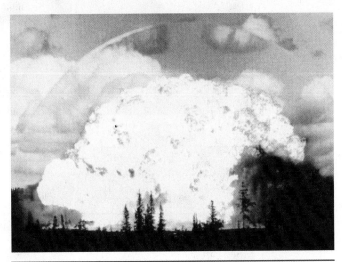

● **Figure 8-2** An explosion releases tremendous amounts of heat energy, generating a pressure wave, blast wind, and projection of debris. (*Reproduced from Bombing: Injury Patterns and Care. Office of Public Health Preparedness and Response. www.CDC.gov*)

CONTENT REVIEW

▶ Examples of Incendiary Agents

- Napalm
- Gasoline
- White phosphorus
- Magnesium

secondary explosives set intentionally to disrupt rescue and to injure emergency responders. After the blast, emergency responders are left to locate, extricate, and provide medical care for the victims. (See Volume 5, Chapter 2, Blunt Trauma, for a detailed explanation of the blast process, the associated mechanisms of injury, and assessment and care of the blast victim.)

Incendiary agents are a special subset of explosives with less explosive power and greater heat and burn potential. Napalm, used extensively during the Vietnam War, is a military example, whereas the Molotov cocktail or gasoline bomb is more of a terrorist weapon. Some incendiary agents are of special concern. White phosphorus may spontaneously combust when exposed to air and may be a part of military munitions or a terrorist weapon. It can be very difficult to extinguish when it contacts the skin. Often, fire-resistant oil is used to exclude the air and extinguish any flame. Another example is magnesium, a metal that burns vigorously and at a high temperature (3,000°C). It also is difficult to extinguish. Incendiary agents are likely to cause severe and extensive burn injuries. (For more information on burn injuries and their care, see Volume 5, Chapter 6, Burn Trauma.)

Terrorists may choose to increase the effectiveness of their weapons by incorporating other agents with explosives. In some cases, they surround the explosive charge with old auto batteries, thereby contaminating the explosion scene with both lead and sulfuric acid. They may also surround the charge with scrap metal, nails, or screws that act as shrapnel. In some cases in the Middle East, terrorists have surrounded the explosive with nails coated with a form of rat poison, a derivative of warfarin (Coumadin), to increase the severity of wound hemorrhage associated with shrapnel wounds.

NUCLEAR DETONATION

Nuclear detonation is the release of energy that is generated when heavy nuclei split (fission) or light nuclei combine (fusion) to form new elements. The unleashed energy is tremendous and creates an explosion of immense proportion. In addition to the extremes of the injury-producing mechanisms associated with conventional explosions, radiant heat is likely to incinerate everything in the immediate vicinity of the blast and induce serious burn injury to exposed skin even at great distances from the blast epicenter. Burn injuries are likely to be the most lethal and debilitating injuries associated with a nuclear detonation.

The damage associated with a typical nuclear detonation is extreme and results in concentric circles of total destruction and mortality, severe destruction and very high mortality, heavy destruction and moderate mortality, and light destruction and limited mortality (Figure 8-3 ●). The explosive energy disrupts communications, power, water and waste service, travel, and the medical, emergency medical, and public safety infrastructures. The destruction also disrupts access to the scene and limits the ability of the EMS system to identify, reach, and care for the seriously injured. It is an extreme disaster with great loss of life and injury and presents a great challenge to emergency responders.

The nuclear reaction also generates particles of debris and dust that give off nuclear radiation. Gases, heated by the explosion, draw these particles high into the atmosphere, where upper

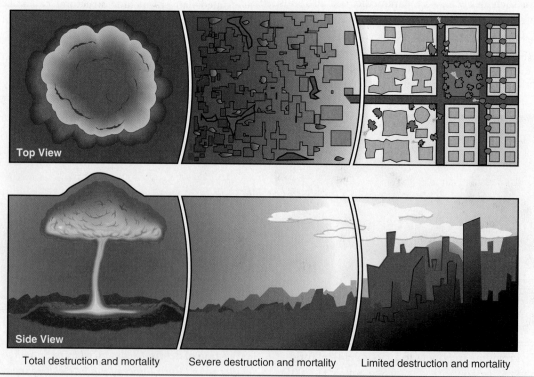

Top View

Side View

Total destruction and mortality   Severe destruction and mortality   Limited destruction and mortality

● **Figure 8-3** The concentric circles of destruction following detonation of a nuclear weapon.

air currents carry the contamination until it falls to Earth as fallout. This uplifting of irradiated debris leaves the scene almost radiation free from moments after the blast until about 1 hour post-ignition. Thereafter, there is a serious danger from fallout at the scene and downwind for many, many miles.

Nuclear radiation cannot be felt, seen, or otherwise detected by any of our senses. However, it damages the cells of the human body as it passes through them. Radiation passage changes the structure of molecules and essential elements of the cells. Damaged cells then go on to repair themselves, to die, or to produce altered or damaged cells (cancer). As the intensity and duration of exposure increases, so do the degree and extent of cell damage and the risk to life. Nuclear radiation from the sun and other natural sources bombards us constantly. This exposure is very limited and the damage caused by it is minimal. However, the initial radiation produced by the nuclear chain reaction (the blast) and **fallout** can produce serious and life-threatening exposure. (See Volume 5, Chapter 6, Burn Trauma, for the types of radiation, mechanisms of injury, and the assessment and care of the irradiated patient.)

A Nuclear Incident Response

The first hour post-ignition is generally spent moving the injured into structures that will protect them from fallout. Ideally, they are moved into the central areas of large, structurally sound buildings or at least to some cover from the falling contaminated dust. Simultaneously, emergency responders organize, determine the direction of fallout movement, and begin to extricate the walking wounded and seriously injured from the outer perimeter of the explosion. During this time, evacuation of those in the anticipated path of fallout occurs. (They should remain outside the fallout pathway for at least 48 hours and until radiologic monitoring determines it is safe to return.) Entry into the scene is made from upwind and laterally to upper air movement in order to limit radioactive fallout exposure to rescuers.

As the response is organized, egress and evacuation routes are cleared, the injured are located and evacuated, and the response moves closer and closer to the blast epicenter. In general, some limited medical care is provided where the victims are found, but most emergency medical care is provided at treatment sectors that are remote from the seriously damaged areas and away from where fallout is expected. Patients are brought to a decontamination area, monitored for contamination, and decontaminated as needed before care begins.

Care for victims of a nuclear detonation involves decontamination (as necessary), treatment as for a conventional explosion (compression/decompression, blunt and penetrating injury care), and treatment for thermal burns. Burns are the most common and most immediately life-threatening injuries associated with a nuclear detonation and will likely be the focus of most care.

Before victims of a nuclear detonation arrive at an emergency medical treatment sector, someone must monitor them for radioactive contamination. This monitoring is accomplished using a device called a **Geiger counter**. The Geiger counter measures the passage of radioactive particles or rays through a receiving chamber and requires some training to use properly. (Usually, someone specially trained—and other than EMS—provides radioactive monitoring and decontamination.) If any significant radioactivity is noted, the patient's clothing is removed and he is washed with soap, water, and gentle scrubbing and then rinsed. All contaminated clothing is bagged, and the wash water is collected for proper disposal. A properly decontaminated patient does not pose a radiation threat either to himself or to you. During a response to a suspected nuclear incident, you will likely wear a **dosimeter**, a pen-like device used to record your total radiation exposure. This device is then monitored to determine when your exposure level is such that you should leave the scene for your own safety. Specially trained scene responders or health physicists will monitor dosages and determine how long you, as a care provider, can safely work at the scene.

If the risk of fallout and continuing radiation exposure is serious, paramedics may be asked to help distribute potassium iodide (KI) tablets. These tablets reduce the uptake of radioactive iodine (a common component of radioactive fallout) by the thyroid, which reduces the risk of thyroid injury or cancer. You may also be involved in the effort to evacuate the public from the expected fallout path.

Generally, patients with serious radiation exposure present with nausea, fatigue, and malaise (a general ill feeling). Treatment for these patients is limited to support, such as keeping them warm and well hydrated. The sooner these symptoms appear after the incident, the more serious the exposure. Generally, if symptoms occur earlier than 6 hours after the detonation, the exposure was very high. However, the effects of radiation exposure differ widely among individuals, so early diagnosis of the exposure extent and survivability from symptoms is unreliable. Because of the severity and nature of a nuclear detonation, disaster triage is necessary and many serious-to-critical burn and radiation-exposure patients will not survive—in part because of the inability of a medical system to care for the sheer number of victims.

Radioactive Contamination

Radioactive contamination may also be spread using conventional explosives (the "**dirty bomb**"). This type of blast is of conventional origin and does not cause the great magnitude of destruction that a nuclear detonation would. However, the explosion distributes radioactive material over a large area and into the surrounding air. The result is an explosion site with radioactive material contaminating the immediate vicinity. The greatest danger of this terrorist weapon is that the nature of the risk (the radiation) may not be recognized until well after the incident. Consequently, many more individuals and rescuers may be exposed or contaminated. Emergency care for victims of a recognized dirty bomb ignition includes radioactive decontamination and treatment (at a remote sector) for injuries that would be expected from a conventional bomb blast.

CHEMICAL AGENTS

Another terrorist WMD is the release of chemical agents. Potential chemical weapons range from simple hazardous materials common in our society, such as chlorine gas, to sophisticated chemicals, such as nerve agents specifically designed to harm

CONTENT REVIEW

► Classifications for Chemical Weapons

• Nerve agents
• Vesicants
• Pulmonary agents
• Biotoxins
• Incapacitating agents
• Other hazardous chemicals

humans. Because these chemical weapons are often gases or aerosols that will disperse in an open or windy area, the more common targets for their use are confined spaces such as subways or large buildings, which have central heating or air conditioning, or areas where many people congregate, such as arenas, shopping malls, and convention centers.

The concepts of volatility (vapor pressure) and specific gravity are important to understanding how chemical weapon agents are distributed. **Volatility** is the ease with which a chemical changes from a liquid to a gas. Most chemical weapons are liquids that are moderately volatile. They are often deployed by an explosion or sprayed into the atmosphere, creating an aerosol. A chemical that remains a liquid is said to be *persistent* and poses a contact or absorption threat, whereas vapors, gases, or aerosols present an inhalation danger. An example of a persistent chemical weapon is mustard agent. An example of a volatile, inhalable chemical weapon is lewisite.

Specific gravity refers to the density or weight of the vapor or gas as compared with air. A vapor or gas with a specific gravity less than air rises and quickly disperses into the atmosphere. This limits the effectiveness of the agent as a weapon. A gas with a specific gravity greater than air sinks beneath it, stays close to the ground, and accumulates in low places. Closed spaces, such as a basement, or low areas, such as a river valley, resist dispersal of the vapor and maintain the danger. Common chemicals with high specific gravity include chlorine and phosgene.

Environmental conditions affect the dispersal of chemical weapons. In strong winds, the gas or vapor mixes with large quantities of air and dilutes and disperses very quickly, limiting its concentration and effectiveness. Light wind moves the cloud downwind as a unit, increasing its effectiveness and the area involved. In windless conditions (which are infrequent) the cloud remains stationary, decreasing the area affected by it. Trees and buildings retard dispersion, whereas open spaces enhance dispersal. Precipitation, especially rain, may deactivate or absorb some agents, such as chlorine. Early morning and the time just before sunset are best for agent release because the winds are usually at their lowest velocity. The interior of a building with few open windows, especially when being heated or air conditioned, is an especially controlled environment. Confined within a building, a chemical agent remains concentrated and deadly for a prolonged period.

Chemical weapons are classified according to the way they cause damage to the human body. These chemicals include nerve agents, vesicants, pulmonary agents, biotoxins, incapacitating agents, and other hazardous chemicals.

Nerve Agents

Nerve agents and some insecticides damage nervous impulse conduction. These agents generally inhibit the degradation of a neurotransmitter (acetylcholine) and quickly cause a nervous system overload. This results in muscle twitching and spasms, convulsions, unconsciousness, and respiratory failure. Some common examples of nerve agents include GB (sarin), VX, GF, GD (soman), and GA (tabun). Although not designed as weapons, organophosphate (malathion, parathion) and carbamate (sevin) insecticides share a similar mechanism of action to nerve agents. They are much less potent, but they are still dangerous.

Nerve agents present as either vapor or liquid and are capable of being absorbed through the skin or inhaled and absorbed through the respiratory system. Exposure quickly leads to a series of signs and symptoms remembered as SLUDGE, or **S**alivation, **L**acrimation, **U**rination, **D**iarrhea, **G**astrointestinal distress, and **E**mesis. In addition to these signs, the patient may experience dyspnea, **fasciculations** (these are prominent), **rhinorrhea**, blurry vision, **miosis**, nausea, and sweating. Ultimately, the patient may become unconscious, seize, stop breathing, and die.

The actions of nerve agents can generally be reversed if the antidote is administered shortly after exposure. However, many nerve agents permanently bind to the agents, reabsorbing the neurotransmitters, and their effects become more difficult to reverse. The prognosis for a patient exposed to a nerve agent is good with aggressive artificial ventilation and quick administration of the antidote.

Treatment for nerve agent exposure includes the administration of atropine and then pralidoxime chloride. The military currently has these medications available in a two-part auto-injector set called a **Mark I kit**. As the threat of nerve agent release to the civilian population becomes greater, these kits may become increasingly available to the EMS provider. The autoinjectors are designed for self-administration or buddy-administration (mainly for military personnel) or may be administered by rescue personnel. They are quick to use and may be necessary when confronted with numerous patients exposed to a nerve agent. The antidote combination is often followed by the administration of diazepam to reduce seizure activity. The autoinjector is a convenient way to administer this regimen of medications; however, the intravenous route is more rapid and preferred when available and as time permits.

The Mark I kit contains 2 mg of atropine and 600 mg of pradoxime chloride. It is administered for the first and mild symptoms of exposure (blurry vision, mild dyspnea, and rhinorrhea) and repeated in 10 minutes if symptoms do not improve. If serious signs and symptoms are present, three doses of both atropine and pralidoxime chloride may be administered. Intravenous administration should provide 2 mg of atropine every 5 minutes (until drying of secretions or 20 mg is administered) and 1 g of pralidoxime chloride every hour (until spontaneous respirations return). A pediatric version of the Mark I kit is available.[3]

Vesicants (Blistering Agents)

Vesicants are agents that damage exposed tissue, frequently causing vesicles (blisters). They are capable of causing damage to the skin, eyes, respiratory tract, and lungs, and are able to induce generalized illness as well. The mustard gas of World War I is an example of a vesicant. Other examples include sulfur mustard (HD), nitrogen mustard (HN), lewisite (L), and phosgene oxime (CX). With the exception of phosgene oxime, the vesicants are thick oily liquids that create a toxic vapor threat in warm temperatures. The liquid form, however, is highly toxic to the touch. Lewisite and phosgene oxime induce immediate irritation on contact or inhalation, whereas the mustards produce only slight discomfort that becomes more severe with time. The slow progression of signs and symptoms may prolong contact and increase the severity of exposure.

Patients exposed to vesicants present with the signs and symptoms of injury to the skin, mucous membranes, and lungs. Exposed skin exhibits the signs of a chemical burn, including pain, **erythema**, and eventually blistering. The eyes and upper airway display a burning or stinging sensation, with tearing and rhinorrhea. Respiratory tract exposure results in dyspnea, cough, wheezing, and pulmonary edema. Systemic signs and symptoms include nausea, vomiting, and fatigue. Signs and symptoms occur slowly with the mustard agents, which may prolong exposure.

Emergency care for the patient exposed to a vesicant is immediate decontamination. Exposure of even a few minutes can result in permanent injury. The exposed areas should be irrigated immediately with water from a hose (using limited pressure if possible). Also irrigate the eyes, with a preference for saline over water, but do not delay irrigation to await the proper fluid. If blistering has occurred, treat the lesions as you would any chemical burn. Apply loose sterile dressings, gently bandage affected eyes, and medicate the patient for any serious pain.

Pulmonary Agents

Pulmonary agents are those that cause chemical injury primarily to the lungs. They include phosgene, chlorine, hydrogen sulfide, and similar agents, and some of the by-products that are created when synthetics such as plastic combust. These agents attack the mucous membranes of the respiratory system from the oral pharynx and nasal pharynx to the smaller respiratory bronchioles and alveoli. They produce inflammation and pulmonary edema, resulting in dyspnea and hypoxia. Early signs and symptoms of pulmonary agent exposure are related to irritation of the upper airway. They include rhinorrhea; nasal, oral, and throat irritation; wheezing; and cough. The victim may also experience tearing and eye irritation. Pulmonary edema is generally a late sign of exposure.

Emergency care for the individual exposed to a pulmonary agent is removal from the environment; exposure to fresh air; high-concentration oxygen; and rest. Endotracheal intubation and ventilation may be required. In cases of moderate to severe respiratory distress, consider 0.5 mL of albuterol by nebulized inhalation.

Biotoxins

Another type of agent that is classified as a biological agent but behaves more like a chemical agent is the **biotoxin**.[4] These toxins are produced by living organisms but are themselves not alive. Such agents include ricin, staphylococcal enterotoxin B (SEB), botulinum toxin, and trichothecene mycotoxins (T2). Ricin, a by-product of castor oil production, inhibits the body's ability to synthesize proteins. It may be either aerosolized and inhaled or ingested. Ricin causes pulmonary edema when inhaled and gastric symptoms when ingested. Poisoning by both routes may cause shock and multiple organ failure.

Staphylococcal enterotoxin is produced by a bacterium, *Staphylococcus aureus,* and is the agent most commonly responsible for food poisoning. Contamination may occur either orally, causing nausea and vomiting, or by inhalation, causing dyspnea and fever. Though only a small amount of toxin may cause symptoms and 50 percent of those contaminated may be incapacitated, SEB is rarely fatal.

Botulinum, the most toxic agent known, is an infrequent result of improper canning technique. It is 15,000 times more potent than VX, the most lethal nerve agent. Fortunately, the botulism toxin is very unstable, which limits its usefulness as a weapon of mass destruction. Like the nerve agents, botulinum attacks the nervous system. It interferes with impulse transmission and interrupts the central nervous system's control of the organs. The result is weakness, paralysis, and death by respiratory failure. Botulinum can be ingested or inhaled.

Trichothecene mycotoxins are a group of biotoxins produced by fungus molds. They prohibit protein and nucleic acid formulation and affect body cells that divide rapidly first. T2 acts very quickly, causing skin irritation (pain, burning, redness, and blistering), respiratory irritation (nasal and oral pain, rhinorrhea, epistaxis, wheezing, dyspnea, and hemoptysis), eye irritation (pain, redness, tearing, and blurry vision), and gastrointestinal symptoms (nausea, vomiting, abdominal cramping, and bloody diarrhea). T2 is most effective when absorbed through the skin. Generalized signs and symptoms include central nervous system signs, hypotension, and death.

Management of a victim of a biotoxin is supportive; antitoxins are generally not available. A special concern is directed to careful decontamination because even a very small amount of biotoxin can endanger rescuers and others.

Incapacitating Agents

Incapacitating agents include the riot control agents used by police and for personal protection, as well as newer agents being investigated by the military. These agents are intentionally selected or designed to incapacitate, not injure or harm, the recipient.

Riot control agents include CS, CN (mace), capsaicin (pepper spray), and CR. You may come into contact with these agents when they are released by police to suppress a large public disturbance or to subdue an assaultive or violent individual or are released by an individual for personal protection or possibly in the commission of a crime. These agents may, in the future, be used by those who wish to disrupt the public and incite terror.

The exposed patient often complains of eye irritation and tearing as well as rhinorrhea. If the agent is inhaled, these symptoms are often accompanied by airway irritation and dyspnea. These signs and symptoms are relieved by removal from the source, exposure to fresh air, and the administration of oxygen, when needed. The signs and symptoms further diminish with time.

The anticholinergic agents (atropine-like drugs) BZ and QNB are the prototype incapacitating agents for the military. The primary method of distribution of these agents is through the detonation of a mixture of explosive and agent. This explosion produces an aerosolized cloud. Exposure to BZ and QNB produces inappropriate affect, dry mucous beds, dilated pupils, slurred speech, disorientation, blurred vision, inhibition of the sweating reflex, elevated body temperature, and facial flushing. These effects become apparent after about 30 minutes of inhalation and last for up to 8 hours. The most dangerous effects of exposure include dysrhythmias and hyperthermia from the loss of the sweating reflex. The actions of BZ and QNB may be reversed by the administration of physostigmine.

Other Hazardous Chemicals

Any toxic chemical has a potential for use as a weapon of mass destruction. Industry produces countless hazardous materials with the potential to cause great harm if released into the air or water supply or ignited to release toxic gases. The only difference between an accidental release and one that is intended to incite terror is that the intentional release will likely be optimized to affect the greatest number of people. It may also be more difficult to identify the agent used by a terrorist because the container will likely not identify the agent. The Department of Transportation's *Emergency Response Guidebook,* which should be carried on every ambulance and fire apparatus, is a good guide to most common hazardous materials that might be used as a weapon as well as information on other WMD agents. It can also be helpful in denoting isolation and evacuation distances and suggesting specific care management steps.

Recognition of a Chemical Agent Release

A chemical weapon release may be visible as a cloud of mist, vapor, dust, or as puddles, or it may be completely unrecognizable. There may be an associated smell such as that of newly mown grass (phosgene), rotten eggs (hydrogen sulfide), or other strange or unusual odors. Suspect a chemical release if there are chemical odors when and where chemicals are not used or expected. However, never search out such an odor or touch any suspect liquid or material. You may also notice clusters of patients with chemical exposure symptoms or injured, incapacitated, or dead insects, birds, or animals. (You might remember that parakeets have been used in mines to detect toxic gas levels.) Given that the terrorist may be intent on optimizing the effect of the release, be especially wary of large public gatherings or large but confined spaces such as public buildings and low spaces that limit dissipation such as subway terminals. Terrorists may also target food or water supplies with either chemical or biological agents. This may result in very widespread effects.

A cardinal sign of a chemical release is the manifestation of similar signs and symptoms occurring rapidly among a group of individuals. Common signs of a chemical release include inflamed mucosa (eye, nasal, oral, or throat irritation), exposed skin irritation, chest tightness, burning and/or dyspnea, gastrointestinal signs (nausea, abdominal cramping, vomiting, and diarrhea), and central nervous system disturbances (confusion, lethargy, nausea/vomiting, intoxication, headache, and unconsciousness).

Management of a Chemical Agent Release

Approach the scene from upwind and higher ground and remain a good distance away from the site. Generally, evacuate the immediate area if the release is small and contained. However, if the release involves a great quantity of material, such as that in a railway tank car or large commercial storage container, evacuate the general population for a radius of 700 to 2,000 feet and 1.5 miles downwind during the day. If the release occurs at night, then evacuate a 2,000-foot radius and as much as 6 to 7 miles downwind (Figure 8-4 ●).

Once the public danger is reduced by scene isolation, make sure the injured are properly decontaminated before you begin care. Rescuers coming out of the danger zones must also be decontaminated. The agency that provides spill containment and decontamination at the hazardous materials incident generally provides decontamination for both nuclear and chemical weapons of mass destruction. This service is most commonly the fire department. (See Chapter 5, Hazardous Materials.)

In addition to the specific emergency care steps noted earlier, most patients require decontamination, exposure to fresh air, oxygen administration, and possibly respiratory support. As a precautionary measure, use personal protective equipment (PPE), including a well-fitting HEPA filter mask, nitrile gloves (latex gloves do not offer much protection against chemical agents), and a Tyvek® disposable suit. Be careful of leather clothing items. Belts, watchbands, and shoes made of leather absorb many chemical agents and will present a continuing exposure danger once contaminated. These precautions provide very minimal protection against chemical agents and do not constitute the PPE necessary to work in a warm or hot zone.

BIOLOGICAL AGENTS

Biological agents are either living organisms or toxins produced by living organisms that are deliberately distributed to cause disease, incapacitation, and death. Generally, these agents are grouped as noncontagious (anthrax and biotoxins) or as contagious and capable of spreading from human to human (smallpox, Ebola, plague). Contagious agents are of greatest concern because the people originally infected can spread the disease, often before the medical community has recognized that a biological weapon attack has occurred. EMS and other medical systems are especially vulnerable because they are called to treat those who first display the disease's signs and symptoms, possibly before the nature and significance of the disease is known. Noncontagious agents affect only those who received the initial dose, thus limiting the scope of the disease and making it somewhat easier to identify when and where the contact took place.

Identification of a biological agent release is difficult because there is often no noticeable cloud of gas or any noticeable odor.

Hot, Warm, and Cold Zones Associated with a Hazardous Materials Release

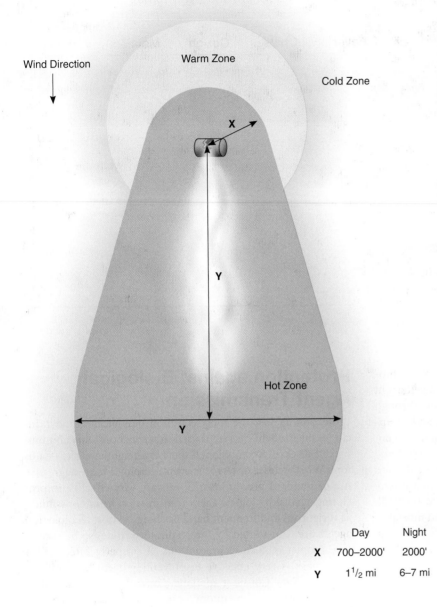

	Day	Night
X	700–2000'	2000'
Y	1½ mi	6–7 mi

● **Figure 8-4** Hot, warm, and cold zones associated with a hazardous materials release.

health department begin to work to identify the disease's nature and when and where the exposure most likely happened. By the time the disease outbreak is recognized as a bioterrorism event, secondary exposures from those affected by contagious agents may already be occurring. These secondary exposures may include family members, friends, workmates, and the medical system, including EMS, emergency department personnel, and other health care providers.

Mother Nature may be the most sinister of all bioterrorists. Mutant strains of common diseases, such as the more serious variations of influenza, multiple-drug-resistant strains of tuberculosis, or the recent cold-like virus called *severe acute respiratory syndrome (SARS)*, may emerge and create epidemics of massive proportions. Outbreaks of naturally occurring disease may be more likely and more severe than a terrorist's use of a biological weapon. Tracking the origin and combating these naturally occurring diseases is exactly like tracking and combating a biological weapon used by terrorists.

Currently the list of potential WMD diseases is extensive and contains pneumonia-like agents, encephalitis-like agents, and others.

Pneumonia-Like Agents

Pneumonia-like bioterror agents include anthrax, plague, tularemia, and Q fever and are the most likely agents for a terrorist attack.[5] They generally cause cough, dyspnea, fever, and malaise. Anthrax and plague are the most deadly, with 90 to 100 percent mortality. Anthrax is a very effective biological agent, though it is not contagious, which limits any human-to-human transmission. The strain of plague most likely used for bioterrorism is pneumonic, which carries not only a very high mortality (100 percent untreated and about 57 percent when treated), but also has minimum victim survival when left untreated for the first 18 hours after signs and symptoms appear. Pneumonic plague incubates over one to four days and can be spread through droplets and inhalation. Tularemia (also known as rabbit fever or deerfly fever) may be aerosolized and presents with signs and symptoms in two to ten days. It carries a mortality rate of up to 5 percent. Q fever may appear in 10 to 20 days after contact and lasts from two days to two weeks; however, it is more of an incapacitating disease with a very low death rate.

Encephalitis-Like Agents

Smallpox and Venezuelan equine encephalitis (VEE) are influenza-like diseases with headache, fever, and malaise and a higher mortality, probably because these diseases attack

This identification is especially challenging because any signs and symptoms of the disease occur at the end of the incubation period, often days or weeks after the initial contact. Rapid identification is further complicated because many potential biological weapons present with signs and symptoms typical of influenza or many other common and general illnesses (Table 8–1).

Most commonly, the existence of a biological attack is recognized when numerous patients report to the emergency department or medical clinic with similar signs and symptoms or when a health care provider notices a geographic cluster of patients. Care providers may also notice a disease occurring out of season (many patients with flulike symptoms during the summer) or a disease outside its normal geographic regions (tropical disease in the northern latitudes). Only then can the

TABLE 8–1 | Characteristics of Biological Agents

Disease	Incubation Period	Mortality	Signs and Symptoms				
			Fever	Chills	Cough	Malaise	Nausea/ Vomiting
Anthrax	1–6 days	90%	√		√	√	
Pneumonic plague*	1–6 days	57–100%	√	√	√	√	
Tularemia	3–5 days	35%	√		√	√	
Q fever	2–14 days	1%	√		√	√	
Smallpox*	12 days	30%	√			√	√
Venezuelan equine encephalitis	1–5 days	1%	√	√	√	√	√
Cholera	1–3 days	50%					√
Viral hemorrhagic fever	3–7 days	5–20%	√			√	
Ebola*	3–7 days	80–90%	√			√	

*Human-to-human contagious disease.

the central nervous system. They are very effective as biological weapons because small amounts of aerosolized agent can cause the disease. Smallpox is very contagious through airborne droplets via the respiratory route. Signs and symptoms usually appear after about 12 days in about 30 percent of those exposed, with about a third of that number dying within five to seven days. Smallpox is considered eradicated as a naturally occurring disease, but it is thought that it may exist in the WMD programs of some countries. With VEE, human-to-human transmission does not occur, and mortality is generally less than 20 percent.

Other Agents

Cholera is a common disease in underdeveloped countries and is frequently linked to poor sanitation. It is most commonly transmitted by the fecal–oral route and primarily causes severe dehydration and shock because of profuse diarrhea. It is one of the few agents that is not transmitted by the inhalation route and may be delivered as a weapon by way of contamination of food or untreated water.

Viral hemorrhagic fever (VHF) is a class of disease that includes the deadly Ebola virus. As the name suggests, hemorrhagic fever attacks the bloodstream and damages blood vessels, causing them to leak and the patient to bleed easily. The patient may bruise easily and display petechiae (tiny red patches of dermal hemorrhage). Most diseases of this class can be spread through the inhalation route or through direct contact with infectious material. VHFs may carry a high mortality rate (90 percent) and are aerosolized easily, though they are difficult to cultivate.

Protection against Biological Agent Transmission

Protection against the most common biological weapons includes the prudent care steps used to prevent ordinary communicable disease transmission. If there is a heightened alert status for a WMD release or terrorist event, employ a more aggressive use of standard precautions. Gloves are very effective in protecting against biological agent transmission from body fluids, as is rigorous and frequent hand washing. Almost all biological agents are transmitted by the respiratory route, so be sure to take droplet inhalation precautions. A properly fitted HEPA filter mask is very effective in preventing agent transmission (Figure 8-5 ●). Consider applying a mask to your patient if he displays any signs or symptoms of respiratory disease. A sodium

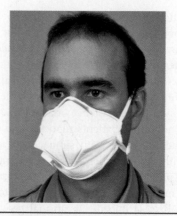

● **Figure 8-5**   A HEPA filter mask.

hypochlorite solution (0.5 percent) or other disinfectants are very effective in killing many biological agents. The ambulance interior and any equipment used or possibly contaminated should be cleaned vigorously with the solution.

Immunizations against many biological agents are not available. Those immunizations that are available usually carry a small risk of associated reaction. Hence, the prophylactic administration to a very large number of health care workers may not be warranted unless or until a significant risk becomes apparent. Consult with your medical director for your system's recommendations and the method used to provide you with immunizations if the need arises.

Emergency care for most patients affected by biological weapons is limited to supportive care—maintain body temperature, administer oxygen, and provide hydration (and, in some cases, IV fluids). Because some of the biological agents may produce respiratory compromise, protocols may call for an albuterol or other nebulized treatment. If practical, consider the use of metered-dose inhalers (MDIs) rather than nebulization, because MDIs limit aerosolized-droplet formation and subsequent risk of contaminating inhalation. Once the exact organism is isolated (after prehospital care), then a regimen of antibiotic therapy may be prescribed.

If a biological attack is suspected, health officials will interview the victims carefully. They will try to determine when the patients first noticed symptoms and identify any close personal contacts since that time. These people may be infected if the agent is indeed contagious. The public health approach to biological terrorism may also involve isolation and quarantine. The patient or caregiver exposed to a highly contagious disease may be quarantined through a restriction to home or may be confined within a commandeered facility such as a motel. A person with the signs and symptoms of the disease may be isolated through a similar arrangement. There is a danger associated with placing affected patients or caregivers in a hospital or other medical facility because they can then endanger other patients or care providers who are receiving or providing care there.

GENERAL CONSIDERATIONS REGARDING TERRORIST ATTACKS

Scene Safety

One in every five victims of the World Trade Center collapse on September 11, 2001, was a member of an emergency response team. This great number of emergency personnel deaths underscores the need to recognize the dangers to EMS providers and ensure that safety is an active concern during the response to any potential act of terrorism.

Terrorists in other countries often set secondary explosive devices with the intent to disrupt any rescue attempt. A chemical release or radioactivity can linger and affect those who attempt unprotected rescue of patients. Biological agents are likely to affect the EMS provider as well. It is imperative that you carefully analyze a scene to determine the risk to you and other rescuers. Then

ensure that the scene is entered only by those properly equipped and trained to enter a hazardous or deadly environment.

Recognizing a Terrorist Attack

It is relatively easy to recognize a nuclear or conventional explosion. However, remember that radioactive fallout travels with the upper wind current (not just currents at ground level), so watch cloud movement. Stay upwind. Remember, too, that terrorists may use the conventional explosion to distribute radioactive or other hazardous material (the "dirty bomb"), and they may set secondary detonations through booby traps or timers that are designed to target rescuers. Also be aware of structural collapse, because the explosion may weaken a building's structure. Do not enter the scene until you are sure it is safe from all hazards.

A chemical release may not be as obvious. There may or may not be a cloud of gas or aerosolized material. There also may or may not be any unusual odors. However, groups of victims will be complaining of similar symptoms, although symptom development may take some time. Suspect a chemical incident when you notice incapacitated small animals, birds, and insects. You may also be alerted to a possible chemical incident when confronted with chemical-exposure-like symptoms where chemicals are not usually used. Stay upwind and uphill of the site and request that victims and potential victims evacuate (or be evacuated) to you. Only personnel who are specially trained and equipped to deal with hazardous materials should enter the scene. However, to protect yourself, don nitrile gloves, a well-fitting HEPA filter mask, and a Tyvek® coverall when caring for a patient who has been decontaminated. These precautions provide only limited protection while working on decontaminated patients. They are not considered adequate for entry into the scene (warm or hot zone).[6, 7]

Identifying a biological agent at the time of release is probably impossible. There might be a cloud of dust or aerosolized material but there are no immediate signs and symptoms from those exposed. Such contamination also may be distributed by the mail (anthrax-laced letters, for instance) or other mechanisms. The incident is likely to be recognized after the incubation period and only after several patients report to the emergency departments or clinics with the disease. Then the local health department will investigate what all victims have in common to identify where the biological agent release took place. If you happen to notice many patients presenting with signs and symptoms of illness at or around the same time, consider a possible biological attack. As with any potential disease, don gloves and a well-fitted HEPA filter mask. (See Volume 4, Chapter 10, Infectious Diseases and Sepsis.) It is important to remember that you may be inadvertently exposed to a contagious agent, contract the disease, and then become a carrier. If you become aware of possible exposure or notice the signs and symptoms of a contagious disease, contact the proper health resource (your medical director, service infection control agent, or other person, according to protocols or your service policies) and ensure that you do not transmit the disease to others.

Responding to a Terrorist Attack

Your first role in responding to a possible act of terrorism is to ensure your own safety and that of your patient, other rescuers, and the public. Once safety is ensured, make certain all patients are properly decontaminated (if need be) and then begin to provide the appropriate emergency medical care.

Your role as an emergency care provider for a terrorist attack is very similar to the other emergency responses you are more likely to encounter during your career. A nuclear incident is handled as a conventional explosion with a hazardous material (radiation) involved. The release of a chemical agent is a hazardous material incident. A biological weapon release is handled like an infectious disease outbreak. Although the location of the attack may maximize the number of people it affects, it is still a hazardous material incident (chemical or radiation agent), an infectious disease incident (biological event), a conventional explosion, or a combination. Use the training you already have for these situations and follow your system's protocols and disaster plans for each.

Once a WMD incident is identified, begin preparing for the casualties. Often this will entail instituting the incident command system and establishing extrication, decontamination, triage, treatment, and transport sectors. Carefully match the available resources against the nature, number, and severity of injuries. Review Chapter 3, Multiple-Casualty Incidents and Incident Management.

CHAPTER REVIEW

SUMMARY

Many of the mechanisms of injury used by terrorists (toxic gases, radiation contamination, or biological agents) induce their damage subtly so that there is little scene evidence. Your responsibility is to maintain an enhanced lookout for any signs of CBRNE release or exposure and limit the contact that you, the general population, and your patients have to such an agent. In general, it is not the role of EMS to deal with CBRNE agents. Your role as a paramedic is likely to be providing supportive care after patient decontamination.

YOU MAKE THE CALL

You are dispatched to "an explosion with possible injuries." Your emergency vehicle is the first to arrive at a synagogue with smoke pouring from broken windows and obviously injured people on the lawn.

1. What special safety considerations would you observe for this scene?

2. What are the likely injuries to expect from this mechanism of injury?

3. Should you enter the synagogue?

See Suggested Responses at the back of this book.

REVIEW QUESTIONS

1. _____ are the most common method by which terrorists strike.
   a. Explosives
   b. Chemical weapons
   c. Anthrax exposures
   d. Poisonings of public water supplies

2. After an initial explosion, associated dangers include _____.
   a. fire
   b. electrical hazard
   c. structural collapse
   d. all of the above

3. _____ are likely to be the most lethal and debilitating injuries associated with a nuclear detonation.
   a. Burn injuries
   b. Inhalation injuries
   c. Blunt trauma injuries
   d. Penetrating trauma injuries

4. If there is serious risk of fallout and continuing radiation exposure, paramedics may be asked to help distribute _____ tablets.
   a. iron
   b. magnesium
   c. potassium iodide
   d. sodium chloride

5. Which of the following is not a common example of a nerve agent?
   a. GB (sarin)
   b. GD (soman)
   c. GA (tabun)
   d. carbamate (sevin)

6. Emergency care for the patient exposed to a vesicant is immediate _____.
   a. triage
   b. fluid therapy
   c. oxygenation
   d. decontamination

7. Which of the following agents is not considered contagious?
   a. Ebola
   b. anthrax
   c. plague
   d. smallpox

8. _____ is a common disease in underdeveloped countries and is frequently linked to poor sanitation.
   a. Cholera
   b. SARS
   c. Tularemia
   d. VEE

See Answers to Review Questions at the back of this book.

REFERENCES

1. Stevens, G., A. Jones, G. Smith, et al. "Determinants of Paramedic Response Readiness for CBRNE Threats." _Biosecur Bioterror_ 8 (2010): 193–202.

2. Grace, M. B., K. D. Cliffer, B. R. Moyer, et al. "The U.S. Government's Medical Countermeasure Portfolio Management for Nuclear and Radiological Emergencies: Synergy from Interagency Cooperation." _Health Phys_ 10 (2011): 238–247.

3. Sandilands, E. A., A. M. Good, and D. N. Batemen. "The Use of Atropine as a Nerve Agent Response with Specific Reference to Children: Are Current Guidelines Too Cautious?" _Emerg Med J_ 26 (2009): 690–694.

4. Aas, P. "The Threat of Mid-Spectrum Chemical Warfare Agents." _Prehosp Disaster Med_ 18 (2003): 306–312.

5. Daya, M. and Y. Nakamura. "Pulmonary Disease from Biological Agents: Anthrax, Plague, Q Fever, and Tularemia." _Crit Care Clin_ 21 (2005): 747–763.

6. Castle, N., R. Owen, S. Clark, et al. "Comparison of Techniques for Securing the Endotracheal Tube while Wearing Chemical, Biological, Radiological, or Nuclear Protection: A Manikin Study." _Prehosp Disaster Med_ 25 (2010): 589–594.

7. Castle, N., Y. Pillay, and N. Spencer. "Comparison of Six Different Intubation Aids for Use while Wearing CBRN-PPE: A Manikin Study." _Resuscitation_ 82(12) (2011): 1548–1552.

FURTHER READING

Bevelacqua, A., and R. Stilp. _Terrorism Handbook for Operational Responders._ 3rd ed. Clifton Park, NY: Delmar Cengage Learning, 2009.

Buck, G. _Preparing for Biological Terrorism: An Emergency Services Guide._ Albany, NY: Delmar Publishing, 2002.

Byrnes, M. E., D. A. King, and P. M. Tierno. _Nuclear, Chemical, and Biological Terrorism: Emergency Response and Public Protection._ Chelsea, MI: Lewis Publishers, 2003.

De Lorenzo, Robert A., and Robert S. Porter. _Tactical Emergency Care: Military and Operational Out-of-Hospital Medicine._ Upper Saddle River, NJ: Pearson/Prentice Hall, 1999.

Emergency Response Guidebook (ERG2008). Washington, DC: U.S. Department of Transportation, 2008.

Marks, M. E. _Emergency Responder's Guide to Terrorism._ Chester, MD: Red Hat Publishers, 2003.

Sachs, G. _Terrorism Emergency Response: A Workbook for Responders._ Upper Saddle River, NJ: Pearson/Prentice Hall, 2003.

Sidell, F. R., W. C. Patrick III, and T. R. Dashiell. _Jane's Chem-Bio Handbook._ 2nd ed. Alexandria, VA: Jane's Information Group, 2003.

PRECAUTIONS ON BLOODBORNE PATHOGENS AND INFECTIOUS DISEASES

Prehospital emergency personnel, like all health care workers, are at risk for exposure to bloodborne pathogens and infectious diseases. In emergency situations it is often difficult to take or enforce proper infection control measures. However, as a paramedic, you must recognize your high-risk status. Study the following information on infection control carefully.

Infection control is designed to protect emergency personnel, their families, and their patients from unnecessary exposure to communicable diseases. Laws, regulations, and standards regarding infection control include:

- *Centers for Disease Control and Prevention (CDC) Guidelines.* The CDC has published extensive guidelines on infection control. Proper equipment and techniques that should be used by emergency response personnel to prevent or minimize risk of exposure are defined.
- *The Ryan White Act.* The Ryan White Act of 1990 allows emergency personnel to find out if they were exposed to an infectious disease while rendering patient care. Employers are required to name a "designated officer" to coordinate communications with the treating hospital.
- *Americans with Disabilities Act.* This act prohibits discrimination against individuals with disabilities, including those with contagious diseases. It guarantees equal employment opportunities and job protection if the infected individual can perform essential job functions and does not pose a threat to the safety and health of patients and coworkers.
- *Occupational Safety and Health Administration (OSHA) Regulations.* OSHA has enacted a regulation entitled Occupational Exposure to Bloodborne Pathogens that classifies emergency response personnel as being at the greatest risk of occupational exposure to communicable diseases. This regulation requires employers to provide hepatitis B (HBV) vaccinations free of charge, maintain a written exposure control plan, and provide personal protective equipment. These requirements primarily apply to private employers. Applicability to local and state governmental employees varies by locality. Many states have developed their own OSHA plans.
- *National Fire Protection Association (NFPA) Guidelines.* This is a national organization that has established specific guidelines and requirements regarding infection control for emergency response agencies, particularly fire departments and EMS services.

STANDARD PRECAUTIONS AND PERSONAL PROTECTIVE EQUIPMENT

Emergency response personnel should practice Standard Precautions by which ALL body substances are considered to be potentially infectious. To practice Standard Precautions, all emergency personnel should utilize personal protective equipment (PPE). Appropriate PPE should be available on every emergency vehicle. The minimum recommended PPE includes the following:

- *Gloves.* Disposable gloves should be donned by all emergency response personnel BEFORE initiating any emergency care. When an emergency incident involves more than one patient, you should attempt to change gloves between patients. When gloves have been contaminated, they should be removed as soon as possible. To properly remove contaminated gloves, grasp one glove approximately 1 inch from the wrist. Without touching the inside of the glove, pull the glove halfway off and stop. With that half-gloved hand, pull the glove on the opposite hand completely off. Place the removed glove in the palm of the other glove, with the inside of the removed glove exposed. Pull the second glove completely off with the ungloved hand, only touching the inside of the glove. Always wash hands after gloves are removed, even when the gloves appear intact.
- *Masks and Protective Eyewear.* Masks and protective eyewear should be present on all emergency vehicles and used in accordance with the level of exposure encountered. Masks and protective eyewear should be worn together whenever blood spatter is likely to occur, such as during arterial bleeding, childbirth, endotracheal intubation, invasive procedures, oral

suctioning, and cleanup of equipment that requires heavy scrubbing or brushing. Both you and the patient should wear masks whenever the potential for airborne transmission of disease exists.

- *HEPA and N-95 Respirators.* Due to the resurgence of tuberculosis (TB), prehospital personnel should protect themselves from TB infection through use of an N-95 or a high-efficiency particulate air (HEPA) respirator, as approved by the National Institute of Occupational Safety and Health (NIOSH). It should fit snugly and be capable of filtering out the tuberculosis bacillus. An N-95 or HEPA respirator should be worn when caring for patients with confirmed or suspected TB. This is especially true when performing "high-hazard" procedures such as administration of nebulized medications, endotracheal intubation, or suctioning on such a patient.
- *Gowns.* Gowns protect clothing from blood splashes. If large splashes of blood are expected, such as with childbirth, wear impervious gowns.
- *Resuscitation Equipment.* Disposable resuscitation equipment should be the primary means of artificial ventilation in emergency care. Such items should be used once, then disposed of.

Remember, the proper use of personal protective equipment ensures effective infection control and minimizes risk. Use ALL protective equipment recommended for any particular situation to ensure maximum protection.

Consider ALL body substances potentially infectious and ALWAYS practice Standard Precautions.

The following are suggested responses to the "You Make the Call" scenarios presented in each chapter of Paramedic Care, Volume 7, Operations. Each represents an acceptable response to the scenario but should not be interpreted as the only correct response.

Chapter 1—Ground Ambulance Operations

1. *Should you drive down the open eastbound right lane with your lights and siren on? Explain.*

No—you should always use the left to pass vehicles. Motorists are taught to "move to the right when you see the lights" and by attempting to pass on the right, there is a potential that motorists may move to the right, into your path, as they try to make room.

2. *Should you enter the oncoming traffic by going around the left side of the vehicle that is currently stopped in the left-hand, eastbound lane? Explain.*

Yes—passing to the left is the safest place to pass. By cautiously moving into the oncoming traffic lane, you will be able to capture the westbound traffic's attention and move around other vehicles in the eastbound lane safely. Remember, this should be done cautiously and at a rate of speed slow enough to allow you to stop and maneuver as necessary to avoid obstacles.

3. *How can you best deal with this very dangerous intersection?*

The best method for dealing with this intersection is to make sure all your warning devices are operating (lights, siren, air horn). If your unit is equipped with an emergency horn, such as an air horn or horn on the siren, you should sound it as you approach the intersection. Changing the siren function from wail to high/low, yelp, or even phaser (depending on the type of siren) will also help to capture attention.

Begin to move to the left lane slowly so that all vehicles (that are aware of you) see where you are moving to. Slow down to a contained, slow, safe speed as you approach the intersection. Watch in all directions for traffic movement and be prepared to stop. When you get to the intersection, you should stop, make sure traffic has stopped in all directions, and then proceed through the intersection slowly.

Chapter 2—Air Medical Operations

1. *Would you go ahead and allow the patient to be transported by helicopter when her condition clearly does not warrant helicopter transport?*

Not based on the current findings. If the patient was showing signs of shock or decomposition, then it might be an option, but currently she is not showing those signs and does not require the use of an emergency helicopter service.

2. *What would you tell her husband and the first responders to explain your decision to not transport by helicopter?*

You must be very diplomatic in these situations to avoid upsetting the squad/fire department and/or the family. Explain to the family and squad the indications for helicopter transport and the importance of keeping the helicopter available for other emergencies. You can also explain to them your ability and commitment to keep the patient comfortable for the duration of the ride.

3. *What options are available to you to assist in dealing with the situation?*

If necessary, you can contact medical control to help you in making these decisions. Your medical director may very well talk with the family member if necessary to help mitigate the situation.

Additionally, based on your protocols, you can provide this patient with pain relief medications that will help with her comfort for the ride.

Chapter 3—Multiple-Casualty Incidents and Incident Management

1. *What two roles in the Incident Management System will you and your partner fill, as you are first on scene?*

One of you will be incident command while the other will begin size-up and triage as necessary.

2. *How would you size up the incident?*

You need to determine a safe location to stage the EMS units, as well as how many confirmed patients and how many suspected patients/victims you have. Determine the number of resources that are on the way and how many additional resources you are going to need. Make a radio call to give a brief report of what you have determined and what you have found.

3. *What additional resources would you anticipate, and what instructions would you provide for them?*

You can anticipate the need for more ambulances, medical first responders, and fire units. Let the ambulances and medical first responders know where the staging area will be and who the contact will be for that area so they can receive orders when they arrive.

4. *How would you use the Incident Management System to organize this incident?*

At this point you know that you will need an incident commander, medical operations chief, and fire operations chief. Under the medical operations you will need triage, treatment, and transport divisions. Depending on the number of resources, you can assign those to different people or overlap roles. Additionally, you will need a safety officer and potentially a public information officer.

5. *What would your initial radio report sound like in this incident?*

Medic One is on scene assuming command. We have a multiple-story motel with heavy smoke showing from the back. We have reports of twenty-plus victims. Requesting an additional eight transport units. Have all EMS stage at [give the staging location].

Chapter 4—Rescue Awareness and Operations

1. *What are your immediate considerations as you size up the scene?*

Immediate considerations include safety, hazards, number of patients, control of traffic and bystanders, and need for additional resources (implementation of the IMS).

2. *Why would you consider this a rescue operation?*

Because the patient is unconscious and entrapped in a potentially unstable vehicle/environment.

3. *What additional resources would you request?*

Additional resources might include police, fire department, another EMS unit, and possibly a low-angle rescue team to help move the patient up the embankment.

Chapter 5—Hazardous Materials

1. *What do you suspect has happened based on your quick scene size-up?*

You suspect hazardous materials are involved in the incident. The tractor-trailer is carrying a placard, it is leaking some kind of liquid, and occupants are drooling, tearing, sweating, and experiencing respiratory distress.

2. *What are your initial priorities?*

Your initial priorities are life safety, incident stabilization, and property conservation.

3. *How will you identify the substance involved in the accident?*

Identification of the substance can be performed by interpreting the placard that indicates some kind of poison. An NAERG will identify the specific chemical. Based on the poison placard and the SLUDGE symptoms exhibited by the occupants of the truck, you suspect an organophosphate insecticide. Positive identification can be made using the shipping papers found with the driver of the truck or in the cab. You might also consult one or more of the computerized data banks or telephone hotlines mentioned in this chapter.

4. *What additional resources would you request?*

You will ask for a hazmat team and special fire apparatus. These units will be needed for entry, removal of the patient from the car, hazard control, and decontamination. You will also request three additional ambulances. Counting your unit, there will be one ambulance for each patient and one for the hazardous materials team.

5. *Is this a fast-break or a long-term incident? Explain.*

This is a fast-break incident. Two patients exhibiting critical symptoms have self-rescued and brought themselves to your ambulance.

6. *What are your first actions?*

Your first actions are to secure the scene, set up a perimeter to prevent further decontamination, and request assistance. On arrival of fire apparatus, available PPE can be donned, and two-step decontamination performed on the two occupants of the truck who are near your ambulance.

Chapter 6—Crime Scene Awareness

1. What is your evaluation of this situation from a safety perspective?

There is a significant potential for danger. The son's apparent intoxication, combined with the patient's warning that he "isn't quite right when he's drinking," clearly indicates the need for immediate action.

2. What are your options?

The two immediate options both involve retreat. You either retreat with the patient or without the patient. In this case, both you and the son want the same thing—for you to leave. However, unless you can calm down the son, you may have to leave the patient behind, at least temporarily. Even though this action may be tactically and legally correct, thoughts of abandonment charges can be haunting. You may try to buy some time until the police arrive, but your main priority is personal safety. You also know that further agitation may only worsen the patient's condition. No matter how unsatisfactory, you may have to leave the scene until the police arrive to take charge of the situation.

Chapter 7—Rural EMS

1. What apparatus or support are you going to need to perform this rescue?

As soon as the mechanism of injury and scene environment are known, additional personnel should be summoned. Because the water is surrounded by high cliffs and is remote, you should request a water rescue team. Following the request for adequate support and specialized rescue teams, you determine whether to transport the patient by helicopter or a ground unit. The transport time to the trauma center, the weather, the difficulty accessing the patient, and the overall time from the onset of the injury should be considered. It is better to ask for help that you may not need than to need help and realize it has not been requested.

2. Based on the mechanism of injury, what injuries should you suspect?

The victim jumped into the water from a 50-foot cliff and landed in water of unknown depth, but apparently shallow. The history that he "jumped" rather than "dove" into the water indicates that the patient may have lower extremity injuries in addition to head and chest injuries. Because the patient is unresponsive, it is likely that he has sustained a head injury. A chest injury is possible, as is the possibility of barotrauma if he held his breath when he jumped. If the patient landed on his feet, you should expect lower extremity injuries, including possible calcaneal fractures, lumbar spine fractures, and a cervical spinal injury. Always assume the worst and hope for the best.

3. What will you do to stabilize this patient?

Stabilization of this patient is primarily surgical. However, you can attempt "field stabilization" while rescue resources prepare for egress from the quarry. The airway should be controlled if the GCS is less than or equal to 8. Full spinal immobilization should occur. Special attention should be paid to the chest because the patient is at risk for direct trauma and barotrauma. The on-scene time could be prolonged. Therefore, initiate fluid therapy per protocols and splint any fractures. If the patient has a neurologic deficit consistent with a spinal cord injury, consider beginning high-dose methylprednisolone therapy. Be sure to protect body temperature.

4. What factors made it impossible for you to meet response, treatment, and transport times in the rural setting when compared with the urban or suburban setting?

The location, mechanism of injury, required rescue resources, distance to the trauma center, and many other factors indicate that this patient will not be in a trauma center within an hour, much less an operating room. You may have to provide extended care while extrication is carried out. You have to do the best you can with what you have available. This victim undertook a high-risk exposure with some knowledge that transport to a hospital might be quite prolonged. He has to accept those risks.

Chapter 8—Responding to Terrorist Acts

1. What special safety considerations would you observe for this scene?

In addition to concerns about broken glass, structural collapse, smoke inhalation, electricity, and fire dangers, you should have concerns about secondary explosives that may have been set to injure rescuers and about possible chemical or radioactive contamination associated with the blast.

2. What are the likely injuries to expect from this mechanism of injury?

Suspect pressure injuries to the hollow organs—ears, bowel, sinuses, and lungs—with a special concern for injury to the lungs. Anticipate penetrating trauma from debris thrown by the blast or injury secondary to the patient being thrown by the blast. Smoke inhalation may also affect patients as may the emotional stress of the incident.

3. Should you enter the synagogue?

No, await the fire service because of the smoke and advise them to use caution in case there are secondary explosive devices. Treat patients upwind and at a safe distance from the incident.

ANSWERS TO REVIEW QUESTIONS

Below are the answers to the Review Questions presented in each chapter of Volume 7.

CHAPTER 1—GROUND AMBULANCE OPERATIONS

1. c
2. b
3. c
4. d
5. c
6. a

CHAPTER 2—AIR MEDICAL OPERATIONS

1. a
2. d
3. a
4. d
5. c
6. d
7. a
8. b
9. a
10. d
11. b
12. b
13. c
14. b
15. b
16. d
17. d
18. a
19. a

CHAPTER 3—MULTIPLE-CASUALTY INCIDENTS AND INCIDENT MANAGEMENT

1. b
2. b
3. d
4. c
5. b
6. b
7. a
8. a
9. c
10. a

CHAPTER 4—RESCUE AWARENESS AND OPERATIONS

1. d
2. b
3. a
4. c
5. b
6. a
7. d
8. a
9. c
10. c

CHAPTER 5—HAZARDOUS MATERIALS

1. c
2. b
3. d
4. b

5. c
6. d
7. a
8. a

CHAPTER 6—CRIME SCENE AWARENESS

1. b
2. b
3. d
4. b
5. c
6. c
7. c
8. b

CHAPTER 7—RURAL EMS

1. b
2. c
3. d
4. d
5. b
6. d

CHAPTER 8—RESPONDING TO TERRORIST ACTS

1. a
2. d
3. a
4. c
5. d
6. d
7. b
8. a

acetylcholinesterase (AChE)   enzyme that stops the action of acetylcholine, a neurotransmitter.

active rescue zone   area in which special rescue teams operate; also known as the "hot zone" or "inner circle."

acute effects   signs and/or symptoms rapidly displayed on exposure to a toxic substance.

ADAMS   Atlas and Database of Air Medical Services, created by the Center for Transportation Injury Research and the Association of Air Medical Services that includes information on air medical service providers, their communication centers, base helipads, rotor and fixed wing aircraft, and receiving hospitals.

aeromedical evacuation   transport by helicopter.

air bags   inflatable high-pressure pillows that when inflated can lift up to 20 tons, depending on the make.

air-purifying respirator (APR)   system of filtering a normal environment for a specific chemical substance using filter cartridges.

biological agents   either living organisms or toxins produced by living organisms that are deliberately distributed to cause disease and death.

biotoxins   poisons that are produced by a living organism but are themselves not alive.

biotransformation   changing a substance in the body from one chemical to another; in the case of hazardous materials, the body tries to create less toxic materials.

blood spatter evidence   the pattern that blood forms when it is splattered or dropped at the scene of a crime.

body armor   vest made of tightly woven, strong fibers that offer protection against handgun bullets, most knives, and blunt trauma; also known as "bulletproof vests."

branches   functional levels within the IMS based on primary roles and geographic locations.

CAMEO®   Computer-Aided Management of Emergency Operations; website developed by the EPA and NOAA as a source of information, skills, and links related to hazardous substances.

C-FLOP   mnemonic for the main functional areas within the IMS command: finance/administration, logistics, operations, and planning.

CBRNE   acronym for chemical, biological, radiological, nuclear, and explosive, developed following the increase in terrorism; refers to situations in which any of these five hazards is or may be present.

CHEMTEL   Chemical Telephone, Inc.; maintains a 24-hour, toll-free hotline at 800-255-3024; for collect calls and calls from other points of origin, dial 813-979-0626.

CHEMTREC   Chemical Transportation Emergency Center; maintains a 24-hour, toll-free hotline at 800-424-9300; for collect calls and calls from other points of origin, dial 703-527-3887.

closed incident   an incident that is not likely to generate any further patients; also known as a contained incident.

cold zone   location at a hazmat incident outside the warm zone; area where incident operations take place; also called the green zone or the safe zone.

command   the individual or group responsible for coordinating all activities and who makes final decisions on the emergency scene; often referred to as the incident commander (IC) or officer in charge (OIC).

command staff   officers who report directly to the incident commander; officers who handle public information, safety, and outside liaisons, also known as management staff.

compartment syndrome   condition that occurs when circulation to a portion of the body is cut off; after a period of time toxins can develop in the blood, leading to shock when circulation is restored.

concealment   hiding the body behind objects that shield a person from view but that offer little or no protection against bullets or other ballistics.

consensus standards   widely agreed-on guidelines, such as those developed by the National Fire Protection Association and others.

CONTOMS   Counter-Narcotics Tactical Operations; program that manages the training and certification of EMT-Ts and SWAT-Medics.

cover   hiding the body behind solid and impenetrable objects that protect a person from bullets.

cribbing   wooden slats used to shore up heavy equipment.

crush points   mechanisms of injury in which two or more objects come together with enough weight or force to crush the affected appendage.

cytochrome oxidase   enzyme complex, found in cellular mitochondria, that enables oxygen to create the adenosine triphosphate (ATP) required for all muscle energy.

delayed effects   signs, symptoms, and/or conditions developed hours, days, weeks, months, or even years after the exposure.

demobilized   released for use outside the incident, as occurs when resources including personnel, vehicles, and equipment are no longer needed at the scene.

demographic   pertaining to population makeup or changes.

Department of Homeland Security (DHS)   a cabinet-level department of the U.S. government, created in response to the terrorist attacks of September 11, 2001. It is charged with protecting the United States and its territories from terrorist attacks and overseeing the response to terrorist attacks, man-made accidents, and natural disasters.

deployment   strategy used by an EMS agency to maneuver its ambulances and crews in an effort to reduce response times.

dirty bomb   a conventional explosive device that distributes radioactive material over a large area.

disaster management   management of incidents that generate large numbers of patients, often overwhelming resources and damaging parts of the infrastructure.

disentanglement   process of freeing a patient from wreckage, to allow for proper care, removal, and transfer.

dosimeter   an instrument that measures the cumulative amount of radiation absorbed.

DOT KKK 1822E specs   the manufacturing and design specifications produced by the Federal General Services Administrative Automotive Commodity Center.

due regard   legal terminology found in the motor vehicle laws of most states that sets up a higher standard for the operators of emergency vehicles.

eddies   water that flows around especially large objects and, for a time, flows upstream around the downside of an obstruction; provides an opportunity to escape dangerous currents.

emergency operations center (EOC)   a site from which civil government officials (municipal, county, state, and/or federal) exercise direction and control in an emergency or disaster.

EMS communications officer   notifies hospitals of incoming patients from a multiple-casualty incident; reports to the transportation officer; may also be called the EMS COM or MED COM.

EMT-Tacticals (EMT-Ts)   EMS personnel trained to serve with a technical emergency medical service or a law enforcement agency.

erythema   general reddening of the skin due to dilation of the superficial capillaries.

essential equipment   equipment/supplies required on every ambulance.

explosives   chemical(s) that, when ignited, instantly generate a great amount of heat resulting in a destructive shock wave and blast wind.

extrication   use of force to free a patient from entrapment; also a group or branch responsible for removing patients from entanglements and transferring them to the treatment area, also known as rescue group.

facilities unit   selects and maintains areas used for rehabilitation and command.

fallout   radioactive dust and particles that may be life threatening to people far from the epicenter of a nuclear detonation.

fasciculations   involuntary contractions or twitchings of muscle fibers.

finance/administration section   responsible for maintaining records for personnel, time, and costs of resources/procurement; reports directly to the IC.

fixed-wing aircraft   vehicles capable of flight that use fixed wings to generate lift; airplanes.

Geiger counter   an instrument used to detect and measure the radiation given off by an object or area.

gold standard   ultimate standard of excellence.

hate crimes   crimes committed against a person solely on the basis of the individual's actual or perceived race, color, national origin, ethnicity, gender, disability, or sexual orientation.

hazardous materials (hazmat)   any substance that causes adverse health effects on human exposure.

heat escape lessening position (HELP)   developed by Dr. John Hayward, it is an in-water, head-up tuck or fetal position designed to reduce heat loss by as much as 60 percent.

hot zone   location at a hazmat incident where the actual hazardous material and highest levels of contamination exist; also called the red zone or the exclusionary zone.

incendiary agents   a subset of explosives with less explosive power but greater heat and burn potential.

incident command post (ICP)   place where command officers from various agencies can meet with each other and select a management staff.

Incident Command System (ICS)   a management program designed for controlling, directing, and coordinating emergency response resources; sometimes used as a synonym for **Incident Management System (IMS).**

incident commander (IC)   the person responsible for coordinating all activities at a multiple-casualty scene.

information officer (IO)   collects data about the incident and releases it to the press or media.

instrument flight rules (IFR)   regulations that permit an aircraft to operate in instrument meteorological conditions.

liaison officer (LO)   coordinates all incident operations that involve outside agencies.

local effects   effects involving areas around the immediate site; should be evaluated based on the burn model.

lock-out/tag-out   locking off of a machinery switch, then placing a tag on the switch stating why it is shut off; method of preventing equipment from being accidentally restarted.

logistics section   supports incident operations, coordinating procurement and distribution of all medical resources.

Mark I kit   a two-part auto-injector set the military uses as treatment for nerve agent exposure; involves the administration of atropine and then pralidoxime chloride.

material safety data sheet (MSDS)   easily accessible sheet of detailed information about chemicals found at fixed facilities.

medical supply unit   coordinates procurement and distribution of equipment and supplies at a multiple-casualty incident.

minimum standards   lowest or least allowable standards.

miosis   abnormal contraction of the pupils; pinpoint pupils.

morgue   area where deceased victims of an incident are collected.

morgue officer   person who supervises the morgue; may report to the triage officer or the treatment officer.

multiple-casualty incident (MCI)   incident that generates large numbers of patients and that often makes traditional EMS response ineffective because of special circumstances surrounding the event; also known as a mass-casualty incident.

mutual aid agreements   agreements or plans for sharing departmental resources.

mutual aid coordination center (MACC)   an aspect of the NIMS system that oversees the coordination and utilization of resources from outside the local public safety entity.

National Incident Management System (NIMS)   national system used for the management of multiple-casualty incidents, involving assumption of responsibility for command and designation and coordination of such elements as triage, treatment, transport, and staging.

nerve agents chemicals that inhibit the degradation of a neurotransmitter (acetylcholine) and quickly facilitate a nervous system overload.

night vision goggles (NVG) electro-optical goggles used to detect visible and infrared energy to provide a visible image in the dark.

nuclear detonation the release of energy that is generated when heavy nuclei split (fission) or light nuclei combine (fusion) to form new elements. The unleashed energy is tremendous and creates an explosion of immense proportion.

open incident an incident that has the potential to generate additional patients; also known as an uncontained incident.

operations fulfills directions from command and does the actual work at an incident.

particulate evidence evidence such as hairs or fibers that cannot be readily seen with the human eye; also known as microscopic or trace evidence.

peak load the highest volume of calls at a given time.

pinch points mechanisms of injury in which two objects come together and catch a portion of the patient's body in between them.

planning provides past, present, and future information about an incident.

primary area of responsibility (PAR) stationing of ambulances at specific high-volume locations.

primary contamination direct exposure of a person or item to a hazardous substance.

primary triage triage that takes place early in the incident, usually on first arrival.

prompt care facilities hospital agencies that provide limited care and nonemergent medical treatment.

pulmonary agents chemicals that primarily cause injury to the lungs; commonly referred to as choking agents.

rapid intervention team ambulance and crew dedicated to stand by in case a rescuer becomes ill or injured.

recirculating currents movement of currents over a uniform obstruction; also known as a "drowning machine."

reportable collisions collisions that involve more than $1,000 in damage or a personal injury.

reserve capacity the ability of an EMS agency to respond to calls beyond those handled by the on-duty crews.

rhinorrhea watery discharge from the nose.

rotor-wing aircraft vehicles that use rotating blades (rotors) to provide lift and propulsion; helicopters.

rust out an inability to keep abreast of new technologies and standards.

safety officer (SO) monitors all on-scene actions and ensures that they do not create any potentially harmful conditions.

SALT acronym for a mass triage system that reflects the components of the assessment: **S**ort, **A**ssess, **L**ifesaving Interventions, and **T**reatment/Transport.

scene-authority law legal state or local statute specifying who has ultimate authority at a multiple-casualty incident.

scrambling climbing over rocks and/or downed trees on a steep trail without the aid of ropes. This can be especially dangerous when the surface is wet or icy.

scree loose pebbles or rock debris that can form on the slopes or bases of mountains; sometimes used to describe debris in sloping dry stream beds.

secondary contamination transfer of a hazardous substance to a noncontaminated person or item via contact with someone or something already contaminated by the substance.

secondary triage triage that takes place after patients are moved to a treatment area to determine any change in status.

section chief officer who supervises major functional areas or sections; reports to the incident commander.

sector interchangeable name for a branch, group, or division; does not, however, designate a functional or geographic area.

semi-decontaminated patient another name for field-decontaminated patient.

shear points mechanisms of injury in which pinch points meet or pass, causing amputation of a body part.

shipping papers documents routinely carried aboard vehicles transporting hazardous materials; ideally should identify specific substances and quantities carried; also known as bills of lading.

short haul a helicopter extrication technique in which a person is attached to a rope that is, in turn, attached to a helicopter. The aircraft lifts off with the person attached to it. Obviously this means of evacuation requires highly specialized skills.

silo gas toxic fumes (oxides of nitrogen, or NO_2) produced by the fermentation of grains in a silo.

singular command process in which a single individual is responsible for coordinating an incident; most useful in single-jurisdictional incidents.

span of control number of people or tasks that a single individual can monitor.

special weapons and tactics (SWAT) team a trained police unit equipped to handle hostage holders and other difficult law enforcement situations.

specific gravity refers to the density or weight of a vapor or gas as compared with air.

spotter the person behind the left rear side of the ambulance who assists the operator in backing up the vehicle.

staff functions supervisory roles in the Incident Management System.

staging area location where ambulances, personnel, and equipment are kept in reserve for use at an incident.

staging officer supervises the staging area and guards against premature commitment of resources and freelancing by personnel; reports to the branch director.

START acronym for the most widely used disaster triage system; stands for **S**imple **T**riage **a**nd **R**apid **T**ransport.

strainers a partial obstruction that filters, or strains, the water such as downed trees or wire mesh; causes an unequal force on the two sides.

synergism a standard pharmacological principle in which two substances or drugs work together to produce an effect that neither of them can produce on their own.

system status management (SSM) a computerized personnel and ambulance deployment system.

systemic effects effects that occur throughout the body after exposure to a toxic substance.

tactical emergency medical service (TEMS) a specially trained unit that provides on-site medical support to law enforcement.

terrorist act the use of violence to provoke fear and influence behavior for political, social, religious, or ethnic goals.

tiered response system system that allows multiple vehicles to arrive at an EMS call at different times, often providing different levels of care or transport.

transportation unit supervisor coordinates operations with the staging officer and the transportation supervisor; gets patients into the ambulance and routed to hospitals.

treatment group supervisor controls all actions in the treatment group/sector.

treatment unit leaders EMS personnel who manage the various treatment units and who report to the treatment group supervisor.

triage act of sorting patients based on the severity of their injuries.

triage group supervisor person who supervises a triage group or triage sector at a multiple-casualty incident.

triage officer the person responsible for triage, or sorting patients into categories based on the severity of their injuries.

UN number a four-digit identification number specific to a given chemical; some UN numbers are assigned to a group of related chemicals, but with different characteristics, such as the UN 1203 designation for diesel fuel, gasohol, gasoline, motor fuels, motor spirits, and petrol. (The letters UN stand for "United Nations." Sometimes the letters NA for "North American" appear with or instead of the UN designation.)

unified command process in which managers from different jurisdictions—law enforcement, fire, EMS—coordinate their activities and share responsibility for command.

vesicants agents that damage exposed skin, frequently causing vesicles (blisters).

visual flight rules (VFR) regulations under which a pilot operates an aircraft in weather conditions clear enough for the pilot to see where the aircraft is going.

volatility the ease with which a chemical changes from a liquid to a gas; the tendency of a chemical agent to evaporate.

warm zone location at a hazmat incident adjacent to the hot zone; area where a decontamination corridor is established; also called the yellow zone or contamination reduction zone.

warning placard diamond-shaped graphic placed on vehicles to indicate hazard classification.

weapons of mass destruction (WMDs) variety of chemical, biological, nuclear, or other devices used by terrorists to strike at government or high-profile targets; designed to create a maximum number of casualties.

windshield survey a survey of the emergency scene conducted by the incident commander through the windshield of his vehicle as it arrives at the scene.

wrap points mechanisms of injury in which an appendage gets caught and significantly twisted.

Absorption, 106
Acetylcholinesterase (AChE), 104
Acids, 104
Active rescue zone, 70
Acute effects, 103
ADAMS (Atlas and Database of Air Medical Services), 26
Agricultural emergencies, 132
    mechanisms of injury, 134–135
    patient care, 135–136
    safety considerations, 132–133
    trauma potential, 133–134
Air bags, 133
Air medical operations
    approach, 28–29
    controversies, 26
    departure, 30
    fixed-wing aircraft, 18
    guidelines, 21–25
    history, 17
    landing zone, 27–28
    limitations, 21, 25
    loading, 29–30
    patient handoff, 29
    in recreational emergencies, 138–139
    rotor-wing aircraft, 18–20
    staffing, 25–26
    uses, 15–16, 20–21
Air-purifying respirator (APR), 109
Alkalis, 104
Alpha radiation, 102
Ambulance collisions, 6–7
Ambulance operations. *See also* Air medical operations
    collision reduction, 7
    deployment, 5–6
    design, 2–3
    due regard standard, 8–9
    escorts, 9
    intersection safety, 10
    lights and sirens, 9
    multiple-vehicle responses, 9
    parking and loading, 9–11
    provider education, 6–7
    staffing, 6
    standard operating procedures, 8
    standards, 2–4
    vehicle/equipment checklist, 4–5
Anthrax, 149, 150
Asphyxiants, chemical, 105
Atropine, 146

Basket stretcher, 85–86
Beta radiation, 102
Biological agents, 148
    characteristics, 150
    cholera, 150
    encephalitis-like, 149–150
    identification of release, 148–149
    pneumonia-like, 149
    protection against, 150–151
    viral hemorrhagic fever, 150

Biotoxins, 147
Biotransformation, 104
Blankets, protective, 65
Blood spatter evidence, 123–124
Body armor, 121
Boiling point, 101
Botulinum, 147
Branches, 45
Bullying, 113
BZ, 148

C-FLOP mnemonic, 39
CAMEO®, 99
Carbon monoxide exposure, 105
Cave-ins, 79–80
Cervical collar, in-water application, 76
Chemical, biological, radiologic, nuclear, and explosive (CBRNE) weapons, 143. *See also* Terrorist acts
Chemical weapons, 145–146
    biotoxins, 147
    incapacitating agents, 147–148
    management of release, 148, 149
    nerve agents, 146
    pulmonary agents, 147
    recognition of release, 148
    vesicants, 146–147
CHEMTEL, 99
CHEMTREC, 99
Cholera, 150
Clandestine drug laboratories, 118–119
Closed incident, 41
Cold zone, 101, 149
Command, 39. *See also* Incident Management System (IMS)
    establishing, 40
    incident communications, 42
    incident size-up, 40–41
    operations functions, 45–46
    procedures, 42–43
    resource utilization, 42
    singular vs. unified, 41
    staging area identification, 41–42
    structure, 59
    termination, 43
Command staff, 43–45
Compartment syndrome, 133
Concealment, 120
Confined spaces, 78–79
Consensus standards, 38
Contact and cover, 120–121
Contamination. *See* Hazardous materials (hazmat) incidents
CONTOMS (Counter-Narcotics Tactical Operations), 122
Corrosives, 104
Cover, 120
Cribbing, 133
Crime scene awareness, 113–114
    approach, 114–116
    clandestine drug laboratories, 118–119
    domestic violence, 119

drug-related crimes, 117–118
evidence documentation, 124
evidence preservation, 122–123
evidence types, 123–124
highway encounters, 116
legal considerations, 123
police operations, 122
safety tactics, 119–121
street incidents, 116–117
tactical patient care, 121–122
Crowds, dangerous, 117
Crush points, 134
Cyanide exposure, 105
Cytochrome oxidase, 105

Dams/hydroelectric intakes, 73. *See also* Water rescues
Decontamination, 105–106
    decision making, 106–107
    eight-step process, 107
    methods, 106
    transportation considerations, 107–108
    two-step process, 107
Delayed effects, 103
Demobilized, 43
Demographic, 5
Department of Homeland Security (DHS), 38
Deployment, 2, 5–6
Dilution, 106
Dirty bomb, 145
Disaster, 37
Disaster management, 56
Disentanglement, 67
Distraction, 120
DNA identification, 123
Domestic incidents, 39
Domestic violence, 119
Dosimeter, 145
DOT KKK 1822F specs, 2
Drowning, 74–75. *See also* Water rescues
Drug-related crimes, 117–118. *See also* Crime scene awareness
Due regard standard, 8–9

Ebola virus, 150
Eddies, 74
Emergency operations center (EOC), 39
Emergency Response Guidebook (ERG), 98–99
EMS communications officer, 56
EMS system
    rural. *See* Rural EMS
    scientific basis, 10
    tactical, 114, 121–122
EMT-Tacticals (EMT-Ts), 122
Erythema, 147
Essential equipment, 2
Evasion, 120
Evidence preservation and documentation, 122–124
Explosives, 143–144

Extrication, 55, 69. *See also* Rescue awareness and operations
Eye protection, 64, 65

Facilities unit, 45
Fallout, 145
Farm machinery, 132–135
Fasciculations, 146
Finance/administration section, 45
Fingerprints, 123
Fixed-wing aircraft, 17. *See also* Air medical operations
Flammable/explosive limits, 101
Flash point, 101
Foot protection, 64

Gamma radiation, 102
Geiger counter, 145

Hate crimes, 117
Hazardous materials (hazmat), 93
   agricultural, 133–134
   cycles and actions, 103–104
   NFPA 704 System, 97–98
   placard classifications, 96–97
   terminology, 101–103
   in terrorist acts, 93, 94, 96. *See also* Terrorist acts
Hazardous materials (hazmat) incidents
   contamination types, 103
   exposure routes, 103
   incidence awareness, 95–96
   incident management system, 94–95
   medical monitoring of personnel, 109–110
   paramedic role, 93–94
   patient treatment, 104–105. *See also* Decontamination
   protective equipment, 108–109
   skills practice, 110
   substance identification, 98–99
   terminology, 101–103
   zones, 99, 101
Hazardous terrain rescues, 84
   environmental issues, 88
   extended care assessment, 87–88
   patient access, 85
   patient packaging, 85–86
   patient removal, 86–87
   types, 84
Hearing protection, 64, 65
Heat escape lessening position (HELP), 72
Helicopters. *See also* Air medical operations
   advantages, 20
   characteristics, 18–19
   in hazardous terrain rescues, 87
   limitations, 19–20
   in wilderness rescues, 138–139
Helmets, 64, 65
High-angle rescue, 85–87. *See also* Hazardous terrain rescues
Highway operations/rescue
   automobile features, 82
   danger warning signs, 116
   hazards, 80–81
   hybrid vehicle features, 84

   skills practice, 84
   strategies, 83–84
   vehicle stabilization, 83
Hot zone, 101, 149
Hybrid automobiles, 84
Hydrocarbon solvent exposure, 105
Hydroxocobalamin, 105

Ignition temperature, 101
Immediately dangerous to life and health (IDLH), 103
Incendiary agents, 144
Incident command post (ICP), 41
Incident Command System (ICS), 37–38
Incident commander (IC), 39–40
Incident Management System (IMS), 38–39. *See also* Multiple-casualty incident (MCI)
   command. *See* Command
   command staff, 43–45
   finance/administration section, 45
   functional divisions, 45–46
   at hazardous materials incidents, 94–95
   logistics section, 45
   operations section, 45
   planning/intelligence section, 45
   preplanning, drills, and critiques, 57
   rehabilitation, 55
Information officer (IO), 44
Instrument flight rules (IFR), 20
Isolation/disposal, 106

JumpSTART Pediatric MCI Triage Tool, 49, 51

Landing zone (LZ), 27–28
Legal considerations
   evidence preservation, 123
   National Incident Management System, 39
   nontraditional roles in terrorist attacks, 151
   safety issues in rescue calls, 68
Lethal concentration/lethal dose (LCt/LD), 103
Liaison officer (LO), 44
Local effects, 104
Lock-out-tag-out, 133
Logistics section, 45
Low-angle rescue, 85–87. *See also* Hazardous terrain rescues

Mark I kit, 146
Mass-casualty incident. *See* Multiple-casualty incident (MCI)
Material safety data sheets (MSDSs), 99–100
Medical evacuation, 17. *See also* Air medical operations
Medical supply unit, 45
Mental health support, 44–45, 57–58
Minimum standards, 2
Miosis, 146
Morgue, 51–52
Morgue officer, 52
Motor vehicle collisions. *See* Highway operations/rescue

Multiple-casualty incident (MCI), 36–37. *See also* Incident Management System (IMS)
   closed, 41
   command. *See* Command
   common problems, 57
   communications, 55–56
   extrication/rescue, 55
   high-impact, 37
   low-impact, 37
   open, 41
   staging, 54
   transport, 54–55
   treatment, 52–54
   triage. *See* Triage
Mutual aid agreements, 45
Mutual aid coordination center (MACC), 39

Napalm, 144
National Incident Management System (NIMS), 38, 39
Nerve agents, 146
Neutralization, 106
NFPA 704 System, 97–98
Night vision goggles (NG), 16
911 system, 129
Nuclear detonation, 144–145

Occupational Safety and Health Administration (OSHA), 3
Open incident, 41
Operations section, 45

Particulate evidence, 124
Parts per million/parts per billion (ppm/ppb), 103
Patho Pearls
   hazmat and terrorism, 93
   rural EMS quality considerations, 128
   scientific basis of EMS, 10
Peak load, 5
Personal flotation device (PFD), 65, 72, 75
Pesticides, 10–105
Pinch points, 134, 135
Placard classifications, hazardous materials, 96–97
Planning/intelligence section, 45
Pneumonic plague, 149, 150
Poisons. *See* Hazardous materials (hazmat)
Ppm/ppb, 103
Pralidoxime chloride, 146
Primary areas of responsibility (PARs), 5
Primary contamination, 103
Primary triage, 46–47
Prompt care facilities, 131
Pulmonary agents, 147
Pulmonary irritants, 104

Q fever, 149, 150
QNB, 148

Radiation, 102
Rapid intervention team, 55
Recirculating currents, 72–74
Recreational emergencies, 137–139
Rehabilitation unit, 55
Reportable collisions, 6

Rescue awareness and operations, 62
    in confined spaces, 76–80
    crew assignments, 66
    in hazardous terrain. *See* Hazardous
        terrain rescues
    highway. *See* Highway operations/
        rescue
    legal considerations, 66
    paramedic's role, 63
    patient protection, 65
    phase 1 (arrival/size-up), 67
    phase 2 (hazard control), 67–68
    phase 3 (patient access), 68
    phase 4 (medical treatment), 68–70
    phase 5 (disentanglement), 70
    phase 6 (patient packaging), 70–71
    phase 7 (removal/transport), 71
    preplanning, 66
    rescuer protection, 64–65
    standard operating procedures, 66
    in water. *See* Water rescues
Reserve capacity, 6
Retreat, 119
Rhinorrhea, 146
Riot control agents, 147
Rotor-wing aircraft, 17. *See also* Air medical
    operations
Rural EMS, 128, 130–131
    agricultural emergencies, 132–137
    challenges, 128–130
    distance factor, 131–132
    problem solving, 130–131
    quality considerations, 128
    recreational emergencies, 137–139
    scenarios, 132, 137, 138
Rust out, 129

Safety glass, 82
Safety officer (SO), 44
Safety tactics, 119–121
SALT (sort–assess–lifesaving
    interventions–treatment/transport)
    triage, 48–50
Scene-authority law, 38
Scrambling, 87
Scree, 84
Search and rescue, 16
Secondary contamination, 103
Secondary triage, 47
Section chief, 43
Sector, 46
Semi-decontaminated patient, 107

Severe acute respiratory syndrome
    (SARS), 149
Shear points, 134
Shielding, protective, 65
Shipping papers, 98–99
Short haul, 87
Silo gas, 133
Singular command, 41
Situational awareness, 40
SLUDGE, 104, 146
Smallpox, 149–150
Span of control, 40
Special weapons and tactics (SWAT)
    team, 121
Specific gravity, 101, 146
Spinal immobilization, in-water, 76
Spotter, 6
Staff functions, 44
Staging area, 41–42, 54
Staging officer, 54
Staphylococcal enterotoxin B (SEB), 147
START system, 47–48
Stokes basket, 85–86
Strainers, 73, 74
Street gangs, 117
Structural collapses, 79–80
Submerged victims, 76. *See also* Water rescues
Surface water rescues. *See* Water rescues
Synergism, 104
System status management (SSM), 6
Systemic effects, 104

Tactical emergency medical service (TEMS),
114, 121–122
Tempered glass, 82
Terrorist acts, 143
    biological agents. *See* Biological agents
    chemical agents. *See* Chemical
        weapons
    explosive agents, 143–144
    hazardous materials, 93, 94, 96. *See
        also* Hazardous materials (hazmat)
        incidents
    nontraditional EMS roles in, 151
    nuclear detonation, 144–145
    recognition, 151–152
    response, 152
    scene safety, 151
Threshold limit value/ceiling level limit
    (TLV-CL), 103
Threshold limit value/short-term exposure
    limit (TLV/STEL), 103

Threshold limit value/time weighted average
    (TLV/TWA), 103
Tiered response system, 6
Traffic hazards, in highway rescues, 80
Transportation unit supervisor, 54
Treatment group supervisor, 52–53
Triage, 46
    JumpSTART system, 49, 51
    morgue, 51–52
    primary and secondary, 46–47
    SALT system, 48–50
    speed, 51
    START system, 47–48
    tagging/labeling, 51, 53
Triage group supervisor, 46
Triage officer, 40
Trichothecene mycotoxins, 147
Tularemia, 149, 150
Type I ambulance, 3
Type II ambulance, 3
Type III ambulance, 3

UN number, 96
Unified command, 41

Vapor density, 101
Vapor pressure, 101
Venezuelan equine encephalitis, 149–150
Vesicants (blistering agents), 146–147
Violent street incidents, 116–117. *See also*
    Crime scene awareness
Viral hemorrhagic fever (VHF), 150
Visual flight rules (VFR), 19
Volatility, 146

Warfarin, 144
Warm zone, 101, 149
Warning placard, 95, 96–97
Water rescues
    basic techniques, 72, 73
    causes, 71
    in flat water, 74–76
    in moving water, 72–74
    patient immobilization, 76–77
    preparation, 71–72
    self-rescue techniques, 73–74
    water temperature and, 72
Water solubility, 11
Weapons of mass destruction (WMDs), 96,
    143. *See also* Terrorist acts
Windshield survey, 40
Wrap points, 134